The Voice Diagnostic Protocol

A PRACTICAL GUIDE TO THE DIAGNOSIS OF VOICE DISORDERS

Shaheen N. Awan, PhD, CCC-SLP
Professor
Department of Audiology & Speech Pathology
Bloomsburg University
Bloomsburg, Pennsylvania

AN ASPEN PUBLICATION®
Aspen Publishers, Inc.
Gaithersburg, Maryland
2001

The author has made every effort to ensure the accuracy of the information herein. However, appropriate information sources should be consulted, especially for new or unfamiliar procedures. It is the responsibility of every practitioner to evaluate the appropriateness of a particular opinion in the context of actual clinical situations and with due considerations to new developments. The author, editors, and the publisher cannot be held responsible for any typographical or other errors found in this book.

Library of Congress Cataloging-in-Publication Data

Awan, Shaheen N.
The voice diagnostic protocol: a practical guide to the diagnosis of voice disorders/ Shaheen N. Awan.
p. cm.
Includes bibliographical references and index.
ISBN 0-8342-1717-1
1. Voice disorders—Diagnosis. 2. Medical protocols. I. Title.
RF512 .A936 2000
616.8′55075—dc21
00-045095

Orders: (800) 638-8437
Customer Service: (800) 234-1660

About Aspen Publishers • For more than 40 years, Aspen has been a leading professional publisher in a variety of disciplines. Aspen's vast information resources are available in both print and electronic formats. We are committed to providing the highest quality information available in the most appropriate format for our customers. Visit Aspen's Internet site for more information resources, directories, articles, and a searchable version of Aspen's full catalog, including the most recent publications: **www.aspenpublishers.com**
Aspen Publishers, Inc. • The hallmark of quality in publishing
Member of the worldwide Wolters Kluwer group.

Editorial Services: Erin McKindley
Library of Congress Catalog Card Number: 00-045095
ISBN: 0-8342-1717-1

Printed in the United States of America

1 2 3 4 5

To my children, Rachel and Jordan,
and
To my wife Karen—my counselor and
best friend, who makes all things possible.

Contents

Acknowledgments

To my assistants Kelly Byrne, Cara Dellinger, Dominica DiRocco, and Amy Montgomery, who provided invaluable help in the collection of information and analysis of data used in this project.

To Dr. Nelson Roy, for his gracious assistance and advice concerning key aspects of this book.

To my students, past, present, and future, who have always challenged and inspired me.

To my family, for their support and encouragement.

To Karen J. Awan, for her tireless work in manuscript review, collection and typing of references, and overall project management, which made the last stages of manuscript preparation much less difficult.

CHAPTER 1

Introduction: The Voice Diagnostic Protocol and Initial Stages of the Diagnostic Process

The goal of this book is to provide detailed information regarding the rationale and procedures for an array of relatively low-cost and readily available methods of voice analysis that will be collectively referred to as the *Voice Diagnostic Protocol (VDP)*. A *protocol* may be defined as a set of methods or procedures by which a clinical study may be carried out. By stressing the use of relatively low-cost methods, it is the intention of this book to provide detailed information and instruction on methods that can be used by *any* speech pathologist in *any* situation or environment. Although it is hoped that all readers interested in the study of voice evaluation procedures will benefit from the content of this book, it is particularly designed as a resource for (1) graduate students in speech-language pathology and (2) practicing speech-language pathologists interested in expanding their skills in voice diagnosis.

The *VDP* provides the clinician with a detailed and comprehensive assessment of voice function, incorporating elements of patient history, perceptual assessment, acoustic methods, and important estimates of physiological activity. By focusing solely on voice diagnostic procedures, it is the intention of this book to illuminate methods that are often "buried" or discussed in a cursory manner in more general voice texts. However, focus on a single topic necessarily means that certain associated areas of study *will not* be included:

- This is not a book dealing with resonance-based disorders such as velopharyngeal inadequacy/incompetence and associated speech characteristics such as hypernasality and hyponasality and nasal emission. This book deals with "voice" as a phonatory event, with focus primarily on laryngeal and respiratory mechanisms.
- Although aspects of this book will necessarily deal with elements of laryngeal anatomy, phonatory physiology, and acoustic principles, it is not an anatomy or speech science text.

- It is not a book dealing with the method and interpretation of laryngoscopy or stroboscopy. Although these are important elements of a voice diagnostic, most clinicians do not have the training and/or the equipment to carry out these procedures. In addition, when done for diagnostic purposes, it is essential that visualization of the larynx be carried out by an otolaryngologist familiar with laryngeal disorders, who will then make an appropriate medical diagnosis and recommendations. It is expected that the clinician reading this book will seek appropriate referral sources for laryngoscopic evaluation (as well as stroboscopy, if necessary).
- This is not a book dealing with instrumentation methods such as electroglottography (EGG), advanced aerodynamic assessment, or electromyography (EMG). Although these methods may add valuable information to our assessment of vocal function, they require an expense and expertise with instrumentation that may make them clinically unfeasible in many situations.

Although many of the tasks discussed in this protocol will appear "simple" or uncomplicated on the surface, review of the theoretical background of these tasks, descriptions in the literature, issues of validity and reliability, etc., make even "simple" procedures quite complex in terms of clinical use and interpretation. Therefore, the background information provided in this book is believed to be necessary if the clinical information gathered from these tasks is to be reasonably interpreted and used with maximum effectiveness. Even though many of the tasks incorporated in the *VDP* use instrumentation methods, they cannot really be judged to be objective in nature. True objective measures would be independent of human error, judgment, perceptions, and bias of the clinician (Behrman & Orlikoff, 1997; Nicolosi, Harryman, & Kresheck, 1989). In addition, an ideal objective test would also be independent of influence from patient behavior (i.e., the patient would not be able to influence test results as a function of his or her immediate behavior). In the case of many instrumental tasks of vocal function, the ways in which measures are obtained and interpreted are subjective in nature and affected by both clinician and patient (Behrman & Orlikoff, 1997).

THE CONCEPT OF DIAGNOSIS VS. ASSESSMENT/ EVALUATION

The title of this book clearly indicates that the procedures described herein are to be components of a *diagnostic* protocol. The term *diagnostic* has been specifically used to indicate that the outcome of this process will achieve several important goals:

1. Our diagnostic decisions will be based on a synthesis of information from diverse areas all dealing with aspects of voice function, such as anatomy and physiology, acoustics, perception, psychometrics, and knowledge of norms and testing techniques.
2. The final diagnosis will be derived from the ability to distinguish the patient's problem from a large field of possibilities (Haynes, Pindzola, & Emerick, 1992). This process is referred to as *differential diagnosis*, a process that takes into account all significant variables contributing to the disorder and attempts to differentiate the presenting problem from related or dissimilar problems (Weinberg, 1983).
3. The final diagnosis will actually be the beginning of a continuous venture that will be open to revision on the basis of the patient's future behavior.

Some may object to the use of the term *diagnosis* or *diagnostic* as used by speech-language pathologists, perhaps because of (1) the association of the term with the medical profession and (2) the possible implication that the speech-language pathologist will be carrying out a medical procedure. Some would prefer the use of terms such as *assessment* or *appraisal* to describe our methods. However, these terms are *not* synonymous with *diagnosis* and describe only the procedures used within the overall diagnostic method. In contrast, "diagnosis requires placing measurements and other observational data into context and perspective in order to decide whether a problem exists and to differentiate one problem from others which may have similar performance aspects" (Peterson & Marquardt, 1990, p. 4). It is my belief that the term *diagnosis* is a universal term that describes a process of investigation and deduction that cannot be reserved for a particular field or profession.

A PHYSIOLOGICAL VIEW OF VOICE DIAGNOSIS

The various sections of this book will stress the possible relationships between perceptual, acoustic, and other measures of voice and the underlying physiology of phonation. It is not enough to simply recognize that a patient has a rough-sounding voice, higher than expected fundamental frequency, or short maximum phonation time—the clinician must develop a rational hypothesis as to *why* the patient has certain characteristics. This is where application of our knowledge of the underlying physiology or pathophysiology affecting voice production comes into play. A number of previous works dealing with diagnosis of voice disorders have also stressed this point. Murry (1982) stated that "the assessment of the vocal mechanism…encompasses a detailed analysis of the abnormal physiologic behavior of the laryngeal mechanism, specifically, and the relationship between the behavior of the laryngeal mechanism and the patient's general speech and voice production" (p. 478). Bless and Hicks (1996) stated that "assessment of vocal function has evolved to mean deriving a description of voice production…that allows clinicians to make inferences about the functioning of the underlying anatomical and physiological condition of the larynx" (p. 124). Behrman and Orlikoff (1997) go so far as to stress that "the underlying pathophysiology *is* [italics added] the voice disorder that the clinician must seek to understand" (p. 10).

Once the clinician can hypothesize the possible causative factors (behavioral or organic) underlying the patient's voice disorder, the development of treatment goals becomes evident. A physiological approach to diagnosis should lead to physiological voice therapy, in which "the management approach is a direct modification of the inappropriate physiologic activity" (Stemple, 1993, p. 4). It is clear that the success of voice therapy is highly dependent on the skill and inferences of the voice clinician derived from the initial diagnosis.

AVOIDANCE OF MEDICAL DIAGNOSTIC TERMS

The focus of the speech pathologist involved in the voice diagnostic should be to assess voice production, identify possible underlying factors (behavioral and/or organic) that may be responsible for the cause and maintenance of the voice problem, and determine the severity of the voice problem (Behrman & Orlikoff, 1997; Colton & Casper, 1996; Murry, 1982). It is *not* the speech pathologist's responsibility to determine the specific existence and type of pathological condition that may be affecting the phonatory function of the patient (Behrman & Orlikoff, 1997; Murry, 1982). Although the literature is ripe with the perceptual and acoustic description of various pathological states, the voice clinician should focus his or her diagnostic conclusions on possible physiological mechanisms that may be responsible for the various perceptual, acoustic, and other signs observed in the particular patient rather than on diagnostic labels. This description is much more informative and potentially useful to the speech pathologist and the patient than applying a medical term or label to the patient's disorder. The use of medical diagnostic terminology should be avoided for the following reasons:

1. It is outside the realm of the speech pathologist to make medical diagnoses. An appropriate referral must be made to the attending physician or otolaryngologist, who will apply the "label" to the patient's organic pathological condition.
2. A multitude of different disorders with different labels can result in similar perceptual, acoustic, etc., characteristics. As an example, vocal nodules, polyps, and other lesions that affect the margin(s) of the fold(s) and restrict glottal closure may all have some degree of breathiness. Therefore, it can be seen that the chance for error in applying a medical diagnostic term solely on the basis of perceptual and/or acoustic information is a strong possibility.
3. As in other areas of speech pathology, *we do not treat labels*. Instead, we must treat each patient as a unique entity with his or her own unique physiological disturbances (both primary and secondary [i.e., compensatory] in nature). Therefore, diagnosis should accentuate the underlying physiology of the patient and the voice disorder rather than a particular label or category to which they may belong.

THE USE OF INSTRUMENTATION: OBJECTIVE EVALUATION OF THE VOICE WITH METHODOLOGY AVAILABLE TO ALL VOICE CLINICIANS

Traditionally, the major component of a voice evaluation dealt solely with a perceptual description of voice characteristics. Although perceptual characterization of the voice is still an essential component of any voice diagnostic, it can no longer be the only parameter to be included in a complete voice diagnostic. There are several important reasons why perceptual judgments alone are not adequate:

1. Variability in training and experience between therapists inevitably leads to a lack of reliability and validity in the perceptual judgments that are made. Discussion with colleagues will often reveal that even such commonly used severity terminology such as mild, moderate, and severe may have very different meanings for different therapists.
2. Perceptual judgments alone do not allow for objective comparison with normative groups. One of the fundamental diagnostic decisions made in any evaluation is one of "normal" vs. "abnormal." One of the valuable aids we have in making this decision is a measure of the average performance for a target group

in conjunction with a measure of the average deviation. Unfortunately, perceptions cannot be compared with measurable norms in any valid manner.
3. Progress in therapy sessions may not be gauged effectively with perceptions alone. Perceptual judgments may not detect relatively small but significant changes in voice characteristics that may indicate that a treatment procedure is having a positive effect on the patient. In addition, perceptual judgments alone may not provide the data required to justify continuation of therapy and reimbursement for treatment.

It can be seen that the effective gauging of the patient's voice characteristics in both diagnosis and treatment is somewhat lacking if perceptual judgments are used alone. Therefore, a key component of the *VDP* is the addition of instrumental measures wherever possible. Behrman and Orlikoff (1997) define instrumental measures as "those obtained using electronic or computer-based equipment" (p. 9). There are several key reasons why the addition of instrumental measures strengthens our diagnostic protocol (Behrman & Orlikoff, 1997):

1. Rapid evolution of the environment in which speech-language pathologists' practice has demanded greater sophistication from the clinician in terms of diagnostic methods.
2. Health-care delivery and reimbursement issues have required the voice clinician to quantify patient characteristics both in diagnosis and through the course of therapy.
3. Instrumentation procedures may be able to tell the clinician how a patient is making use of and coordinating the various subsystems (respiratory, phonatory, articulatory) of the speech mechanism.
4. Instrumental measures may help form a more solid foundation for clinical judgments.
5. Instrumental measures allow for the comparison of vocal performance to appropriate normative data.

It can be seen that instrumental measures help to verify clinical judgments and hypotheses. If clinical experience, expertise, and perceptual judgments form the basis of diagnostic hypotheses, then instrumental measures are a key factor in the acceptance or rejection of these hypotheses.

RATIONALE FOR ACOUSTIC METHODS

A key element of the *VDP* is that perceptual signs of the voice will be verified and supported by means of acoustic methods. Acoustic analysis of the voice represents an area of instrumental analysis that presents a number of distinct advantages to the clinician.

Clinician Experience and Familiarity

All master's degree–level speech-language pathologists generally have one or more courses in basic speech science and acoustic methods as part of their academic training. Therefore, many of the concepts of frequency, intensity, periodicity vs. aperiodicity, etc., that underlie the acoustic methods used in the voice diagnostic will be relatively familiar to the clinicians using them.

Noninvasive

Acoustic methods are noninvasive and therefore may be used with all patients by any clinician. In addition, most patients are relatively familiar with the use of microphones and will be comfortable speaking into them. These benefits do not necessarily extend to other instrumental methods of voice analysis.

Good Availability and Relatively Low Cost

The equipment necessary for high-quality acoustic analysis is readily available to most clinicians for a relatively modest cost. The advent of low-cost multimedia computers in recent years, in conjunction with the proliferation of software for acoustic analysis, has made acoustic analysis methods widely available.

Correspondence with the Underlying Physiology of Voice Disorders

The acoustic signal is the by-product of phonation (the oscillation of the vocal folds as determined by aerodynamic and myoelastic forces). Because the acoustic signal is determined, in part, by movements of the vocal folds, "there is a great deal of correspondence between the physiology and acoustics, and much can be inferred about the physiology based on acoustic analysis" (Colton & Casper, 1996, p. 21). It must be noted that the relationships between phonatory physiology and acoustics are certainly not perfect. The voice signal "is a complex product of the nonlinear interaction between aerodynamic and biomechanical properties of the voice production system" (Behrman & Orlikoff, 1997, p. 10). Because this interaction is nonlinear, accurate predictions regarding underlying phonatory physiology cannot always be made on the basis of the acoustic signal alone. However, when acoustic analysis results are placed within the context of a complete VDP, very powerful inferences may be made.

Good Applicability to Future Therapy

Acoustic methods lend themselves well to both diagnostic procedures and treatment methods. It has been my experi-

ence that most patients, even relatively young children, are able to easily understand (in a simple, but effective manner) many of the measures displayed in voice analysis programs (e.g., jitter values "should go down"; F_0 values "should go up"; displayed F_0 contours should flatten). In this way, acoustic methods provide a valuable link between the voice diagnostic and voice therapy.

Wide Body of Literature

Acoustic analysis methods have an extensive history of use with a wide range of voice-disordered populations. This provides the clinician with a vast body of literature that may be accessed to aid in the interpretation of diagnostic findings.

THE VOICE DIAGNOSTIC PROTOCOL DEFINED

The *VDP* provides the voice clinician with an array of test procedures by which reasonable and accurate diagnostic hypotheses may be made regarding the presenting voice disorder. The *VDP* incorporates a wide range of analysis methods (perceptual, acoustic, and selected physiological methods) that meet the following criteria (Hirano, 1991):

- They present minimum discomfort to the patient.
- They are noninvasive techniques.
- In most cases, they require minimal amounts of time to complete the procedure.
- They provide relatively immediate test results.
- They require minimum expense.

The various procedures in the *VDP* are shown in Figure 1–1.

The *VDP* can be described as a method of *voice profiling*. Voice profiling allows the clinician the opportunity to derive influences regarding the underlying anatomical and physiological status of the phonatory mechanism (Bless & Hicks, 1996). An accurate profile of voice function requires the acquisition of multiple measures and observations derived from a wide range of methods. Several important reasons for this method of voice profiling are shown below.

- Bless and Hicks (1996) state that single tests or measures must be considered as part of a larger battery of tests of vocal function. Diagnostic hypotheses should not be made on the basis of one test or measure because "one cannot look at an isolated phenomenon without running the risk of misinterpreting results" (Titze, 1991 in Bless & Hicks, 1996).
- Colton and Casper (1996) believe that the most complete information regarding the patient's vocal functioning cannot be obtained by means of only one or two

Assessment Areas of the VDP

The Voice Diagnostic Protocol

Background Information
Presession information
Case history re: patient dysphonia
Speech and hearing mechanism results

Pitch/Frequency
Perceptual determination (habitual pitch, pitch variability)
Mean speaking F_0
F_0 variability (F_0 standard deviation/pitch sigma)
F_0 range (total phonational range and speaking range)

Loudness/Intensity
Perceptual determination (habitual loudness, loudness variability)
Mean/modal speaking intensity
Intensity range—phonetogram
"High-quiet" phonation

Quality
Perceptual determination (primary quality deviations, instability, strain, diplophonia)
Quantitative analysis of perturbation and noise (jitter, shimmer, HNR)

Duration—Respiratory/Phonatory Control
Perceptual determination (including "five for five" testing and reading of a standard passage on one breath)
Vital capacity
Maximum phonation time
S/Z ratio
Phonation quotient

Evaluation of Muscle Tension Dysphonia (MTD)
Effects of laryngeal reposturing and massage
Effects of sustained speech production (rapid counting)

Figure 1–1 Outline of the Tasks Incorporated into the *Voice Diagnostic Protocol*

procedures. "Each procedure adds to our understanding of normal voice production and the deviations that alter the normal state" (Colton & Casper, 1996, p. 197).

- Kent, Kent, and Rosenbek (1987) state that "particularly when performance is deficient compared to norms, data should be taken from repeated trials, or other tasks should be used to complete the interpretative framework" (p. 383). In addition, Kent et al. (1987) indicate that the relationship and consistency of test results within a category of testing may tell the clinician something about the type and severity of a disorder.

- Gerratt and Kreiman (in Orlikoff et al., 1999) state that acoustic measures of vocal quality may be accounted for by many physiological conditions and affected in similar ways by various types of laryngeal behavior and pathological conditions. This fact exemplifies the notion that acoustics must be part of a comprehensive diagnostic protocol that includes detailed case history information, perceptual assessment, and physiological measures.

- Hirano (1991) notes that voice function is multidimensional in nature, and, therefore, we need a set of tests to evaluate vocal function in its entirety.

REQUIRED EQUIPMENT AND MATERIALS FOR THE *VDP*

The following items are necessary to complete the various tasks incorporated in the *VDP* (see Appendix A):

- A Pentium-level multimedia computer, incorporating Microsoft Windows 95 or higher (Microsoft Corporation). A multimedia computer generally includes a 16-bit sound card and speakers necessary for the recording and playback of speech samples.
- Voice analysis software. Several of these packages are available for use on a Windows-based PC. Examples are *CSpeechSP* (P. Milenkovic, Madison, WI); *Dr. Speech* (Tiger DRS Inc., Seattle, WA); *EZVoicePlus* (VoiceTek Enterprises, Nescopeck, PA); and *Multi-Speech Model 3700* (Kay Elemetrics Corp., Lincoln Park, NJ). All these programs will use the sound card already installed in a multimedia computer for recording and playback. When obtaining voice analysis software, make sure that the program is able to provide perturbation and noise analyses from sustained vowel samples, as well as continuous speech analysis (some programs require add-on packages to provide all these analysis options).
- A good quality microphone (unidirectional dynamic or condenser). Ideally, this microphone will have a frequency response between 50 Hz and 15 kHz.
- Microphone preamplifier or mixer (see Figure 1–2). This item is not a necessity but is useful because many

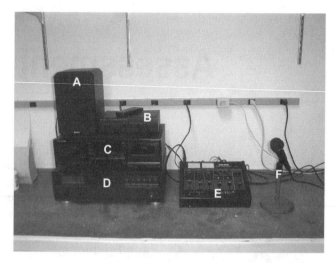

Figure 1–2 Standard Recording and Playback Equipment Used in Voice Evaluation. (A) Speaker for Playback; (B) Amplifier; (C) Cassette Deck; (D) Digital Compact Cassette (DCC); (E) Preamplifier Mixer; (F) Unidirectional Microphone.

cassette, DAT (Digital Audio Tape), DCC (Digital Compact Cassette), and MD (MiniDisc) decks do not have microphone inputs. Therefore, the microphone can be input into the preamplifier mixer and then fed into the line input of the recording deck. In addition, a mixer is useful to input the signal into the computer. Although most sound cards have a microphone input, the line input of the sound card often provides better quality recording (Huang, Lin, & O'Brien, 1995). Therefore, the microphone would be plugged into the microphone input of the mixer, and the line out from the mixer would be connected to the line in of the sound card.

- A sound level meter (SLM). This is necessary to make measurements of vocal intensity. Most Radio Shack stores carry low-cost SLMs in either analog (Model 33-2050) or digital (Model 33-2055) models. The digital display is often easier to read than the meter display of the analog model. The SLM may also be used as a microphone by connecting its line out to the mixer microphone input.
- A spirometer. This is necessary for measurements of vital capacity and estimates of airflow. A number of relatively low-cost hand-held models are available.
- Stopwatch.
- Ruler (for measuring mouth-to-microphone distance).
- Good quality cassette, DAT, or MD. Most voice recording in the *VDP* is done directly into the computer. In fact, this is preferable because it removes possible detrimental effects of tape noise, multiple external amplifiers, etc. However, in the event that a portable recorder is

necessary for voice recording away from the computer (e.g., case history interviews that may take place in a room different from that which houses speech/voice instrumentation), I suggest the use of a portable MD unit. MD is a digital recording medium that provides many benefits over standard recording methods (no tape noise; no need for tape bias setting; no tape deterioration; ability to index samples for immediate recall; samples may be erased, combined, moved, named; up to 148 minutes of mono recording time on a single disc). In addition, portable MD units generally contain a microphone input, removing the necessity for a preamplifier mixer. A study by Winholtz and Titze (1998) indicated that MD units are more than adequate for voice analysis purposes and do not introduce any significant distortions into the record/playback process.

The most expensive item in this equipment list will most probably be the computer. However, because most clinical settings (hospital, school, private office) will already have access to a computer with multimedia capabilities, the actual costs for the equipment used in the *VDP* are relatively low. Figure 1–3 shows a standard equipment setup as may be used during voice diagnostic testing.

THE BENEFITS OF REDUNDANCY

Voice profiling as conducted by means of the *VDP* incorporates an extremely important facet of accurate diagnostic decision making—redundancy. Most would consider redundancy a form of inefficiency, in which procedures and observations are simply repeated in an identical manner.

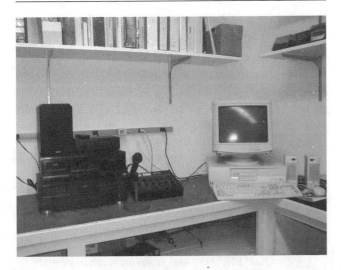

Figure 1–3 Voice Recording Equipment Set Up Next to a Pentium-Level Personal Computer. Digitization and analysis of voice samples will be conducted by use of the computer.

However, in the case of diagnostic testing as discussed here, the redundant addition of observations to our overall voice profile is done according to slightly different procedures. Redundant data are not collected as exact copies but as associations of an underlying behavior or process. De Callatay (1986) states, "Because there are slight variations in possible solutions, there will be an increase in the number of pattern recognitions, increasing the chances of finding a best choice" (p. 97). In this form of redundancy, (1) a larger weight will be given in the development of clinical hypotheses to signs of underlying behaviors that have been frequently repeated, and (2) a more comprehensive view of the underlying behavior will be provided.

Redundancy is used for improved development of clinical hypotheses and for reliability (i.e., repeatability) purposes. However, redundancy in diagnostic testing does not have to be inefficient. Many of the redundant tests used in the voice diagnostic protocol are conducted on the same speech sample. As an example, the same continuous speech sample may be analyzed perceptually and acoustically. In terms of acoustics, several different but associated procedures can be conducted on the same recorded speech sample (e.g., computations of jitter, shimmer, and harmonics-to-noise ratio). Therefore, redundancy can be incorporated as a beneficial aspect of clinical decision making without impeding the efficient completion of the voice diagnostic.

KEY PARAMETERS FOR CONSIDERATION BEFORE BEGINNING THE DIAGNOSTIC SESSION

Before beginning the voice diagnostic, the clinician must be clear on three particular parameters that will be evaluated during the case history interview and throughout the diagnostic session:

- What is normal vs. disordered voice?
- If a voice is disordered, how may we describe its severity?
- Once we have identified a disordered voice, what are the primary voice disorder types by which we may categorize it?

Normal vs. Disordered Vocal Quality

To distinguish between *normal* and *disordered* behaviors, it is essential that we define our terms. Unfortunately, there is difficulty in actually defining what a *normal* voice is, even though most people, laypersons as well as professionals, are often able to identify voices that "sound different." This point was emphasized in a study by Anders, Hollien, Hurme, Sonninen, and Wendler (1988), in which trained practitioners in clinical voice analysis (speech-language pathologists, speech scientists, phoneticians) and laymen controls were asked to identify samples of normal vs. hoarse phonation and also rank the severity of the disordered samples. Anders et al. (1988) observed that the disordered samples could be easily identified and ranked by trained and untrained groups alike—the hypothesis that training could enhance the accuracy of perceptual identification was not supported.

Fex (1992) states that "normal voice quality is a conception based on subjective opinion, may vary with different cultures, and certainly is difficult to define; a vast number of people are supposed to have normal but nevertheless individually differentiated voice" (p. 155). So, what is it that the listener detects in the voice signal that allows for the discrimination between normal and disordered voice? It appears that there are a number of characteristics (age, gender, racial type, body size/type, etc.) that determine a range for normal voice type and quality. As we are exposed to the range of normal voice types throughout our lives, we gain experience as to the limits of normal voice and, thereby, develop a mental scale by which normal is gauged. *As long as a particular voice does not deviate substantially from this internal gauge in terms of parameters such as pitch, loudness, quality, and duration, it will be considered within the normal range.* When a voice is perceived as deviating from the normal range, it may be characterized as being *dysphonic.* The term *dysphonia* literally means "abnormal/difficult/impaired voice."

METHODS FOR RATING SEVERITY OF DYSPHONIA

Having some definition by which we may distinguish normal from disordered/dysphonic voices, the clinician should also enter the diagnostic situation with some working knowledge of basic terminology by which we will categorize our patient's characteristics and communicate them to others. In each of the following chapters of this book, the reader will be introduced to definitions for primary voice characteristics and disturbances that have been well established and can be agreed on by most voice scientists and clinicians. However, much of the difficulty in accurately defining the perceptual attributes of the voice comes not in applying the categorical label but in accurately describing the severity of the observed disorder. When we judge the severity of a disorder, we are recognizing that the condition may exist along a continuum. This continuum extends in growing proportions from an absence or minor amount of the observed deviant voice characteristic to an extreme amount. The lower end of this continuum should probably be best acknowledged as being a "minimal" level, because even normal voice signals are not necessarily perfect. On the other end of the continuum, an extreme level of voice deviation may overpower the normal

voice signal and, most probably, has a significant effect on patient and listener alike.

Several methods have been described by which the severity of voice deviations may be described or quantified (Kreiman, Gerratt, Kempster, Erman, & Berke, 1993):

1. Categorical ratings: In this method, voice samples are assigned to discrete categories such as mild, moderate, severe.
2. Equal-appearing interval (EAI) scales: The severity of a perceived voice characteristic is assigned a number (most commonly between 1 and 7), with the higher numbers representing increased amounts of perceived disruption in the voice signal.
3. Visual analog (VA) scales: Instead of scaling the voice by use of specified incremental levels of voice disruption (as in EAI scales), VA scales provide the judge with an undifferentiated line on which a mark is placed to indicate the level of voice severity or deviation. Only the extremes of the line are labeled (e.g., minimal vs. extreme). The use of this type of scaling procedure may be helpful in reducing bias in the rating process.
4. Direct magnitude estimation (DME): In this method, a number is assigned to indicate the degree of voice deviation. Numbers may be assigned in an unrestricted manner (i.e., any number possible) or restricted fashion (anchored DME in which numbers are assigned in relation to a reference voice sample with a preassigned magnitude).
5. Paired comparison: Two voice samples are judged as to the extent of difference on single or multiple dimensions of the voice signal.

Pros and Cons of Perceptual Assessment of Disordered Voice

Various methods have been described by which the severity of a deviant voice type may be documented. However, there has been considerable controversy as to the overall benefit and usefulness of perceptual assessment of the voice. An article by Orlikoff et al. (1999) presents various viewpoints dealing with the appropriate use of auditory-perceptual judgments of voice (and in particular, voice quality) in the assessment of dysphonia. The pros of perceptual assessment may be summarized as shown below.

- Perceptual assessment methods are available to all clinicians and may provide a global measure of vocal performance.
- Perceptual judgment and assessment are of primary relevance to most voice patients. The patient is often most concerned with how others perceive his/her voice.

- The perceptual severity and quality of the voice are often the impetus for the voice evaluation in the first place and, therefore, must be confirmed, evaluated, and described by the clinician.
- Perceptual rating is the "gold standard" for assessing the clinical relevance of subsequent acoustical analyses.
- Perceptual judgments provide a comprehensive impression of the voice that includes aspects of voice not captured by acoustic measures.
- Perceptual judgments are important in determining the ultimate success or failure of voice therapy.

Unfortunately, a number of factors are involved with the perceptual assessment of the voice that may make the process nebulous (Murry, 1982) and error prone. The cons of perceptual assessment of the voice may be summarized as shown below (Orlikoff et al., 1999).

- Perceptual assessment of the voice appears to be affected by problems of scale validity and reliability.
- Perceptual assessment does not provide an awareness of the physiological details that result in the acoustic product.
- Perceptual quality may be difficult to characterize and communicate in terms of quantified results and, therefore, may not be as credible as numerical test procedures. In this regard, results of perceptual assessment may not be sufficient for medicolegal purposes.

Although more pros than cons have been presented, the possible deficiencies in the perceptual assessment process are important for us to consider in more detail. In particular, we will focus on a discussion of the reliability and validity issues involved with perceptual assessment of the voice.

Reliability

Reliability of an assessment procedure focuses on the ability to repeat one's measurements or observations. The ability to repeat measurements is directly related to the precision and accuracy of measurements (Schiavetti & Metz, 1997). Kreiman et al. (1993) provide a comprehensive review of studies that have been concerned with the assessment of speech and voice quality. Their review indicates that, although average levels of intra-judge and inter-judge reliability are generally high, average reliability measures tend to mask considerable variability in perceptual judgments. In addition, the use of correlational statistics to substantiate the presence of reliability only indicates that judgments (whether intra-judge or inter-judge) may vary in a consistent manner; they do not necessarily indicate that judgments are in agreement (i.e., judgments were exactly the same).

The variability in ratings may be due to several factors:

- The severity of the perceived voice disturbance may affect intra-judge and inter-judge reliability. Kreiman et al. (1993) have observed that quality ratings vary more for pathological than normal voices and more for mid-scale voices (i.e., mild to moderate voice disturbances) than for voices at scale extremes (i.e., normal or severe voices).
- The type of scaling procedure used may result in variability in ratings, with EAI scale ratings observed to produce more drift in test-retest comparisons than VA scales.
- Because judges are exposed to more and different examples of voice productions, their internal gauge of what defines normal versus disordered may change, resulting in a lack of precision in their test versus retest ratings of voice quality.

It should be recalled that reliability does not ensure validity of measurement procedures but is a necessary prerequisite for validity (Schiavetti & Metz, 1997). Therefore, the aforementioned factors affecting reliability of perceptual assessment also contribute to the next section dealing with factors that affect the validity of perceptual assessment of the voice.

Validity

The validity of a test procedure refers to the ability to measure what we intend to measure. Validity implies a satisfactory and consistent definition or set of definitions for the characteristic behavior we are attempting to measure or rate. In terms of perceptual assessment of the voice, if the characteristics we are attempting to identify and rate are poorly defined, defined differently from person to person, or have shifting definitions, then validity will be affected in addition to reliability. Several issues possibly affecting the validity of perceptual judgments of the voice may be summarized as follows:

- Quality judgments that attempt to rate the severity of the voice deviation are characteristically poorly defined. Although it is common for working definitions or examples to be provided for scale anchors (normal and severe), there is generally little or no definition provided for the mid-scale ratings. With this in mind, it is no wonder that mid-scale ratings have been seen as the location of greatest variability and disagreement between judges rating voice quality (Kreiman et al., 1993).
- Quality judgments that are unidimensional in nature may have poor content validity because they do not account for the multidimensional nature of voice. It has been said that, "The voice is a multi-dimensional phenomenon, comprised of a number of elements that

contribute to overall voice quality and voice effectiveness" (Orlikoff et al., 1999, p. 90). Hammarberg, Fritzell, Gauffin, Sundberg, and Wedin (1980) showed that samples of pathological voices could be perceptually summarized in terms of five bipolar factors: (1) unstable-steady, (2) breathy-overtight, (3) hyperfunctional-hypofunctional, (4) coarse-light, and (5) head vs. chest register. Gelfer (1993) indicated that five dimensions of the voice signal accounted for the similarity or dissimilarity of normal female voices. The perceptual correlates of the five dimensions were: (1) perceived pitch, (2) perceived loudness, (3) perceived age and rate, (4) variability in perceived pitch, and (5) perceived voice quality. With this in mind, rating the voice by use of a single scale factor (e.g., "roughness") may not account for other key voice characteristics that should be included in the description.

- In addition to various voice characteristics, our perceptual measurements may be swayed by other extraneous sources. For example, severity of vocal roughness may be influenced by coexisting hypernasality or some other nonvoice source information (de Krom, 1994).

Overall, two key factors can be seen that may be the sources of reduced validity and reliability in perceptual assessment of the voice: (1) variation in definition for measurement terms and (2) variation in experience of the listeners. These factors may be seen to change the calibration of the judge on test-retest measurements or to affect the similar calibration of different judges (remember that calibration can refer to observers or scorers in addition to machines/instruments). These changes in calibration produce changes in the obtained measurements (i.e., voice ratings) (Campbell & Stanley, 1966). Both validity and reliability may be affected by changes in calibration.

HOW TO DO IT: RATING DYSPHONIC SEVERITY

Perhaps the challenge in selecting a method of perceptual assessment of voice quality is to find one that is complex enough to portray the multidimensional nature of voice quality deviation and yet be understandable enough that (1) clinicians may easily learn and use the system with limited training, and (2) results may be communicated easily among colleagues and other professionals. This book proposes that the severity of a particular voice disruption (pitch, loudness, quality, etc.) be rated on a 7-point categorical/EAI rating scale ranging from 0 to 6. A 0 rather than a 1 is suggested as the lower anchor of the scale to represent the absence or minimal nature of the perceived voice disorder. (See Appendix B.)

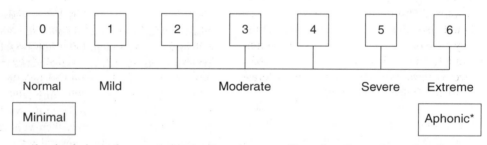

*Lack of phonation—may be due to extremes of hypofunction or hyperfunction.

Within this scale, certain points (1, 3, 5) are labeled with the commonly used severity terminology of mild, moderate, and severe. These are our severity categories, which are ranked on an EAI scale of increasing magnitude. These terms are freely used by speech pathologists to describe various disorders. Yet, the next time a colleague uses one of these terms or you use one yourself, ask yourself, "What does mild, moderate, or severe really mean?" You will probably find (1) great difficulty in defining these terms and (2) a substantial amount of variation in definition from person to person. Of course, lack of agreement in definition is one of the key elements that results in reduced reliability and agreement in perceptual judgments of voice quality. Review of the voice literature finds very little in terms of definition for these commonly used severity terms. It is common that definitions are provided for the end points of the severity continuum, but not for the intermediate points. As an example, de Krom (1994) describes a 10-point EAI scale in which the left side of the scale (number 1 in this example) represented "not present at all," and the right side of the scale (number 10) represented "maximally present." Askenfelt and Hammarberg (1986) used a 5-point EAI scale, with 0 representing no deviance and 4 representing a high degree of deviance from normal. In studies using both 7-point EAI scales and VA scales, Kreiman et al. (1993) only provide definitions of the end points of each scale (e.g., "not rough at all" versus "extremely rough"). It is this lack of definition, particularly for the intermediate points of the severity continuum, that contributes to the increased variability and decreased reliability and agreement in perceptual ratings. Kreiman et al. (1993) confirm the variability or ratings in the midrange of vocal quality scales and conclude that "If the quality to be rated is poorly defined or lacks perceptual reality, listeners will not be able to rate it consistently" (p. 32).

Severity Terminology Defined

It seems that one of the major problems in judging voice is its multidimensional nature. Voice is composed of numerous characteristics that may be weighted differently by different judges (de Krom, 1994; Higgins, Chait, & Schulte, 1999). As an example, while listening to the same disordered voice sample, one judge may be focusing on aspects of pitch, whereas the other puts more emphasis on vocal quality. In addition to the perceptual characteristics of the voice, severity definitions should also take into account "the impact the voice problem may have on the speaker's ability to communicate and obtain employment" (Higgins et al., 1999, p. 103). The following severity terminology attempts to incorporate a number of the possible diverse effects of dysphonia.

- *Mild:* Although the listener experienced in the perceptual characteristics of the disordered voice would consider the voice abnormal, the untrained listener may consider the voice to be only unusual in nature and within normal expectations. The voice characteristic is not distracting, and the ability to effectively communicate is not affected. The dysphonia does not interfere with phonation.
- *Moderate:* Both trained and untrained listeners would consider the voice abnormal. There may be intermittent periods in which the voice characteristic is highly distracting. The ability to effectively communicate is noticeably affected under certain conditions (e.g., noisy environments). The dysphonia may occasionally cause phonation to cease or become highly effortful.
- *Severe:* Both trained and untrained listeners would consider the voice extremely abnormal. The voice characteristic is highly distracting. The ability to effectively communicate is consistently affected. The dysphonia

causes phonation to be mainly absent or extremely effortful.

The clinician is encouraged to closely compare the perceived abnormal voice characteristic(s) to all parts of these definitions. It may be that a disordered voice does not show all the characteristics mentioned under each definition, or it may show characteristics crossing definitions. In these cases, intermediate ratings (e.g., mild-to-moderate) may be appropriate. In addition, certain dysphonia types (e.g., inappropriately high pitch) may be considered abnormal but not necessarily disrupt the ability to phonate.

It can be seen that these severity definitions emphasize the noticeability and communicative effectiveness of the patient. These factors get to the heart of what may be considered "abnormal" voice production. As previously stated, the degree of deviation from our internal gauge of what normal voice should be is one of the key factors that signals the disordered voice. Therefore, in the severity definitions presented here, we range from a barely noticeable deviation (mild) to one that is so extreme (severe) that the normality of the voice signal is overwhelmed. In addition, these severity definitions take into account the overall effects on communication. As the voice deviation becomes more noticeable, communication between the speaker and the listener will become increasingly impeded. The listener becomes so distracted by the voice deviation that he or she has trouble focusing on and processing the underlying linguistic message. Orlikoff et al. (1999) agree that it is especially important that the attention of the listener is not deviated from the content of the message by a "disturbing voice quality." Prater and Swift (1984) indicated that judgments of intelligibility should be made in addition to judgments of voice severity and aesthetic quality. Andrews (1995) also includes effects on intelligibility in her definitions for mild, moderate, and severe ratings for vocal tremor. Although the listener is affected by the presence of a voice disorder, the speaker also may have increased awareness of the difficulty in communicating and attempt to compensate for the deficit in various ways (behavioral, psychological, social, etc.). Overall, we have the development of a handicapping condition (Haynes et al., 1992) in which the lack of communicative effectiveness begins to have a significant impact on the patient's day-to-day activities.

To account for the multidimensional view of voice production that appears to be so important in describing overall voice character and effectiveness (Gelfer, 1993; Orlikoff et al., 1999), these severity definitions will be applied to all key characteristics of the voice signal (pitch, loudness, quality, and duration). As an example, we may state that a patient has a "mild dysphonia characterized by abnormally low pitch and breathiness." The severity term (in this case, mild) describes the effect of the voice disorder on both listener and speaker—the supporting statements (pitch, quality, etc.) will emphasize the primary characteristics that distinguish this patient's dysphonia. The result is a composite definition (Bless & Hicks, 1996) that accounts for commonly observed voice signal deviations in addition to factors such as consistency, noticeability, and effects on communication.

VOICE DISORDER TYPES

Having identified a possible dysphonia and assigned it a severity rating, the clinician should also form a working hypothesis regarding the type of voice disorder that the patient may have. Traditionally, voice disorders have been separated in two main groups.

Functional Voice Disorders

Commonly, the term functional dysphonia has been used to describe those voice disorders in which dysphonia was observed in the absence of organic pathological condition. However, the term "functional" has been challenged as being vague, with relatively little agreement on criteria by which inclusion into the functional dysphonia category is made (Goldman, Hargrave, Hillman, Holmberg, & Gress, 1996). Numerous varied opinions on what defines this type of voice disorder are found below.

- Koufman and Blalock (1982) believed that functional dysphonias are primarily due to abuse and misuse of a normal laryngeal mechanism, with prolonged abuse resulting in the development of conditions such as nodules, polyps, ulcers, or granulomas of the vocal folds. However, it is characteristic that the observed dysphonia is disproportionately poor compared with the status of the laryngeal mechanism. From a review of 52 functional dysphonia patients, these authors delineated five types of functional dysphonia:
  —Type 1. Hysterical Aphonia/Dysphonia: This type is distinguished by a sudden onset often associated with a distinct precipitating event. The patient typically has a normal laryngoscopic examination, no significant associated symptoms, and no history of prior laryngitis. Voice is characterized by aphonia or whisper, limited pitch range, and variability ("pitch-locked" p. 372); consistent/stable voice dysfunction.
  —Type 2. Habituated Hoarseness: This patient reports persistent hoarseness usually after a preceding bout of viral laryngitis. The patient typically has a normal laryngoscopic examination and no significant associated symptoms. Voice is characterized by breathy, raspy, diplophonic quality; limited pitch range and variability; consistent/stable voice dysfunction.
  —Type 3. Falsetto: This patient reports a sudden or developmental onset with an abnormally high-pitched voice; limited pitch range and variability; consistent/stable voice dysfunction. This patient also typically has a normal laryngoscopic examination and no significant associated symptoms.
  —Type 4. Voice Abuse: This patient reports chronic voice problems, although dysphonia may be intermittent. Vocal abuse or misuse characterized by overuse, inappropriate pitch level, and use of excessive muscle tension are common characteristics. Pain or discomfort in the laryngeal region that worsens with increased voice use may be reported. Laryngoscopy may be normal or show a secondary pathological condition. Voice quality is variable; the patient may initiate voicing with abrupt onsets (hard glottal attack).
  —Type 5. Postoperative Dysphonia: This patient reports dysphonia after an operation. Laryngoscopy may be normal or show ventricular fold compression, ulcers, or granulomas. Presence of pain or discomfort in the laryngeal region and voice characteristics are similar to the Type 4 patient; however, ventricular fold use may be prominent in this patient.
- Boone (1980) stipulated that functional dysphonias were those in which the voice problem was "related to faulty vocal fold approximation" (p. 315) in the absence of organic disease. Patients who were seen with dysphonia but normal vegetative function of the larynx (e.g., normal coughing, throat clearing) were referred to as psychogenic.
- Boone and McFarlane (1988) indicate that the patient is directly responsible for a functional dysphonia by using the laryngeal mechanism in a faulty manner. In these cases, the patient "may approximate the vocal folds in a lax manner," "in a tight manner," "or shut the voice off by bringing the ventricular folds together" (p. 52). In addition, the patient is often observed to have normal laryngeal structures, although "complete supraglottal shutoff (ventricular and aryepiglottic fold adduction)" (p. 53) is often observed.
- Aronson (1990a) sees "functional" as synonymous with "psychogenic," with all associated voice problems attributable to some underlying "psychoneuroses, personality disorders, or faulty habits of voice usage" (p. 8). In addition, Aronson (1990a) believes that the term "psychogenic" has "the advantage of stating positively…that the voice disorder is a manifestation of one or more types of psychological disequilibrium, such as anxiety, depression, conversion reaction, or personality disorder, that interfere with normal volitional control over phonation" (p. 121).
- Unlike Aronson (1990a), Morrison and Rammage (1993) do not believe that "functional" and psychogenic" are synonymous. These authors describe a sub-

type of functional dysphonia that they refer to as "muscle misuse voice disorders" (MMVDs, p. 428). MMVDs may be associated with factors such as misuse of extralaryngeal musculature, poor laryngeal posture and misalignment, poor coordination between respiratory and phonatory functions, and excessive or inadequate laryngeal valving. The term "psychogenic" disorder is associated only with those functional dysphonias in which the observed dysphonia is a direct result of a psychoemotional origin as documented by means of formal psychological testing.

- Peppard (in Stemple, 1993) indicates that certain types of functional dysphonias may be related to altered feedback mechanisms (e.g., hearing impairment).
- Titze (1994) states that functional dysphonias may be related to improper use of the voice, although "some prefer to label all functional dysphonias as idiopathic, indicating that there is no known cause" (p. 307).
- In a review of functional dysphonias in adolescents, Peppard (1996) implies that cases of functional dysphonia (such as functional aphonia or puberphonia) are caused by inappropriate use/misuse of the larynx— "These two non-organically based voice pathologies involve the use by adolescents of relatively simple, often less efficient, modes of phonation" (p. 258). In addition, Peppard (1996) believes that not all functional dysphonias have a psychogenic base, because "some cases…may be the result of habituated patterns that, although inappropriate, were not caused by some underlying psychogenic disorder" (p. 259). According to Peppard (1996) key characteristics associated with functional dysphonia are (1) complete aphonia with very little attempt or struggle to produce phonation, (2) little or no indication of effort, and (3) relatively normal prosodic patterns. Similar to the report of Boone (1980), Peppard (1996) also reports that substantial discrepancies between speaking and vegetative voice use are often observed. In conclusion, Peppard (1996) states that functional dysphonia in adolescents may originate from psychogenic causes, efforts to cope with other communicative disabilities, and/or an habituated, inefficient manner of voice production.
- The multifactorial origins of functional dysphonia were stressed by Roy, Bless, Heisey, and Ford (1997a), who state that, "a disordered voice in the context of a structurally normal larynx is the product of a complex/blend of psychological, social, and physiological factors" (p. 322).
- Roy, McGrory, Tasko, Bless, Heisey, and Ford (1997b) state that, "functional implies a disturbance of physiological function rather than in anatomical structure" (pp. 433–444). However, the heterogeneous nature of functional dysphonia was observed by these authors

in a review of the personality and psychological characteristics of 25 female functionally dysphonic (FD) patients. The overall conclusion by Roy et al. (1997b) was that FD patients "display an array of problems including multiple somatic complaints, diffuse anxiety, and dysphonia" (p. 449).

On the basis of the aforementioned opinions, functional voice disorders are those voice disorders in which (1) the patient's use of the voice mechanism is the underlying cause of the voice problem(s), and (2) the laryngeal mechanism appears normal or shows the development of a secondary pathological condition (i.e., a pathological condition that has developed because of the patient's abuse/misuse of the larynx). The faulty use of the laryngeal mechanism may be related to separate or combined factors of habituated muscle tension and vocal inefficiency, compensatory behaviors, and/or psychological stress. In effect, the patient's use of the vocal mechanism has resulted in the dysphonia—its origin is not attributable to some underlying physical or disease process.

Organic Disorders

Compared with functional disorders, the definition of an organic voice disorder seems to be relatively clear-cut. Organic voice disorders are those in which the underlying cause is a specific lesion affecting the laryngeal mechanism itself or within the neuromotor pathways serving the phonatory mechanism. An underlying physical disruption is responsible for the observed dysphonia, not faulty voice use. Commonality in definition for this term is reflected in the following statements:

- Boone (1980) states that organic problems are "related strictly to organic disease or structural problems" (p. 319).
- Boone and McFarlane (1988) identify organic disorders as those in which "the faulty voice is usually related more to a physical condition than to a vocal abuse-misuse per se" (p. 64).
- Titze (1994) states that "organic voice disorders are those for which a specific lesion can be identified in some organ of the body" (p. 307).

Although the underlying physical disruption is key in identifying organic disorders, it must be remembered that the effects of the physical lesion extend beyond perceptual and acoustic consequences. Bless and Hicks (1996) observe that "organic voice problems are multifarious" with effects that are "biological, psychological, and sociocultural" (p. 120).

Alternative Categories

The terms functional versus organic are not necessarily completely separate entities, because organic disorders can result in improper voice use, and improper voice use can result in organic lesions (Titze, 1994). For reasons such as this, several authors have chosen to categorize voice disorders in alternative categories rather than adhere to the traditional functional versus organic distinction as shown below.

- Weinberg (1983) categorizes voice disorders in terms of (1) abuse/misuse of the larynx; (2) voice disorders resulting from organic disease, physical trauma, or structural change; (3) voice disorders resulting from psychogenic factors; and (4) undetermined causes.
- Titze (1994) prefers to classify voice problems in terms of (1) congenital (structural) disorders; (2) disorders related to tissue change; (3) disorders related to neurological or muscular change; and (4) vocal fatigue.
- Verdolini (1994) distinguishes between physical (organic) and not strictly physical (nonorganic) causes. Within this framework, Verdolini (1994) categorizes voice disorders in terms of (1) discrete mass lesions of the vocal folds; (2) voice disorders caused by distributed vocal fold tissue changes; (3) organically based movement disorders; and (4) nonorganically based disorders.

OUTLINE FOR THE CASE HISTORY SESSION

Having reviewed the basic approach to voice diagnosis, equipment preparation, and definitions of key parameters by which we will describe the disordered voice, we are now ready to begin the diagnostic process. Figure 1–4 presents a flowchart summarizing the key elements of the case history session.

The *VDP* starts with the gathering of background information and significant information regarding the patient's possible voice problem(s) in the case history interview. The following are a number of key areas that should be explored with the patient. Wherever possible, it is best to incorporate these issues into a conversation with the patient/caregiver rather than in a "form-filling" exercise. In addition, the clinician will follow the interview with an examination of the speech and hearing mechanisms to identify any significant characteristics of form or function that may be related to the patient's voice deficits.

Presession Information

Before seeing the patient, it is generally advised to obtain as much background information as possible. Immediate

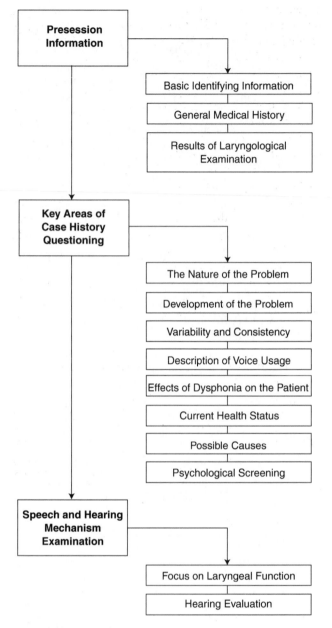

Figure 1–4 Flowchart Outlining the Key Areas of Information Regarding Possible Voice Dysfunction Obtained from the Patient's General Background, Case History, and Speech and Hearing Mechanism Examination

access to information about the prospective patient may be affected by the particular setting in which one works, with the range of initial information extending from simple referral slips with next to nothing in terms of information about the patient's condition to extensive information obtained from medical charts and reports. It must be kept in mind that background information can present something of a double-edged sword to the clinician. On one hand, background information allows the clinician to develop initial hypotheses regarding the patient's condition and underlying deficits. On the other hand, the clinician must be wary of being biased toward a particular clinical hypothesis before the actual collection of patient signs and symptoms has taken place in the diagnostic session. Clinical bias refers to factors that may predispose the clinician to select a particular diagnosis regardless of the actual data observed. The clinician must balance the possibilities presented by background information with the realities of the actual diagnostic session. The background information should spur the clinician on to develop clinical hypotheses, carry out any necessary research regarding the patient's condition before evaluating the patient, and prepare any special tests that may need to be carried out (e.g., although we are focusing on voice evaluation, voice disorders may coexist with other communicative deficits that may also need to be evaluated). However, the clinician must always be prepared for the possibility that the patient may have characteristics that are quite different than background information has led us to believe.

Basic Identifying Information and General Medical History

Before the case history interview, the patient should be given a general case history form to fill out. Numerous examples of these forms are available; however, in using these forms, the clinician is primarily interested in documenting two aspects of the patient's history that do not and should not have to be discussed at length in the interview setting:

1. Identifying information (name, age, date of birth, address, physician name, and contact information, etc.)
2. General medical background; developmental history (in the case of a child patient).

It is *strongly* suggested that the patient (or caregiver) fill out this general case history form before the interview. The general case history form can be reviewed by the speech-language pathologist and, if necessary, key informational points pertinent to the patient's voice disorder can be brought up for clarification in the interview session. The voice clinician is encouraged to carry out a conversation with the patient regarding the key areas of case history questioning and not turn this into a form-filling exercise. It has been my experience that a clinician paying more attention to forms than to the patient appears amateurish. A clinician who appears comfortable with the form and content of the case history interview will be viewed with greater confidence by the patient; with greater confidence, the patient will be more willing to impart information to the clinician.

A review of most general case history forms reveals many areas of questioning that often have no significance to the current patient or the presenting voice disorder. The clinician must not waste time with this material. The clinician must select key areas of questioning that are pertinent to the possible disorder at hand and should always be prepared to answer why they are asking certain questions. This is especially important in certain sensitive areas of health history (e.g., sexual development, illicit drug use).

The Need for Laryngeal Examination Information

In voice disorders, the underlying laryngeal structures may appear normal (as in many functional disorders), show the presence of discrete or distributed benign lesions (e.g., nodules, polyps), or be affected by conditions that have significant, even life-threatening, effects on the patient's overall health (e.g., progressive neurological disease, carcinoma).Unfortunately, all these conditions may have quite similar perceptual and acoustic characteristics. Colton and Casper (1996) demonstrate this fact quite effectively in their reviews of voice disorders related to abuse/misuse, nervous system involvement, and organic disease and trauma. The same perceptual and acoustic signs of hoarseness, increased perturbation levels, and increased spectral noise are reported for disorders as diverse as laryngeal carcinoma, unilateral vocal fold paralysis, laryngitis, and vocal nodules (Colton & Casper, 1996). Peppard (1996) also reports the same perceptual and acoustic signs as possible characteristics of functional dysphonia (with apparently normal larynges in most cases). Of course, perceptual and acoustic signs must be interpreted in light of significant information regarding the patient's health, vocational/social/recreational voice use, etc., obtained by means of the case history interview and medical background. However, the point is clear that the voice clinician (particularly one with relatively little experience) could easily mistake a potentially life-threatening voice problem for one that is functional in nature. With this in mind, I believe that it is essential that referral be made to an otolaryngologist for all voice-disordered cases, with particular emphasis on those in which voice quality deviations are primary characteristics. The referral should occur, ideally, before the voice diagnostic session but definitely before initiation of any voice therapy.

Several authors have made valuable comments on the topic of when and why referral to the otolaryngologist should take place; these are found below.

- Weinberg (1983) described the importance of the laryngeal examination in identifying the possible cause of the voice problem, determining the need for medical treatment, and identification of physical factors that may limit voice change with treatment. The importance of this referral was emphasized by stating that "a(n)...essential part of the diagnostic process for all patients with voice disorders is the completion of a general examination of the head and neck, including the larynx" (p. 159).

- Boone and McFarlane (1988) defer voice therapy until after medical examination because voice therapy may be contraindicated in some cases (e.g., papilloma, carcinoma). "In such cases, the delay of accurate diagnosis of these pathologies could be life-threatening" (p. 80).

- Haynes et al. (1992) emphasize the medical-legal implications and benefits of medical referral. These authors state that "the need for medical diagnosis cannot be overestimated because of the life/health implications for the client, the legal implications for the practicing clinician, and the requirement of third-party reimbursement agencies that services provided be medically necessary" (p. 285).

- Verdolini (1994) states a preference for otolaryngological referral for every voice patient seen. However, "adults older than 50, primarily men, who are hoarse or who have any change in voice for a period of two weeks or more that cannot be reasonably explained... are clearly at risk and should be referred to an otolaryngologist immediately" (p. 290).

- In particular reference to child patients, Case (1996) states that "any child with a voice disorder stemming from abnormal functioning of the vocal folds that produces a difference in voice quality, or in any way makes breathing difficult should be evaluated medically before management by a speech-language pathologist" (p. 72). Case (1996) also stresses that "it is better to err on the side of over-referral" (p. 73) rather than nonreferral, particularly in the situation of the relatively inexperienced voice clinician.

- Even in cases of suspected functional dysphonia (voice disorders in which there is no apparent underlying organic pathological condition and the vocal mechanism appears normal), Peppard (1996) stresses that "ethical practice requires that before any management of voice pathology is started, an otolaryngologist skilled in laryngeal examination and voice disorders must perform a thorough (laryngeal) examination to rule out any possible organic base for the voice disorder" (pp. 259–260).

A complete laryngological examination should involve detailed medical history, head and neck examination, and visual examination of the larynx, with the final result being a medical diagnosis of the problem and recommendations for treatment (Stemple, 1993). Although some speech-language pathologists have acquired skills in laryngeal examination techniques such as mirror laryngoscopy and videostroboscopy, laryngoscopic methods must not be used by the speech-language pathologist for diagnostic purposes. The primary identification and treatment of laryngeal pathological conditions are the clear responsibility of the laryngologist (Boone & McFarlane, 1988). The speech pathologist should review the laryngological examination report for a specific medical diagnosis, description of possible underlying organic pathological condition, and physician recommendations. Although the laryngeal examination report will (generally) provide a diagnostic label for the patient's condition, this does not eliminate the need for the voice diagnostic by the speech-language pathologist. Effective voice therapy recommendations will be made primarily on the basis of the detailed description of the patient's voice characteristics and voice use described in the speech-language pathologist's diagnostic report.

The Nature of the Problem

It is suggested that the clinician start the diagnostic interview with a general open-ended question such as "What can I do for you today?" or "Can you tell me why you are here today?" Several reasons exist for this type of opening question:

1. A general open-ended question provides the patient with the opportunity to describe the possible voice problem(s) in his or her own words. If the clinician began the interview with a closed statement such as "I see here that you have had a hoarse voice," the result would quite possibly be (1) a very limited response from the patient (perhaps even a single word response) and (2) possible clinician and patient bias (the clinician is expecting a certain response, whereas the patient may feel that he or she should provide the expected response).

2. Colton and Casper (1996) have said that patients are often quite accurate in describing their problems. Therefore, we must allow the patient the opportunity and time to describe the problems he or she has been experiencing.

3. As the patient is speaking, the clinician is provided with (1) the first opportunity to observe some of the perceptual characteristics of the voice and (2) a chance to begin verifying some of the patient's complaints (both verbal and what may have been reported in referral statements). Patient complaints are referred to as *symptoms*. One of the primary goals of the voice clinician is to verify as many patient symptoms as possible. Once symptoms are verified (i.e., directly observed by the clinician), they become *signs* (Colton & Casper, 1996). Perceptual judgments regarding the patient's voice characteristics are often the first signs collected by the clinician during the

voice diagnostic—the initial descriptions of the patient about his or her voice problem(s) provide an excellent opportunity for these observations to take place.

4. As the patient is speaking, the clinician is also provided with the opportunity to visualize characteristics that may be accompanying the patient's speech/voice characteristics. These characteristics may include excessive tension in the extralaryngeal region, limited oral movements, and rigidity in the mandibular region.

5. The clinician may start to get some inclination regarding the patient's personality traits and their possible relationship to the perceived voice characteristics and patient symptoms.

This initial aspect of the voice diagnostic interview is often described as an assessment of the nature of the problem (i.e., what is the problem and what are its characteristics). The patient's description of the characteristics of his or her voice problem(s) allows "the clinician to better understand the disorder as the patient sees it" (p. 28, Prater & Swift, 1984). In many cases, the patient's description of the voice problem (e.g., "My voice has had a raspy sound to it for the last few weeks"; "It gets hard to speak at the end of the day.") will correspond closely to the perceptions of the clinician. However, other cases may show a lack of agreement with the views of the speech-language pathologist, with discrepancies caused by factors such as (1) patient misunderstanding of the problem (i.e., reflecting a possible lack of awareness of the disorder), (2) an inability of the patients to deal realistically with their voice deficits (Prater & Swift, 1984), or (3) intermittent voice problems with variable characteristics that may not be in evidence at the time of the interview.

It is hoped that the voice clinician is presented with a patient who is willing to impart information regarding the voice problem(s) relatively freely. However, some patients will require various cues so the nature of their deficits may be grasped. As an example, see below.

Clinician: "Can you please tell me why you are here today?" (general, open-ended question)
Patient: "I have been having trouble speaking lately."
Clinician: "Do you have trouble with the way your speech sounds or in finding the right words to say?" (Focused, leading question)
Patient: "With the way it sounds."
Clinician: "Can you describe for me how your voice sounds when you are having trouble speaking?"
Patient: "It sounds hoarse."

In this example, the patient has answered the initial question regarding the nature of the problem with a short, vague answer. The clinician has responded with a follow-up question that guides the patient to a more descriptive answer that verifies the probable presence of a voice disorder. In the event that the patient is still unable to provide a reasonable description of the problems he or she has been experiencing, it is also useful to ask if the way the voice sounds today (i.e., during the interview) is the way the voice sounds when he or she is having the voice problems. If not, ask the patient to demonstrate the disordered voice.

In addition to the nature of the patient's voice problem, observation of other patient symptoms (i.e., associated symptoms) may provide important information in reaching an appropriate diagnosis. Changes in associated symptoms over time may also be indicators of change in response to treatment (Colton & Casper, 1996). A number of neurological and stress-related symptoms may be associated with factors such as type of voice disorder and onset:

- Dysphagia
- Nasal regurgitation of food and liquids
- Weakness (either bilateral or unilateral) in other parts of the body
- Neurologically related speech and language deficits
- Characteristics of increased musculoskeletal tension
- Increased fatigue
- Heartburn
- Dryness in the mouth and throat

After initial questioning about the nature of the voice problem at hand, the patient must also be questioned in several other key areas so that a complete description of the presenting patient and his or her voice deficit may be acquired.

Development of the Problem

One of the most natural questions after the description of the initial complaint is "How long have you had this problem?" or "When did you first notice your voice problem(s)?" The description of the onset of the voice disorder can be an essential component of case history for both diagnosis and prognosis (Prater & Swift, 1984). The onset of the disorder may be characterized in terms of (1) long duration, gradual onset versus (2) those with sudden onsets. Voice disorders that have developed over a relatively long time generally do not have a specific date of onset that the patient can recall. Various types of voice disorders (organic and functional) may develop over weeks, months, or years. Types of voice disorders that may have a gradual onset are progressive neurological diseases and most laryngeal growths that affect vocal fold vibration (Colton & Casper, 1996). Patients who have had a slow, gradual onset to their voice problem may show less concern about their voice and/or less overall effect on their daily life because they have learned to cope with and compensate for their deficits. Boone and McFarlane (1988) state that gradually developing dysphonias may suggest developing pathological conditions and that these patients may have a poorer overall prognosis for voice/behavior change.

In contrast to gradual onset disorders, those with a sudden onset are often more disturbing to the patient. Acute, sudden onset problems may pose a severe threat to the patient, certainly in terms of ability to carry out daily activities and possibly in terms of overall health (Boone & McFarlane, 1988). The patient may be able to describe the date and details of the onset of the voice disorder with great detail. Voice disorders that develop over a very short time (1 to 2 days or less) may be due to conditions such as severe laryngitis; psychogenic episode (conversion reaction); specific neurological insult (e.g., cerebrovascular accident, closed head injury); trauma to the larynx (external [e.g., blunt trauma to the neck region] or internal [e.g., sudden trauma to the vocal fold mucosa from a singular shouting/screaming episode]); voice disruption as a result of surgery (e.g., vocal fold paresis resulting from thyroid surgery; vocal fold ulceration resulting from intubation). Colton and Casper (1996) indicate that sudden voice change in the absence of symptoms suggestive of an organic pathological condition is often a key component of the psychogenic diagnosis.

Variability and Consistency

It is important for the clinician to discern whether the patient's voice deficits have been relatively consistent over time or have shown degrees of fluctuation. Fluctuation back and forth between better versus poorer voice function is the hallmark of variability and differs from those patients who report consistent change in the voice in terms of steady improvement or worsening of symptoms (Colton & Casper, 1996). Disordered voices that periodically return to normal or near-normal characteristics may be functional in nature. On the other hand, most disorders that have underlying neurological dysfunction or definitive changes in vocal fold structure (e.g., mass lesions) generally do not improve spontaneously (Prater & Swift, 1984). An exception to this is the case of myasthenia gravis, a deficit of neural transmission affecting the myoneural junction. This disorder is variable over time, with patients showing progressive weakness with muscle use, followed by periods of improvement after rest. In those conditions in which dysphonia fluctuates, it is important to question the patient regarding the conditions that are associated with voice change (environmental effects; effects of vocational, social, recreation situations; specific periods of the day associated with poor vs. improved voice). In particular, the patient should be questioned about periods of emotional stress (personal, familial, work-related) that may cause the voice to worsen.

Several authors have commented on the variability of voice disorders. Boone and McFarlane (1988) indicate that hyperfunctional patients often report improved voice function earlier in the day, with increasing dysphonia with increased voice use. Voice that is worse in the morning versus later in the day may be a symptom of postnasal drip or gastroesophageal reflux disease (Boone & McFarlane, 1988; Colton & Casper, 1996). Haynes et al. (1992) state that factors such as personal habits (smoking, alcohol use), work conditions, or medical conditions may affect the variability of a voice disorder. Colton and Casper (1996) report that patients with psychologically based disorders often report considerable variability in their vocal function.

Description of Voice Use

Many voice disorders arise not from definitive underlying organic pathological conditions but from the manner in which the patient uses the phonatory mechanism. Therefore, it is essential that the clinician get a comprehensive view of how the patient uses his or her voice in various situations that may be found within his or her lifestyle. A description of voice use in vocational, social, and recreational settings is of great importance, with abuse, misuse, and overuse of the voice in these various situations often the cause of many functional voice problems (Boone & McFarlane, 1988; Colton & Casper, 1996). Because it is not always possible for the clinician to directly observe the patient in all the aforementioned situations, the patient may be encouraged to demonstrate the voice use in these various settings for the clinician (Boone & McFarlane, 1988). Haynes et al. (1992) state that the clinician must determine the vocal demands of the patient's profession and also determine whether the patient must produce speech under adverse conditions. Several types of voice use and/or setting have been commonly associated with the development of voice disorders:

- Any work setting that requires the patients to use their voices for their livelihood (i.e., professional voice users [Colton & Casper, 1996]) may be potentially harmful in terms of the development of voice disorders, particularly if these patients have not had any professional voice training.
- Social settings such as gatherings at parties or in bars may present a potentially abusive environment.
- Sporting events present a potentially abusive situation for both spectator and participant. Forceful phonation that is potentially damaging to the vocal fold mucosa may accompany strenuous exercise (Colton & Casper, 1996).
- Singing in various situations (choir, theater, recreational musician) presents a potentially abusive condition for many, particularly if they have not had professional voice training (e.g., high-intensity voice in the presence of high levels of background noise; possibly under adverse conditions such as singing in bars in a smoky atmosphere; poor monitors).

Effects of Dysphonia on the Patient

Colton and Casper (1996) stated that "the severity of the (patient's) reaction is not always proportional to the severity of the voice problem" (p. 190). This may be because voice disorders that affect the patient's vocation or draw negative reactions from others will be of more concern to the patient than those voice disorders that do not adversely affect daily life. When asked about the effects of the dysphonia, some patients may be apprehensive about discussing what may be a potentially humiliating effect on their lifestyle. However, the clinician should ensure that expressions of denial regarding effects of the dysphonia are fully explored (Colton & Casper, 1996; Prater & Swift, 1984). It should be remembered that it may not be the actual reactions to the patient's dysphonia that are as important as how a patient feels about the reactions of others (Prater & Swift, 1984). Feelings of stress, tension, and development of possible negative psychological outlook may arise as a result of reactions to dysphonia.

Health Status

The patient's health history should be assessed to determine any possible relationship to the presenting voice disorder. Voice characteristics reflect not only the emotional state and personality of the patient but also the overall physical status (Colton & Casper, 1996). The voice clinician is particularly interested in health history in the following areas:

- Current health status.
- Injuries or trauma to the head and/or neck region.
- Neurological problems.
- Respiratory deficits.
- Allergy-related problems.
- History of frequent upper respiratory tract infections.
- Surgeries, particularly in which the patient may have been intubated.
- Smoking, alcohol use, illicit drug use.
- Ingestion of caffeinated beverages (coffee, tea, soft drinks).
- Use of prescription and over-the-counter medications (e.g., antihistamines, decongestants, diuretics).
- Endocrine imbalances.
- Previous occurrences of voice dysfunction or "loss" of the voice.
- Hydration status—Degree of internal hydration may affect the viscosity of mucus secretions and aids in lubrication of the vocal fold cover (Stemple, 1993). A well-lubricated cover protects the vocal fold during the vibratory cycle and aids in heat dissipation. Ingestion of six 8-ounce glasses of water or fruit juice per day is generally recommended.

Possible Causes

The voice clinician should ask the patient directly what he or she believes may have been the possible cause(s) of the voice problem(s) (Boone & McFarlane, 1988). Comparison of the patient's response to descriptions of possible causes described by referral sources (e.g., physician, previous speech-language pathologist) may reflect on the knowledge and insight the patient has regarding his or her voice problem. Differing views on the possible cause of a voice disorder between the patient, referral sources, and family members may reflect (1) an inability to adequately understand what may have been explained to the patient, (2) an inability to recognize inner causes of the voice problem, or (3) an inability to accept and cope with the problem. Prater and Swift (1984) believe that differences in perception of what has caused the voice problem versus opinions offered by referral sources must be addressed if the patient is to have a positive prognosis for improvement in voice therapy.

Issues Dealing with Psychological Screening

Several authors have stressed the fact that voice disorders may be symptomatic of factors such as (1) inability to hold satisfactory interpersonal relationships (Boone & McFarlane, 1988), (2) struggle with social aspects of communication (Prater & Swift, 1984), and (3) psychological stress arising from diverse (financial, marital, personal, professional, physical, mental, or emotional) sources (Dworkin & Meleca, 1997). In order that these sources are fully investigated, psychological screening must be a critical aspect of voice diagnosis, particularly in the case of "functional" dysphonias. Aronson (1990b) stresses that a psychosocial history is crucial for successful diagnosis and therapy because it often uncovers "a disturbance in the patient's psychologic equilibrium" (p. 288) that underlies the patient's dysphonia.

"Functional" patients often have the following characteristics (Aronson, 1990b):

1. They describe the development of their voice problems in conjunction with the development of personal problems.
2. They are often reluctant to verbally express their conflicts.
3. They are patients with whom no one has bothered to take a psychosocial history.

In addition, evidence of psychological stress may be reflected in the following nonverbal cues (Andrews, 1995; Boone & McFarlane, 1988; Dworkin & Meleca, 1997; Prater & Swift, 1984):

- Sweaty palms
- Avoidance of eye contact

- Excessive postural adjustments
- Facial tics
- Masked facial expression
- Head and neck muscle tension
- Head and/or hand tremors

Although it is not within the purview of the speech-language pathologist to conduct formal personality testing, it is essential that the clinician derive at least an impression regarding the patient's psychosocial behavior and basic adjustment to life (Aronson, 1990b; Haynes et al., 1992; Murry, 1982). Psychological screening of the patient should involve three key areas of questioning:

- Influence of stressors: Stressors are events that necessitate changes in how an individual conducts his or her life (Holmes & Rahe, 1967 in Goldman et al., 1996). Examples of stressors may be changing jobs, moving to a different part of the country, or going through a divorce.
- Influence of anxiety: Anxiety refers to the presence of an unpleasant emotional state or condition (Spielberger, Gorsuch, Lushene, Vagg, and Jacobs, 1983 in Goldman et al., 1996). Goldman et al. (1996) state that "different individuals may inherently experience different levels of anxiety and/or may react to a given stressor (e.g., life event) with different degrees of anxiety" (p. 45). Anxiety may be separated in two components: state anxiety versus trait anxiety. State anxiety refers to the patient's present feelings of anxiety; trait anxiety refers to an individual's persistent or personality-related level of anxiety (Goldman et al., 1996). Examples of anxiety could be feelings of worry or inadequacy.
- Somatic complaints: These are physical complaints, illnesses, weaknesses, etc. (e.g., headaches, heartburn). In some patients psychological stress and/or anxiety may manifest itself in the development of physical symptoms. Exhibit 1–1 provides an example of a simple survey developed by Goldman et al. (1996) that may be given to the patient to gather background information regarding common somatic complaints.

Several studies have directly examined the presence of factors such as stress, anxiety, and somatic complaints in a variety of voice disorders as shown below.

- Cannito (1991) examined psychometric measures of depression, anxiety, and somatic complaints in 18 female patients with spasmodic dysphonia (SD) and a group of matched normal controls. Results showed that 56% of the SD patients were either clinically anxious or depressed. In addition, the SD subjects demonstrated abnormally elevated levels of somatic complaints that were not observed in the normal control subjects. Cannito (1991) concluded that the identification and relief of emotional disorders in SD patients were critical for their effective management, and that any behavioral voice therapy gains would be temporary in patients who remained clinically anxious and depressed.
- Goldman et al. (1996) compared measures of psychological stress, anxiety, voice use, and somatic complaints in groups of women with vocal nodules. In addition, results were compared with women with functional dysphonia (i.e., presence of dysphonia in the absence of an organic pathological condition), as well as a group of normal controls. The Schedule of Recent Experience was used to obtain estimates of psychological stress, and the State-Trait Anxiety Inventory was used to assess levels of anxiety. Results indicated that both dysphonic groups (nodules and functional dysphonia patients) had greater than normal levels of anxiety (both state and trait) and a significantly greater incidence of somatic complaints than the normal controls. In addition, the functional dysphonia group showed a greater level of adjustment-related stress than the normal controls. These authors concluded that there appears to be "evidence of an association between selected psychosocial factors and hyperfunctional voice disorders" (p. 51). The assessment of psychosocial variables would appear to be an important component of a battery of tests used to assist in differential diagnosis and may be useful in identifying those patients who may benefit from counseling or formal psychological evaluation.
- Roy et al. (1997b) reported on results from the Minnesota Multiphasic Personality Inventory (MMPI) obtained from groups of FD women and a group of control subjects without voice disorders. Results showed that only 32% of the FD patients had "normal" profiles on the MMPI compared with 90% of the controls. In addition, the FD patients were significantly different from the control subjects on 7 of 10 personality scales. Two scales were observed to sufficiently discriminate the FD subjects from the controls: (1) a general index of frequency of somatic complaints and (2) a measure of diffuse anxiety. Roy et al. (1997b) concluded that somatic complaints and anxiety may be characteristic traits of FD patients. These traits "may constitute a persistent vulnerability (diathesis) for the development of tensional or somatic symptoms when under conditions of psychological distress" (p. 449). Failure to recognize the possible presence of underlying psychological stress and tension in FD patients may limit the long-term prognosis of these patients.

Psychological factors may be associated with voice disorders as (1) an underlying cause and/or (2) a result of

Exhibit 1–1 Somatic Complaints Survey

1. Do you ever have trouble with heartburn, gastric reflux, or stomach upset?

   __ Never   __ Infrequently   __ At least once per month   __ At least once per week

2. Do you ever have headaches?

   __ Never   __ Infrequently   __ At least once per month   __ At least once per week

3. (when not exercising) Do you have pain in the chest or does your heart seem to pound or race?

   __ Never   __ Infrequently   __ At least once per month   __ At least once per week

4. Fainting or dizziness?

   __ Never   __ Infrequently   __ At least once per month   __ At least once per week

5. Trouble sleeping?

   __ Never   __ Infrequently   __ At least once per month   __ At least once per week

6. (when not exercising) Do you have shortness of breath?

   __ Never   __ Infrequently   __ At least once per month   __ At least once per week

7. Hot or cold spells? Are you easily chilled?

   __ Never   __ Infrequently   __ At least once per month   __ At least once per week

8. Numbness or tingling?

   __ Never   __ Infrequently   __ At least once per month   __ At least once per week

9. Poor appetite, associated weight loss?

   __ Never   __ Infrequently   __ At least once per month   __ At least once per week

10. Overeating, associated with weight gain?

    __ Never   __ Infrequently   __ At least once per month   __ At least once per week

11. Do you ever feel uncomfortable about eating or drinking in public?

    __ Never   __ Infrequently   __ At least once per month   __ At least once per week

12. Do you ever feel like you have a lump in your neck or throat?

    __ Never   __ Infrequently   __ At least once per month   __ At least once per week

13. Do you notice any tenderness in your back or shoulders?

    __ Never   __ Infrequently   __ At least once per month   __ At least once per week

14. Do you have any pain or trouble swallowing?

    __ Never   __ Infrequently   __ At least once per month   __ At least once per week

Source: Reprinted with permission from S. Goldman et al., Stress, Anxiety, Somatic Complaints, and Voice Use in Women with Vocal Nodules: Preliminary Findings, *American Journal of Speech-Language Pathology*, Vol. 5, No. 1, pp. 44–53, © 1996, American Speech-Language Hearing Association.

coping with an incapacitating voice disorder (Roy et al., 1997b). In this view, psychological factors should be considered with all voice disorder types (organic and functional/psychogenic), because "all disease processes carry components of emotional stress" (Colton & Casper, 1996, p. 196). Although the clinician may believe it necessary to refer the patient for formal psychological testing (Murry, 1982), it would appear valuable to include questions dealing with the presence of stressors, anxiety, and somatic complaints in the case history interview. Although the clinician may be met with some degree of patient resistance to this line of questioning (Aronson, 1990b), the possible value obtained in terms of diagnostic accuracy and success in treatment will be well worth the effort.

SPEECH MECHANISM EXAMINATION—BASIC OVERVIEW AND FOCUS ON ASPECTS OF LARYNGEAL EVALUATION

During a voice evaluation, our attention is primarily focused on the function of the respiratory/laryngeal complex. However, it is important that the speech clinician also assess the form and function of the other components of the speech mechanism (face and lips, mandible, velar function, etc.). In particular, the clinician should pay close attention to signs of possible neurological deficits in which abnormalities (unilateral or bilateral) in muscle strength, speed, range, accuracy, steadiness, and/or tone may be present (Darley, Aronson, & Brown, 1975). Neuromuscular deficits affecting one part of the speech mechanism may also be reflected in phonatory function. The clinician is directed toward a comprehensive oral-facial mechanism examination outline such as the Dworkin-Culatta Oral Mechanism Examination (Dworkin & Culatta, 1980) for an extensive assessment of speech mechanism function.

Several key components of the speech mechanism examination are focused on laryngeal function. Detailed evaluation of factors such as pitch, loudness, quality, and durational capability will be discussed in substantial detail throughout the following chapters and, therefore, will not be considered here:

- The sharp cough: During the speech mechanism evaluation, the patient should be asked to produce a sharp cough. Laryngeal weakness may be indicated by the presence of a weak, "mushy" cough (Prater & Swift, 1984).
- Vocal fold diadochokinesis: Observation of the patient's capability to carry out vocal fold diadochokinesis (VF-DDK, a.k.a. laryngeal diadochokinesis [L-DDK]) refers to the repetition of rapid adductory-abductory movements over time. Renout, Leeper, Bandur, and Hudson (1995) described diadochokinesis "as the action

of arresting one motor impulse and substituting in its place a movement that is diametrically opposed" (p. 74). Patients may be asked to produce the syllable /ʔʌ/ (i.e., initiation of a centralized vowel with a glottal stop production [Verdolini, 1994]) or the syllable /hʌ/ (Renout et al., 1995). Use of the syllable /hʌ/ may be preferable because it requires the patient to shift rapidly between abducted and adducted positions. Patients are asked to repeat the selected syllable as fast as possible on one uninterrupted breath (Renout et al., 1995). The patient's production will ideally be recorded and then closely reviewed for the number of repetitions within a 5-second (Renout et al., 1995) or 7-second (Verdolini, 1994) time period. The VF-DDK is then generally reported as the number of syllable repetitions per second.

Verdolini (1994) mentions three characteristics of VF-DDK that should be observed by the clinician:

1. The rate of glottal plosives per second
2. The strength of the plosives
3. Steadiness (i.e., ability to produce rhythmic repetitions) over time

In terms of rate, normal VF-DDK for adults has been reported in the range of five to six syllables per second (Canter, 1965; Shanks, 1966 in Renout et al., 1995) or similar in nature to the expected diadochokinetic rate for the syllable /kʌ/ (Verdolini, 1994).

- Head twisting during phonation: The action of twisting/turning the head sharply to the side has the effect of compressing the pyriform sinus on the side to which the patient is turning. In addition, this movement may serve to push the vocal fold on the side to which the patient is turning more toward the midline of the glottis. This may be an effective technique of improving voice function, particularly for those patients who show some degree of unilateral vocal fold paralysis/paresis (Boone & McFarlane, 1988; Hutchinson, Hanson, & Mecham, 1979; Logemann, 1998). The patient should be asked to twist/turn the head toward the right shoulder and then phonate (sustain the vowel /ɑ/)—the procedure should be repeated by having the patient turn toward the left shoulder. The clinician should listen closely for changes in voice quality. If unilateral paralysis/paresis is present, the patient may be able to achieve better quality voice with the head twisted toward the weak side.

In addition to the aforementioned laryngeal tasks, the clinician should be aware of signs of excessive muscle tension that may be affecting voice production. Characteristics consistent with increased muscle tension may be head or hand tremors, abnormal breathing patterns, visible tightness in the neck or jaw region, or unusual downward or upward excursions of the larynx during speech (Andrews, 1995; Boone & McFarlane, 1988; Stemple, 1993). The reader is referred to Chapter 6 for a detailed description of evaluation procedures and the possible effects of excessive musculo-skeletal tension on voice production.

Hearing Evaluation

In addition to evaluating the integrity of the peripheral speech mechanism, it is also important to assess the hearing mechanism. Murry (1982) stresses that "under no circumstances should the voice evaluation be completed without information about the patient's hearing ability" (p. 485). Difficulty controlling vocal loudness or use of appropriate loudness levels in speech may result secondary to hearing loss (Colton & Casper, 1996; Murry, 1982; Stemple, 1993). Dworkin and Meleca (1997) state that abnormally quiet/soft voices may accompany cases of conductive hearing loss, whereas sensorineural hearing loss may cause the patient to speak in an abnormally loud voice. In the case of a conductive hearing loss, bone conduction is better than air conduction. Therefore, the patient may believe that he or she is producing an adequately loud voice when it is, in fact, too quiet. In sensorineural losses, both air and bone conduction are detrimentally affected, causing the patient to increase

vocal loudness as compensation. With these possibilities in mind, hearing screening is certainly a necessary aspect of the voice diagnostic. Referral for a full audiological examination may also be necessary in some cases.

SUMMARY

The *Voice Diagnostic Protocol* is a set of clinical methods and procedures by which a comprehensive evaluation of phonatory voice disorders may be carried out. We begin the *VDP* with the gathering of background information and significant information regarding the patient's possible voice problem(s) in the case history interview. During this interview, the clinician should always be listening/observing so the statements that the patient/caregiver is providing may be verified. In this way, a number of the descriptions that we are provided with (symptoms) become verifiable facts (signs) (Colton & Casper, 1996). The clinician will follow the interview with an examination of the speech and hearing mechanisms to identify any significant characteristics of form or function that may be related to the patient's voice deficits. Finally, initial hypotheses dealing with the differential diagnosis of the voice problem are being formed at this point. These hypotheses will eventually be proved or disproved through (1) the addition of the formal observations we will be making in our application of specific tests/procedures and (2) comparisons with normative data.

CHAPTER 2

Evaluation of Vocal Pitch/Frequency

DEFINITION

When listening to a musical or singing passage, most people are able to identify a "high" note versus a "low" note. When making this "high" or "low" distinction, the listener is responding to the *pitch* of the voice or instrument that he or she is listening to. Pitch is the auditory perception of the fundamental rate of vibration of some sound-producing source. Pitch corresponds quite well with *frequency*. In contrast to pitch, frequency is the objective measurement of the fundamental rate of vibration (i.e., a measurement of the number of cycles of vibration per second). The assessment of pitch and frequency is an essential aspect of the voice evaluation. Because the pitch and frequency of the voice are a direct result of changes in factors such as (1) elasticity, (2) mass, and (3) the length of the vocal folds, the speech-language pathologist may discern key insights in reference to the function of the phonatory mechanism from their evaluation.

CONTROL OF VOCAL PITCH/FREQUENCY

The frequency of vocal fold vibration is generally referred to as the vocal fundamental frequency (F_0). The most important factors affecting frequency of vocal fold vibration are (1) effective vibrating mass, (2) tension of the folds, and (3) subglottal pressure (Folkins & Kuehn, 1982). Changes in the physical dimensions and positions of the folds relative to each other may affect all three variables. Among the intrinsic muscles of the larynx, the interaction of the cricothyroid and the vocalis/thyroarytenoid muscles appears to be most important for the control of effective mass, stiffness, and tension of the vocal folds (Sawashima & Hirose, 1983; Titze, 1994). When considering the interaction of the cricothyroid and the vocalis/thyroarytenoid muscles, a number of possibilities regarding the control of vocal F_0 are possible as shown.

- If the cricothyroid contracts and the vocalis/thyroarytenoid complex is inactive, the folds will lengthen. This results in a decrease in the effective mass and an increase in the stiffness of both the body (vocalis/thyroarytenoid) and the cover (epithelium and elastic/collagenous fibers of the lamina propria) of the folds (Sawashima & Hirose, 1983; Titze, 1994). The overall effect on voice is that F_0 will increase.
- If the vocalis/thyroarytenoid contracts and the cricothyroid is inactive, the length of the vocal fold will decrease and effective mass will increase. The result is a decrease in vocal F_0. However, during vocalis/thyroarytenoid contraction, the stiffness of the body may increase while that of the cover decreases, making the combined stiffness difficult to predict. Usually, the stiffness of the cover predominates, and, thus, the F_0 would probably decrease (Sawashima & Hirose, 1983; Titze, 1994).
- If the cricothyroid and vocalis/thyroarytenoid contract simultaneously in such a way that the length is unaltered (isometric contraction), it is likely that F_0 will increase somewhat (Titze, 1994).

Although the cricothyroid and vocalis/thyroarytenoid seem to be the primary muscles of frequency change in the larynx, the other intrinsic muscles of the larynx also may be active in frequency change. The lateral cricoarytenoid muscle also has been observed to participate in the regulation of F_0 and register of voice, although in a supportive role to the cricothyroid and vocalis/thyroarytenoid (Hirano, 1981). The posterior cricoarytenoid muscle usually is inactive during phonation, although it may be activated for high-pitched modal voice (Hirano, 1981). Hirano (1981) suggested that posterior cricoarytenoid action at high frequencies in modal register was necessary to brace the arytenoid cartilages against the anterior pull brought about by cricothyroid. A differing view of posterior cricoarytenoid action is presented by Hollien (1983), who states that the anterior pull of the cricothyroid is not enough to raise pitch to high levels in modal register. It is, therefore, supplemented by posterior cricoarytenoid and interarytenoid muscle activity, which pulls the arytenoids in a posterior direction and increases vocal fold tension.

The frequency of the voice has also been observed to increase with increases in subglottal air pressure (Perkins & Yanagihara, 1968). However, such pressure changes may account only for 2 to 4 Hz per cm H_2O (Hixon, Klatt, & Mead, 1971). Hixon et al. (1971) concluded that control of pitch is primarily the result of laryngeal adjustments and not respiratory activity.

The conclusions about the control of frequency that may be made are found below.

1. Laryngeal adjustments during frequency change affect the effective vibrating mass and the tension of the vocal folds.
2. The cricothyroid and vocalis/thyroarytenoid muscles are the principal laryngeal muscles used in raising the F_0. The cricothyroid is mainly responsible for frequency increases, whereas the vocalis/thyroarytenoid is responsible for register change.
3. Secondary roles in raising the F_0 may be played by the lateral cricoarytenoid and posterior cricoarytenoid muscles. The posterior cricoarytenoid may act to brace the arytenoid cartilages against the anterior pull of cricothyroid or may act in concert with the interarytenoid muscles to further elongate the vocal folds by pulling the arytenoids in a posterior direction during high pitch.
4. Subglottal air pressure has a limited influence on increases in vocal pitch.

VOCAL REGISTERS

The vocal register used during phonation greatly affects the physical dimensions and positions of the vocal folds. Three commonly recognized vocal registers occupy overlapping ranges along the frequency scale (Folkins & Kuehn, 1982). The highest of the three registers is *falsetto*, which is seldom, if ever, used during conversational speech. In falsetto (loft register), the folds may remain somewhat open, although parallel, resulting in a characteristic breathy quality (Boone & McFarlane, 1988). Keidar, Hurtig, and Titze (1987) state that falsetto phonation represents a waveform change from modal register phonation. The middle range is referred to as *modal* register (chest register). Modal register is the most used part of the pitch and F_0 range and is used most frequently for speech and most singing (Keidar et al., 1987). The lowest range is *vocal fry* (pulse register). Vocal fry is not used in most common vocal activities, although it may be used by some individuals during conversational speech (particularly at the end of a phrase or sentence) (Folkins & Kuehn, 1982; Keidar et al., 1987). Boone and McFarlane (1988) describe vocal fry as a low-frequency "sputter" (p. 37). Early photographic and x-ray investigations found a lengthening of the vocal folds with increases in frequency up to falsetto register. In falsetto, the consistent direct relation between frequency and vocal fold length becomes variable (Hollien & Moore, 1960).

Changes in vocal register may lead to differences in control of frequency. The aforementioned descriptions of laryngeal control of frequency relate most closely to modal register, in which a rise in vocal pitch is principally achieved by contractions of both the cricothyroid and vocalis/thyroarytenoid. The most noticeable difference in muscle control between the modal and falsetto registers is in the activity of the vocalis/thyroarytenoid. Sawashima, Gay, and Harris (1969) observed that in falsetto, compared with the modal register, there is a marked decrease in electromyography activity for the vocalis/thyroarytenoid that is accompanied by a slight decrease in cricothyroid activity. The difference in the muscle control for the two registers results in a difference in the physical conditions of the cover and body of the vocal folds. This difference is reflected in the mode of vocal fold vibration. Aronson (1973, p. 60) has described the physiological mechanism of falsetto in terms of both intrinsic and extrinsic muscles of the larynx as follows:

1. Through the action of the thyrohyoid and the suprahyoid musculature the larynx is elevated high into the neck.
2. Through action of the stylohyoid muscles, the larynx is tilted downward, resulting in maintenance of the vocal folds in a state of laxity.
3. Even though the vocal folds are in a flabby state, the contraction of the cricothyroid muscles causes the vocal folds to be stretched thin.
4. The vocal folds are now reduced in mass and offer low resistance to subglottal air pressure.
5. Only the medial edges of the folds vibrate because during phonation, subglottal air pressure is at a minimum.

PERCEPTUAL ASSESSMENT OF PITCH

Perceptual analysis of pitch generally focuses on three key characteristics: (1) habitual pitch level, (2) pitch variability and stability, and (3) total pitch range.

Habitual Pitch

The *habitual pitch* has been defined as the pitch that the patient uses most often in everyday speech (Prater & Swift, 1984) and is the pitch level around which normal pitch inflections/variations occur (Case, 1996). Boone and McFarlane (1988) state that the habitual pitch corresponds to the *modal pitch level* (i.e., the most frequently used pitch), whereas Case (1996) indicates that habitual pitch is synonymous with the *average pitch level*.

Colton and Casper (1996) indicate that the assessment of the habitual pitch level should focus on whether the pitch level is appropriate for the patient's age and gender. The determination of "normal" habitual pitch level is clearly related to knowledge of several key patient characteristics (age and gender, body size/type, race, but also socioeconomic and cultural class [Weinberg, 1983]) other than the characteristics of the voice itself. When gauging the normality of pitch, it appears that we make a mental/internal comparison between the perceived pitch level and our expectations (gained through experience) for the person's/speaker's age, gender, etc. When the speaker's pitch level does not fall within our expected range, an abnormal pitch level is perceived. In addition, listener confusion as to age and gender may also occur.

Pitch Variability and Stability

In addition to the habitual pitch level, the voice clinician should make determinations of the patient's capability to vary/change pitch levels during speech, as well as the patient's ability to control the vocal pitch. Normal continuous speech production may incorporate a relatively wide range of pitch variation (a range of approximately 4 to 10 musical notes [semitones] [Awan, 1993]). These pitch variations make up the normal intonation patterns of speech. Intonation patterns include pitch variations that are used linguistically to vary the meaning of utterances (Colton & Casper, 1996). Increases in pitch level may be used to indicate a particularly informative linguistic unit within the utterance or an interrogative/questioning statement; pitch decreases often accompany unstressed syllable production and the end of declarative statements. The use of pitch variability/intonation patterns allows for more interesting and expressive communication. Continuous speech production that lacks pitch variability (monopitch—a "single" pitch level) may be perceived as dull and uninteresting. If pitch variability (either too little or too much) draws attention to itself, it may be considered to be abnormal (Haynes et al., 1992). In addition, there is evidence that reduced pitch variability and intonation patterns may decrease the intelligibility of the utterance, because the rise and fall of the normal pitch contour direct the attention of the listener to the content words of an utterance (Laures & Weismer, 1999).

An important aspect of pitch variability that must be attended to by the voice clinician is the presence of pitch instability or the lack of control of vocal pitch. This type of pitch instability is relatively easily perceived by the clinician (macroscopic) and should not be confused with the relatively microscopic cycle-to-cycle pitch instabilities measured in jitter (see Chapter 4). Pitch instability may be perceived as a "shakiness" in the voice or observed as unexpected pitch changes/variations during conditions in which we would expect pitch to remain relatively stable. In addition to a "shaky" quality, three other important types of pitch instability may be observed.

Pitch Breaks

In this condition, it is most common to observe a rapid pitch change/break upward. This may occur if the speaker is using an inappropriately low pitch during speech (Haynes et al., 1992) or if a patient attempts to sustain a high-pitch modal register phonation that rapidly shifts into falsetto.

Diplophonia

In this condition, the listener may perceive the simultaneous production of two pitches in the voice signal. Diplophonia is attributed to the differential vibration of two different sound sources with different mass/length/tension characteristics (Prater & Swift, 1984). Monsen (1979) observed that the diplophonic voice was characterized by alternating pitch periods rather than simultaneous production of different pitches and attributed diplophonia to irregularities in glottal vibration pattern in which alternating glottal periods were slightly different in period or shape. Although diplophonia is being discussed as a pitch deviation, it should be noted that this characteristic often gives the impression of roughness in the voice.

Vocal Tremor

Defined as a rhythmic variation in pitch (and often loudness) during conditions in which steadiness of pitch would be expected, this characteristic is most evident during the production of sustained vowels.

Total Pitch Range

One other important aspect of pitch determination is the assessment of the total pitch range of the patient (a.k.a. vocal range, total phonational range). This entails an assessment of the range between the lowest pitch in modal register to the highest pitch in falsetto. Total pitch range has been said to provide an important index of laryngeal health (Case, 1996) and is often one of the first parameters of vocal capability affected in voice disorders.

METHODOLOGICAL CONSIDERATIONS IN PITCH PERCEPTION

As stated, the pitch characteristics of the voice may provide the clinician with important insights regarding the status of the phonatory mechanism. Case (1996) stresses the importance of perceptual pitch assessment by stating

"…regardless of what numbers indicate from objective assessment…if a person's voice pitch draws negative attention, a voice disorder exists" (p. 116). However, several other researchers/authors would question Case's (1996) faith in the perceptual judgment of pitch. Colton and Casper (1996) indicate that other perceptual attributes (particularly quality characteristics) of the voice signal may invalidate perceptual judgments of pitch. This view is also held by Bless and Hicks (1996), who state that the complex nature of the voice signal may fool the clinician attempting to characterize the pitch of the voice. The accuracy of pitch perception may be influenced by (1) instability in vocal pitch and/or (2) the addition of significant noise components to the voice signal. This appears to be particularly true for rough/harsh voices (Wolfe & Ratusnik, 1988) that may contain periods of diplophonia (Prater & Swift, 1984) or *subharmonic* components (Omori, Kojima, Kakani, Slavit, & Blaugrund, 1997). *Harmonics* are integer multiples of the fundamental frequency of the voice and, therefore, are frequencies higher in pitch than the fundamental frequency/average pitch level. In contrast, subharmonics occur at noninteger multiples of the fundamental frequency and, therefore, occur between the true harmonics.

As an example, a voice with a fundamental frequency of 100 Hz would have harmonics at 200 Hz, 300 Hz, 400 Hz. …If a subharmonic were present, it would occur between the true harmonics (e.g., at 150 Hz, 250 Hz…). In this example, the pitch of the voice will be perceived as being lower than a 100-Hz fundamental frequency voice normally would be because the largest integer divisor of the harmonic/subharmonic sequence described (100 Hz, 150 Hz, 200 Hz, 250 Hz…) is 50 Hz. This is an example of the "missing fundamental," in which our brain perceives a lower F_0 and,

therefore, a lower pitch than is actually present in the voice signal. Omori et al. (1997) indicate that the perceived roughness of the voice is related to the presence and power of subharmonics. In turn, the rough voice may also be perceived as having a lower pitch. Although it may appear as if our perceptions are being deceived, it must be asked, is the perception of lower pitch really false in the case of the rough voice? Omori et al. (1997) provide examples showing that periodicity may only be achieved every second or third cycle in cases of rough voice. Therefore, the *true* fundamental frequency *is* a low frequency and would be compatible with the perception of a low pitch. Figure 2–1 provides an example of a rough voice waveform showing subharmonic tendencies.

As with all types of perceptual analysis methods, issues of training and experience of the listener must also be considered when assessing the accuracy of pitch judgments. Colton and Casper (1996) believe that it is unlikely that graduate students or new clinicians with limited experience in identifying and rating characteristics such as pitch or tremor will be able to achieve adequate reliability. With this in mind, Colton and Casper (1996) have a clear preference for objective measurements of frequency over perceptual assessment of pitch.

HOW TO DO IT: PERCEPTUAL ASSESSMENT OF PITCH

Habitual Pitch

Perceptual assessment of vocal pitch may be easily carried out and reported using a multipoint scale. Rat-

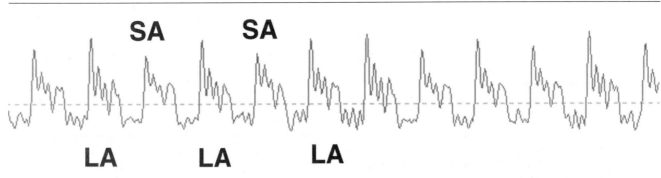

Figure 2–1 Voice Waveform Showing Amplitude Modulation Consistent with the Presence of a Subharmonic. Large-amplitude (LA) and small-amplitude (SA) cycles alternate through portions of the waveform. Periodicity is achieved every second cycle during these portions of the wave.

ings of habitual pitch may be applied to (1) a picture description/spontaneous speech sample and/or (2) a standard reading sample, such as "The Rainbow Passage" (Fairbanks, 1960). Habitual pitch level may be reported using a 7-point categorical/equal-appearing interval rating scale in the following format:

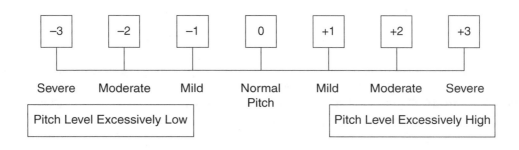

Although the scale incorporates 7 points, note that the central point of the scale is zero (i.e., no substantial difference from normal expectations), with ratings of high pitch (positive numbers) and low pitch (negative numbers) rated on either side of the normal expectation point. Definitions for mild, moderate, and severe are the same as those presented in the Introduction (Chapter 1). Therefore, a moderately high-pitched voice would be one in which both trained and untrained listeners would consider the voice abnormally high, and there may be periods or situations in which the voice characteristic is highly distracting.

Although still requiring the perceptual skills of the clinician, a simple method that can be used to get a more objective determination of the appropriateness of the patient's habitual pitch level is to match the habitual pitch by use of a pitch pipe or musical instrument (e.g., keyboard). Unfortunately, the natural pitch variability (intonation patterns) used in the speaking voice may make it difficult to identify a particular habitual pitch level to match. We can obtain an estimate of the patients' habitual speaking pitch level by having them "chant" a speech utterance (counting), followed by a sustained vowel /ɑ/, which approximates the chanted pitch. The instructions below are given to the patient.

"I want you to repeat the numbers "one, two, three, four." I would like you to chant them like this…":

$\overrightarrow{\text{One}}$, $\overrightarrow{\text{two}}$, $\overrightarrow{\text{three}}$, $\overrightarrow{\text{four}}$

(These words have a horizontal arrow over them to imply a flat intonation pattern.)

🕭 "I want you to sustain the "or" of the number "four" and then match it with a vowel /ɑ/. You will sustain the vowel /ɑ/ for at least 2 to 3 seconds at a comfortable loudness level." (A sample file [1234.WAV] is provided on disk to demonstrate this method.)

During the production of the sustained vowel, the clinician attempts to match (as closely as possible) the pitch of the patient's voice with the pitch pipe, keyboard, etc., and the musical note closest to the patient's habitual pitch level is obtained. According to Boone and McFarlane (1988), the typical male adult voice will have a habitual pitch level near the musical note C_3; the typical female adult voice near musical note A_3; and the typical prepubertal child voice near musical note C_4. Two reasons for using this method of estimating habitual pitch are as follows:

1. Matching a sustained vowel production with a pitch pipe or other musical instrument is much easier and efficient than the method advocated by Boone and McFarlane (1988) and Prater and Swift (1984), in which attempts to match the voice pitch level are made at several random points during a recorded conversational speech sample.
2. A study by Awan, Coy, and Riley (1990) observed no significant difference in pitch (and associated frequency) obtained from the 1, 2, 3, 4 method compared with measures of speaking fundamental frequency obtained by means of the Visi-Pitch.

A note of caution regarding matching vocal pitch with a pitch pipe, etc.—it is my experience that many people (speech/voice clinicians included) have great difficulty in accurately matching tones of different pitch. This observation is supported by studies by Murry (1990) and Weiner, Lee, Cataland, and Stemple (1996), who observed significant errors in matching target pitches by nonsinger judges and graduate students in speech-language pathology, respectively. Obviously, if the clinician cannot make an accurate perceptual judgment as to the true pitch of the patient's voice, estimates of habitual pitch level from a pitch pipe, etc., will be highly questionable. In addition, it has already been mentioned that the complex nature of the voice signal

(particularly when in a disordered state) makes attempts to accurately characterize the pitch of the voice very difficult (Bless & Hicks, 1996; Colton & Casper, 1996).

Perceptual Assessment of Pitch Variability

A similar 7-point categorical/equal-appearing interval rating scale as used for the rating of habitual pitch level may be applied to the rating of pitch variability:

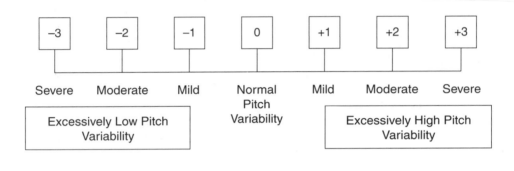

Note that negative numbers on the rating scale represent varying degrees of restricted pitch variability versus positive numbers that represent varying degrees of excessive pitch variability. Again, it is recommended that ratings of pitch variability/intonation be applied to continuous speech samples. As previously stated, observation of tremor is best carried out on a sustained vowel sample. Observation of pitch breaks should also be noted.

Perceptual Assessment of Total Pitch Range

To estimate the total pitch range (i.e., the difference between the lowest pitch in modal register and the highest pitch in falsetto), provide the following instructions to your patient: "I am going to ask you to hold out the sound "ah" (/ɑ/) at several different notes or pitches. Starting at a comfortable pitch level, I would like you to go down in steps to the lowest note you can hold out without your voice breaking or cracking. It will be similar to singing down a scale, such as…" (provide an example for your patient here). When the patient gets to his or her lowest sustainable pitch, have him or her repeat it two to three times so that (1) you can be sure that it is of reasonable quality (do not include vocal fry phonation); (2) you can be sure that it is repeatable; and (3) you can have the opportunity to cue them to lower productions if you believe that they have not truly reached their minimum pitch limit. When you are confident that the

patient has reached the lower pitch limit, attempt to match the vocal pitch using your pitch pipe, keyboard, etc., and identify the musical note that best approximates the vocal pitch. Repeat these steps for the highest pitch (including falsetto register). After finding the high and low pitch levels, simply count the number of semitones in between to arrive at the total pitch range. A 24 to 36 semitone range would be expected for the normal adult. The same caveats should be considered as were mentioned for identification of habitual pitch using the pitch pipe, etc.

QUANTITATIVE EVALUATION OF VOCAL FREQUENCY

Methodology

As previously stated, it is essential that perceptual judgments of voice characteristics be supported and documented by methods of quantitative evaluation. (See Appendix C.) We see that this element of our evaluation is quite important when evaluating pitch because the complexity of the voice signal (particularly when disordered) may lead to inaccurate judgments of pitch levels by the clinician. To quantify our perceptual measures of vocal pitch, we will analyze the acoustic signal of the voice for measures of frequency. During the vibratory cycle, the adducted vocal folds are put into oscillation/vibration by the expiratory airstream. The oscillating motion of the vocal folds "cuts" the outgoing airstream into a series of "puffs." In turn, these "puffs" create disturbances in the surrounding medium of air, which eventually (after undergoing further transformation by the resonating characteristics of the vocal tract) are heard as sound waves by the listener. The pitch of the sound produced is related to the number of vocal fold oscillations/cycles of vibration per unit time, and the term frequency (Hz) refers specifically to the measurement of the number of cycles of vibration per second.

The measurement of the frequency of the voice signal should appear, at least on the surface, to be quite simple to calculate. Basically, we require the following two conditions to be met to make frequency measurements:

1. Some method of (at least temporarily) capturing and storing the voice signal to be analyzed.
2. Some method by which the vibratory cycles of the voice signal may be identified.

Current methods of clinical voice analysis generally use a computer and accompanying analog-to-digital (A-to-D) sound conversion card to record and play back sound waves. These sound cards (e.g., SoundBlaster 16, Creative Labs Inc., Milipitas, CA) are commercially available and are included in most multimedia computers. These A-to-D sound cards commonly allow for sound recording at 16 bits of resolution at sampling rates up to 44,100 Hz. A computer program is required to control the recording and playback process and to graphically display the voice sound wave on the computer screen. A number of programs were mentioned in Chapter 1 that are available for this purpose and will also carry out the various frequency and other measures we require in the voice diagnostic (see Appendix A).

Once the voice signal is captured and stored, it is now possible to estimate the vocal frequency. In particular, we are interested in the fundamental frequency (F_0) of the voice. This term refers to the lowest frequency of vibration in the voice signal, as well as to the frequency spacing between the harmonics of the fundamental frequency. The identification of vocal F_0 is done by identifying the cycle boundaries (i.e., beginning/ending points for each cycle of vibration in the acoustic signal). Computer programs vary in their methods of determining cycle boundaries (Askenfelt & Hammarberg, 1986). Titze and Liang (1993) describe three categories of frequency extraction methods commonly used in acoustic analysis systems:

1. Peak picking: This method defines the period of the cycle as the time interval between two consecutive "pitch" peaks. Analysis can be performed by use of either positive or negative peaks (see Figure 2–2).
2. Zero-crossings: This method defines the period of the cycle as the difference between two consecutive positive-going or consecutive negative-going zero-crossing points. Often, the zero-crossing point is defined as the amplitude closest to zero immediately preceding the peak amplitude of the cycle (see Figure 2–2).
3. Waveform matching: This method evaluates changes of many events from cycle to cycle. The minimal amplitude of the first cycle is located, and the next cycle is found by determining the point at which the mean squared error between the two adjacent cycles is minimized. The procedure is then repeated for each cycle of the waveform.

Various other methods (e.g., autocorrelation) have also been used to identify the cycle boundaries and, thus, the period of the voice signal. Once the period of a cycle is identified, the frequency may be easily computed (because frequency equals the reciprocal of period [in seconds]).

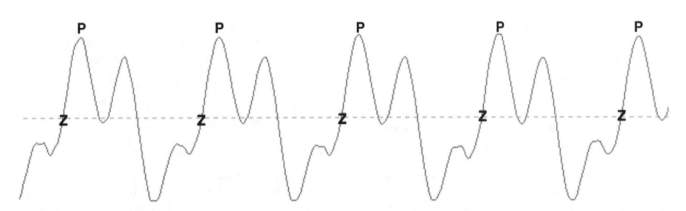

Figure 2–2 Positive Peak (P) and Zero-Crossings (Z) Locations for Several Cycles of a Voice Waveform

The series of mathematical and/or logical steps carried out in a computer program to result in a desired analysis is called an *algorithm*. Unfortunately, regardless of which computer algorithm is used for voice analysis, errors in estimating vocal frequency will inevitably occur under certain situations (Papamichalis, 1987). Voluntary, rapid pitch changes (as in continuous speech production), coarticulatory effects of consonant production, voiced/voiceless transitions, and increased noise in the voice are all situations in which frequency tracking errors may occur. In addition, the parameters that are required by each program to produce an accurate estimate of vocal F_0 must also be monitored closely by the program user. In particular, many programs require the user to provide a frequency range within which the program will search for the true frequency of the voice sample being analyzed. As an example, if one were analyzing the continuous conversational speech of an adult male, one may elect to use a range of 80 to 300 Hz. This range would comfortably allow for the average or habitual frequency of the speaker but also for the frequency changes observed within the intonation patterns of the speaker. Selecting this analysis range is a common parameter of many programs that use algorithms such as autocorrelation or waveform matching. If the range is too wide, the program may produce numerous errors in estimating F_0. If the range is too narrow, the program will be restricted in its ability to identify F_0 fluctuations that are actually present in the signal. The user of a particular program should review its instruction manual closely for instructions on how to set these parameters for optimal F_0 processing.

Although it is often assumed that computer programs will provide accurate estimations of vocal F_0, relatively few studies have objectively assessed the validity and reliability of voice analysis programs and their algorithms. Morris and Brown (1996) evaluated aspects of reliability and agreement among six speech analysis systems in determining vocal F_0. Sustained vowels and reading samples were analyzed from five male and five female adults. Computer analysis results from sustained vowels were also compared to manual estimations of F_0 from sonograms. Results indicated excellent reliability, but considerable variation among analysis systems. Agreement among systems was high for male sustained vowels and female reading samples; poor agreement was observed for male oral readings and female sustained vowels. Due to variability in agreement, these authors concluded that caution must be exercised in comparing F_0 data reported from different software systems. A study by Awan and Scarpino (1999) assessed the accuracy of four commercially available software systems in deriving estimates of vocal F_0 from sustained vowel and continuous speech samples. Subjects included adult males and females as well as children between the ages of five and nine. Results from sustained vowel analysis showed no significant differences in estimations of mean F_0 and F_0 standard deviation among computer programs, as well as no difference between computer calculations and hand-marking estimates. However, results from continuous speech analyses showed significantly lower estimates on mean F_0 as compared to hand marking in a number of the programs used, particularly in the analysis of child voices. In addition, a number of programs were observed to drastically overestimate measures of pitch sigma and speaking range. Awan and Scarpino concluded the following:

> While the voice/speech analysis programs analyzed in this study were highly comparable in terms of their measures of mean F_0 and F_0 standard deviation from sustained vowels, it is evident that the variations in vocal F_0 that accompany the production of continuous speech present difficulties which may result in significant differences between computational results. Each program's ability to distinguish voiced/voiceless distinctions may also result in errors in F_0 tracking. Depending on the voice sample, error correction routines may need to be incorporated prior to the final estimation of signal frequency. There are many instances in which "false" peaks/zeroes are mistaken as "true" cycle boundary markers (p. 330).

Measuring Frequency

With the aforementioned cautions in mind, we are now ready to carry out measures of frequency. These measures of frequency correspond with several of the perceptual measures of pitch we have previously described.

Mean Speaking Frequency

This measure corresponds to the perceptual measure of habitual pitch (Case, 1996). Just as we did with our perceptual measure, the mean F_0 is useful in estimating the appropriateness of frequency level for a patient's age, gender, race, etc. (Colton & Casper, 1996). It is best to make this measurement from a sample of reading or spontaneous speech (i.e., a continuous speech sample). Several authors have indicated that sustained vowel productions may be unnatural for some subjects and may result in productions uncharacteristic of the patients' speaking voice (Askenfelt & Hammarberg, 1986; de Krom, 1994).

Frequency Standard Deviation/Pitch Sigma

Although the mean speaking F_0 is a measure of the central tendency of vocal frequency, it is also useful to objectively measure the variability of vocal frequency. The F_0 standard deviation is a measure of the average variability and is useful in documenting perceived normal/abnormal intonation patterns and pitch instability. F_0 standard deviation may be measured from both continuous speech samples and sustained vowels. F_0 standard deviation is referred to as a measure of *long-term instability*, in which variations in frequency occur more slowly than the glottal vibration itself (Hartelius, Buder, & Strand, 1997).

Although F_0 standard deviation may be reported in Hz, the term *pitch sigma* is used to describe the standard deviation converted to semitones. The following are two key reasons for this conversion:

1. By converting F_0 standard deviation to a musical note scale (semitones), we have an objective measure of variability that has more relation to the perceptual judgment of pitch. Many people will be able to perceive pitch variation in terms of musical tones; on the other hand, what may appear to be large variability in Hz may not be perceptible.
2. By converting to semitones, we "normalize" F_0 variability/deviation for the comparison of different voice types. As an example, it is often observed that, during continuous speech, the F_0 standard deviation is approximately 10% of the mean speaking F_0. Therefore, for a man speaking with a F_0 of 120 Hz, we would expect a F_0 standard deviation of approximately 12 Hz; for a child with a F_0 of 250 Hz, F_0 standard deviation would be approximately 25 Hz. In this example, it appears clear that the child has substantially greater F_0 variability (in Hz) than the adult man (25 Hz vs. 12 Hz). However, when converted to pitch sigma, we would see that both subjects produce approximately the same variability (approximately four semitones) in perceptual/musical tones.

Range—Speaking Range and Total Phonational Frequency Range

Another measure used to document F_0 variation is the *F_0 range*. Range is simply a measure from the lowest F_0 produced in a sample to the highest F_0. Range may be reported in Hz but may also be reported in terms of musical notes (semitones). *Speaking range* is a measure of the frequency or semitone range produced during continuous speech. This measure is also valuable for documenting normal versus abnormal intonation, as well as presence of characteristics such as pitch breaks during speech. An alternative measure of range commonly reported is the range from the lowest F_0 in modal register to the highest in falsetto, referred to as the *total phonational range*. Total phonational range has been said to provide an index of laryngeal health (Case, 1996) and is often one of the first parameters of vocal capability affected in voice disorders.

HOW TO DO IT: EVALUATION OF VOCAL FREQUENCY

To obtain measures of mean speaking frequency, F_0 standard deviation/pitch sigma, and speaking F_0 range, we must obtain a sample of continuous speech. As always, we want our procedures to be standardized so that the same procedures/instructions are provided both intersubject and intrasubject. For the patient who has reading capability, it is recommended that the patient be asked to read "The Rainbow Passage" (Fairbanks, 1960) (see Appendix D). This is a phonetically balanced passage that has been used to elicit continuous speech throughout the speech/voice literature and, therefore, enhances validity when comparing a particular patient's data with those reported in literature dealing with normal/abnormal voice.

The steps in recording your patient's sample will be described in the following. However, we should consider exactly how much/how long of a sample we need to collect. In other areas of speech analysis (e.g., fluency), quite lengthy samples are often required so that the patient is provided with ample opportunity to produce the normal or abnormal speech characteristic the clinician aims to document. However, in voice analysis we are focusing on a behavior (i.e., phonation and associated characteristics of frequency) that is common to even relatively short utterances. Therefore, relatively short samples per recording are often adequate for frequency analysis. With this in mind, it is recommended that we ask our patient to read the entire first paragraph of "The Rainbow Passage," but we will record and analyze only the second sentence of the passage. The following are three reasons supporting this procedure:

1. Research by Horii (1975) indicates that mean F_0 calculated from the second sentence correlates well ($r = 0.985$) with measured F_0 from the entire paragraph (associated standard error of only 3 Hz).
2. By use of an embedded sentence, we hope to retain the naturalness of the patient's speaking style but avoid possible initial or final sentence effects (Horii, 1975).
3. The second sentence is linguistically "simpler" than other sentences in the passage and easily read or repeated by most subjects.

Measures of variability (F_0 standard deviation/pitch sigma) may also be computed for the second sentence of "The Rainbow Passage," but more error may be expected (approximately 10% errors possible in relation to the entire passage; $r = 0.82$). Measures of F_0 variability are better conducted with longer duration samples (Baken, 1987). Horii (1975) showed that F_0 standard deviation from the third sentence of "The Rainbow Passage" (22 words versus 12 words in the second sentence) correlates much better with measures obtained from the entire passage ($r = 0.924$).

The reading of a standard passage is generally useable for most patients. However, we may have patients (e.g., very young children, patients with visual deficits) who may not be able to read effectively. With these patients, we should collect a continuous speech sample of at least 14 seconds in duration (this duration provides an accuracy of ±3 Hz [Baken, 1987; Horii, 1975]). The sample may be elicited by means of open-ended questioning techniques or picture description tasks. Studies by Awan and Mueller (1992, 1996) used the Cookie Theft Picture (Goodglass & Kaplan, 1983) to elicit speech samples from centenarian women with visual problems and from 5-year-old children, respectively. If the patient provides the minimum 14 seconds continuously (i.e., without significant interruption), analysis can be carried out directly. However, if the patient's speech is interrupted for some reason (e.g., cueing from the clinician that occurs on the tape, inordinately long pauses, background noises), then we must analyze the data in one of the following two ways:

1. Edit out the extraneous sounds/noises/pauses to result in a single sound file of at least 14 seconds of contiguous speech.
2. Analyze each of the speech fragments we have collected (e.g., fragment 1 = 4 seconds; fragment 2 = 7 seconds) individually and then compute a weighted mean that will weight longer speech fragments greater than small speech fragments (i.e., greater significance will be given to F_0s from longer duration speech fragments). A weighted mean may be computed following these steps (Awan & Mueller, 1992):
   - Multiply each fragment F_0 by its duration (in seconds). For example, the mean F_0 for a 4-second fragment is 200 Hz. Therefore, $200 \times 4 = 800$. A second fragment has a mean F_0 of 180 Hz over 2 seconds. Therefore, $180 \times 2 = 360$.
   - Sum the products (i.e., each fragment F_0 × duration components). In this example $800 + 360 = 1160$.
   - Divide the sum by the total duration (in seconds). In this example $1160/6 = 193.33$ Hz.

Steps in Recording a Speech Sample for F_0 Analysis (Mean and F_0 SD)—Reading Sample

To record a sample of continuous speech from a standard reading passage, follow the steps below.

1. Place a good-quality microphone a standard distance (approximately 30 cm) from the patient's mouth.
2. Set up your program to record at a sampling rate of 44 kHz with 16 bits of resolution. If your program requires you to set a recording time (i.e., length of time during which the computer will record the sample), set this for at least 10 seconds.
3. Provide your patient with a copy of "The Rainbow Passage" (Fairbanks, 1960). Tell your patient, "I would like you to read this passage in your normal speaking voice."
4. Listen closely to your patient as he or she reads. Just before the start of the second sentence, start recording—stop the recording at the end of the second sentence.
5. Save and name your sample for further analysis.
6. Play back your sample and also review the graphical display of the waveform. Make sure the signal is not distorted as a result of clipping (i.e., the recording level was too strong, and the "tops" of your wave have been clipped/cut off) or too weak as a result of a low recording level. If necessary, rerecord.
7. Edit out any extraneous samples you do not want to analyze (e.g., the end of the first sentence or beginning of the third sentence).
8. Set the appropriate parameters for the program you are using to produce optimal F_0 tracking (F_0 analysis range, polarity, etc.).
9. Compute the F_0 contour/trace (i.e., the graphical image of the changing vocal F_0) for your sample and accompanying statistics. Look closely for significant F_0 tracking errors—these will probably affect the computation of F_0 range most significantly. In the event that F_0 tracking errors are present, consult the user manual of the program you are using to see how the F_0 tracking may be improved (i.e., how the program parameters may be manipulated to improve analysis). In addition, some programs may allow you to manually edit the computed F_0 estimates or manually estimate the "true" F_0 range.

It should be noted that there might be considerable variability in vocal F_0 production both between and within days.

Coleman and Markham (1991) reported on variations in habitual pitch/speaking fundamental frequency (SFF) in various groups of normal speakers. SFF was observed to have an average variation of 2.74 semitones (range: 1.54–4.26 STs) over a 30-day period in a group of young adult females, with SFF expected to be within 3 semitones of their "true" SFF at least 90% of the time. These authors concluded that day-to-day SFF variation by as much as 18% should be considered within normal limits. Mueller and Xue (1996) examined the variability of mean F_0 over an 8-day period. Sixteen female patients were asked to sustain the vowel /ɑ/ at constant pitch and loudness. Vocal F_0 was measured using a VisiPitch 6087 (Kay Elemetrics, Lincoln Park, NJ). Results indicated that mean F_0 fluctuated significantly over the 8-day period. In addition, significant differences in F_0 occurred over three trials. F_0 fluctuated from a minimum of 15 Hz to a maximum of 84 Hz within the 8-day period. In addition, a mean F_0 for the group of 205.85 Hz was observed on day 1 versus a mean F_0 of 217.10 Hz on day 7 (a difference of 11.25 Hz). Although variation in SFF is to be expected, Stone and Rainey (1991) indicate that measures of mean F_0 are "justifiable on the bases that such measures can be expected to be normally distributed, that inter- and intrasubject variability is suitably restricted, and that there would be no significant differences based on at least three trials" (p. 193).

This example has assumed that you will record your patient's speech sample directly into your computer. This method of recording is advocated whenever possible because it avoids the possible sound deteriorating or distorting effects of recording devices and/or amplifiers before digitization. However, in the event that your patient cannot read the standard sample, you may want to compute measures of speaking F_0 from a continuous speech sample.

Steps in Recording a Speech Sample for F_0 Analysis— Continuous Speech Sample

1. Connect a good-quality microphone to an external recording device (high-quality tape recorder, DAT or DCC deck; Minidisc recorder). The use of digital recording methods (DAT, DCC, or Minidisc) is particularly recommended because (1) noise reduction methods (e.g., Dolby) are not necessary; (2) appropriate tape selection and tape bias do not have to be considered; and (3) digital recorders allow for easy marking (time, date, etc.) for particular samples or sections of a sample. If the recording deck you are using does not have a microphone input, you will have to use a preamplifier between the microphone and the line input of the deck (*it is suggested that you not use tape recorders with built-in microphones*, because they generally do not provide the fidelity necessary for adequate voice recording and analysis).

2. I suggest that a continuous speech sample be elicited by means of a picture description task (e.g., the Cookie Theft Picture). Place the picture in front of your patient and provide these instructions: "Look at this picture carefully—I want you to tell me everything that is going on in this picture." Begin recording. Provide cues when necessary to extend the description of all aspects of the picture. The advantage of using a picture description task is that it will elicit similar linguistic responses from all patients and, therefore, provides some degree of standardization both interpatient and intrapatient for test-retest purposes (Awan & Mueller, 1996; Baken, 1987).

3. Continue recording until you are sure that you have at least 14 seconds of your patient's continuous speech to analyze (take into account that you will be editing out your (the clinician's) speech (e.g., if you cued the patient), long periods of silence, etc.

4. When you have collected your sample, you can now digitize it using your computer and analysis program. Connect the output of your recording deck to the input of your sound card (generally, this is a line out from the recording deck to the line in jack on the sound card). Alternately, connect the line out of the recording deck to the line in of a preamplifier mixer, and the line out of the mixer to the line in of the sound card.

5. You can edit and analyze the sample in a number of ways: (1) digitize the entire sample and then use the program's editing functions (i.e., cut, copy, paste) to remove extraneous material. Then, analyze the sample in a similar manner as for the previously described reading passage (starting at Step 5); (2) digitize each sentence/continuous speech section the patient produces and save as individual files. In this way, you have edited out extraneous material before digitizing. You could then paste all the sentences/utterances together and analyze; or (3) if you are using an older voice/speech analysis system (e.g., VisiPitch 6087) in which it may not be possible to store and edit utterances, analyze each utterance individually and copy down all the pertinent F_0 statistics. You can then use the previously described weighted average procedure (Awan & Mueller, 1992) to get the overall F_0 statistics for your patient's multiple utterances.

Steps in Recording Total Phonational Range

When assessing the total phonational pitch/frequency range, it is important for the clinician to be aware of the difference between "physiological" range of phonation versus the "musical" range (Awan, 1991; Awan & Mueller, 1990; Coleman & Mott, 1978; Fairbanks, 1960; Large, 1971; Luchsinger & Arnold, 1965; Van Oordt & Drost, 1963). In assessing physiological range, no constraints are placed on quality, pitch, loudness, or duration of the phonation. Physiological range includes vocal behaviors such as crying, screaming, shouting (i.e., emotional and/or vegetative types of vocal behavior [Awan, 1991]). The physiological limits of vocal pitch/frequency range would rarely (if ever) be used in common or professional vocal situations. In contrast, the musical range develops within the limits of the physiological range and is composed of artistically useable tones (Coleman & Mott, 1978). Awan and Mueller (1990) and Awan (1991) have further described the musical range as entailing "controlled" phonations, in which the patient must (1) sustain both the lowest and highest frequency for a minimum of 2 to 3 seconds, (2) must maintain a relatively steady intensity and frequency level, and (3) must produce a "quality" phonation (i.e., no pitch or phonation breaks; no excessive breathiness, harshness, or hoarseness).

This book suggests that the total phonational pitch/frequency range be assessed in terms of musical range rather than physiological range. Musical range is preferable for the following reasons:

- Musical range provides information in terms of vocal performance and capability used in more realistic vocal conditions.
- Assessment of musical range "stresses" the vocal system by using vocal frequency, intensity, durational, and quality constraints.
- Musical range avoids the possibility of vocal abuse by omitting physiological vocal productions that may be encountered only in vocally demanding situations (e.g., highly emotional situations).

The assessment of musical range has some similarity to Case's (1996) discussion of *vocal idle* (i.e., least effort use of the voice). Case (1996) contends that measures of vocal capability are best evaluated during conditions of less than maximum effort, because it may be argued that even an inefficient larynx can produce voice when enough effort is applied. In a similar manner, it may be argued that even inefficient vocal mechanisms may produce extensive vocal ranges if allowed to produce physiological voice, whereas the actual useable range of vocal pitches and frequencies would be much smaller if evaluated under the conditions of "controlled" phonation. Assessment of musical range has

revealed differences in vocal capability between groups that would not have been revealed if only physiological range had been assessed (Awan, 1991; Coleman & Mott, 1978; Luchsinger & Arnold, 1965; Van Oordt & Drost, 1963).

To record the total (musical) phonational range, follow the steps below.

1. Place a good-quality microphone a standard distance (approximately 30 cm) from the patient's mouth.
2. Set up your program to record at a sampling rate of 44 kHz with 16 bits of resolution. If your program requires you to set a recording time (i.e., length of time during which the computer will record the sample), set this for at least 2 to 3 seconds.
3. To record the patient's minimum pitch level, provide the following instructions to your patient: "I am going to ask you to hold the sound "ah" (/ɑ/) at several different notes or pitches. Starting at a comfortable pitch level, I would like you to go down in steps to the lowest note you can hold out without your voice breaking or cracking. It will be similar to singing down a scale, such as…" (provide an example for your patient here).
4. When the patient gets to the lowest sustainable pitch, have him or her repeat it two to three times so that (1) you can be sure that it is of reasonable quality (do not include vocal fry phonation); (2) you can be sure that it is repeatable; and (3) you can have the opportunity to cue the patient to lower productions if you believe that he or she has not truly reached his or her minimum pitch limit.
5. When you are confident the patient has reached his or her lower pitch limit, record a brief sample on the computer (1 to 2 seconds).
6. Set the appropriate parameters for the program you are using to produce optimal F_0 tracking (F_0 analysis range, polarity, etc.). Compute the F_0 contour/trace (i.e., the graphical image of the changing vocal F_0) for your sample and accompanying statistics. We are primarily interested in the mean F_0 of the production.
7. To record the patient's maximum pitch level, provide the following instructions to your patient: "Starting at a comfortable pitch level, I would like you to go up in steps to the highest note you can hold without your voice breaking or cracking, including falsetto voice—falsetto is a high, thin, reedy voice such as… (provide example). It will be similar to singing up a scale, such as…" (provide an example for your patient here).
8. When the patient gets to his or her highest sustainable pitch, have him or her repeat it two to three

times. When you are confident that the patient has reached the highest pitch limit, record a brief sample on the computer (1 to 2 seconds).

9. Reset the appropriate parameters for the program you are using to produce optimal F_0 tracking (F_0 analysis range, polarity, etc.). Compute mean F_0 of the production.

10. To compute the total phonational range in Hz, simply subtract the lowest pitch/frequency level from the highest. To convert the total range in Hz to semitones, consult a chart of musical note/frequency equivalents (see Exhibit 2–1) and count the number of semitones between the lowest and highest frequency level (you will probably have to "round" the low and high frequency levels to the nearest semitone).

Alternately, the clinician may use the following formula (Baken, 1987) in which the number of semitones (n) between the highest frequency (f_2) and the lowest frequency (f_1) is given by

$$n = \frac{12 \log_{10}(f_2 / f_1)}{\log_{10} 2}$$

✎ A program is provided on disk by which range in semitones may be easily computed (see Figure 2–3 and Appendix E).

WHAT TO EXPECT: NORMAL VOICE

The speaking pitch of the voice primarily depends on the age, gender, and body stature of the patient (particularly as it affects the physical composition of the vocal folds). The normal vocal pitch should be an appropriate physical match

for the speaker and should not present any age or gender confusion for the listener.

Gender

No substantial differences have been found between male and female voices from birth until puberty according to measures of mean fundamental frequency and frequency range. Definitive frequency distinctions between the sexes begin during puberty and continue throughout adolescence. As males and females progress through puberty (often from ages 8 to 13 years, marked by the onset of secondary sex characteristics [Pedersen, Moller, Krabbe, & Bennett, 1986]), both genders will exhibit a lowering of the pitch of the voice, although the lowering is generally not as drastic in the female as the male (Murry, 1982). This lowering may be attributed to changes in vocal fold length, with the length of the male vocal fold increasing approximately 4 to 8 mm from puberty to adulthood, and the female vocal fold increasing approximately 1 to 3.5 mm (Aronson, 1990a). In many cases the adult habitual pitch level has been achieved by the age of 14 to 15 years; however, slight "deepening" of the voice may accompany other growth changes within the vocal tract that affect vocal tract resonances rather than the vibratory frequency of the vocal folds.

The aforementioned differences between male and female laryngeal mechanisms after puberty result in differences between gender groups in mean fundamental frequency used during conversation. Aronson (1990a), in an extensive review of several major studies, indicates that the mean fundamental frequency for 20- to 29-year-old males is 128 Hz (range = 119 to 138 Hz). In contrast, the mean fundamental frequency of the speaking voice in adult females is, on average, approximately 1.6 times higher than that of males (i.e.,

Exhibit 2–1 Semitone-to-Frequency Conversions for the Musical Scale

C_1	$C_1{}^\#$	D_1	$D_1{}^\#$	E_1	F_1	$F_1{}^\#$	G_1	$G_1{}^\#$	A_1	$A_1{}^\#$	B_1
33	35	37	39	41	44	46	49	52	55	58	62
C_2	$C_2{}^\#$	D_2	$D_2{}^\#$	E_2	F_2	$F_2{}^\#$	G_2	$G_2{}^\#$	A_2	$A_2{}^\#$	B_2
65	69	73	78	82	87	92	98	104	110	117	123
C_3	$C_3{}^\#$	D_3	$D_3{}^\#$	E_3	F_3	$F_3{}^\#$	G_3	$G_3{}^\#$	A_3	$A_3{}^\#$	B_3
131	139	147	156	165	175	185	196	208	220	233	247
C_4	$C_4{}^\#$	D_4	$D_4{}^\#$	E_4	F_4	$F_4{}^\#$	G_4	$G_4{}^\#$	A_4	$A_4{}^\#$	B_4
262	277	294	311	330	349	370	392	415	440	466	494
C_5	$C_5{}^\#$	D_5	$D_5{}^\#$	E_5	F_5	$F_5{}^\#$	G_5	$G_5{}^\#$	A_5	$A_5{}^\#$	B_5
523	554	587	622	659	698	740	784	831	880	932	988
C_6	$C_6{}^\#$	D_6	$D_6{}^\#$	E_6	F_6	$F_6{}^\#$	G_6	$G_6{}^\#$	A_6	$A_6{}^\#$	B_6
1047	1109	1175	1245	1319	1397	1480	1568	1661	1760	1865	1976

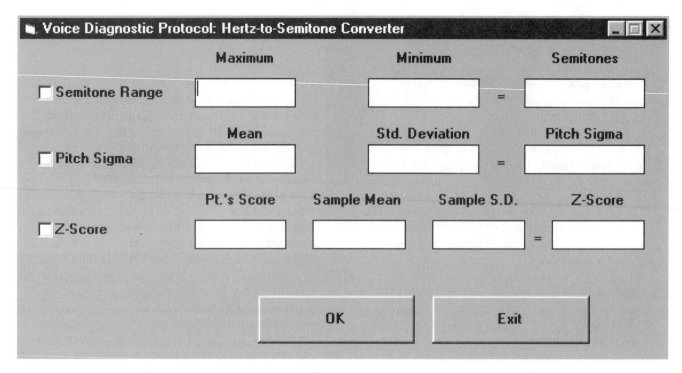

Figure 2–3 Screen Shot of the VDP-UTIL Program

approximately 205 Hz) (Aronson, 1990a). Kelley (1977) found the mean fundamental frequency for 20- to 29-year-old women to be 227 Hz, a slightly higher figure than that speculated by Aronson. Boone and McFarlane (1988) have reported the typical adult male voice to be near 128 Hz (C3), and the typical adult female voice to be near 213 Hz (A4). The pitch of the adult male and female voice is generally expected to remain relatively stable for at least 20 to 30 years after puberty.

Studies of adult pitch/frequency range have generally observed a great deal of similarity between men and women (both genders producing phonational ranges in the vicinity of 24 to 36 semitones), although adult men may have a slightly greater total phonational range than women. Studies by Ptacek, Sander, Maloney, and Jackson (1966), Hollien, Dew, and Philips (1971), and Awan (1989) have observed adult males to produce ranges 1 to 4 semitones greater than adult females, with this difference attributable to the lower fundamental frequencies produced by male subjects.

Race

It has been speculated that there are anatomical differences between racial groups that may result in significant differences in speaking F_0. Boshoff (1945 as cited in Wheat

and Hudson, 1988) observed that the larynges of African-American cadavers were larger than those of Caucasian cadavers, and Krogman (1972) observed that African-American children exhibited more rapid skeletal growth during the first 3 years than comparable Caucasian children. It has been speculated that an increase in the skeletal structure of the body would also result in an increase in the cartilaginous framework of the larynx (Wheat & Hudson, 1988), and a resulting lowering of speaking F_0 levels. However, results from studies on the speaking F_0 of racial groups have been uncertain in this regard. In terms of adult speaking F_0, Hudson and Holbrook (1981) reported on the F_0 characteristics of 200 African-American males (age range = 18 to 29 years). Mean speaking F_0 obtained from "The Rainbow Passage" was 110.15 Hz for the men and 193.10 for the women. The authors concluded that, in relation to previous literature on speaking F_0, African-Americans had lower fundamental frequencies than Caucasian subjects of comparable age. Similar conclusions were made by Hudson and Holbrook (1982), who reported mean speaking F_0s of 108.05 Hz for African-American men and 188.85 Hz for African-American women. In both studies by Hudson and Holbrook (1981, 1982), no direct comparisons to similar age and gender Caucasian subjects were made. A study by Wheat and Hudson (1988) presented normative data on the speaking F_0 of 6-year-old male and female African-Americans. Results showed that the African-American males and females had mean speaking F_0s of 219.50 and 211.30 Hz, respectively. The authors speculated that the observed speaking F_0s were substantially lower than those reported for Caucasian males and females of similar ages, although again direct comparison was not carried out.

In contrast to those studies that have speculated on a lower speaking F_0 for African-American speakers, several studies have observed no significant difference in the speaking F_0s of African-American versus Caucasian subjects as shown below.

- Hollien and Malcik (1967) carried out a cross-sectional study of the voice characteristics of 10-, 14-, and 18-year-old African-American males and compared them with Caucasian males of similar ages. Their results indicated no significant difference between the racial groups in terms of speaking F_0, although the authors did indicate that African-American males showed a trend for lower speaking F_0 levels than Caucasian males, regardless of age group. In addition, frequency variability (as measured by means of pitch sigma) was similar in both racial groups.
- Mayo and Manning (1994) reported on the vocal F_0 characteristics of 20 African-American and 20 European-American young adult male subjects. Results from sustained vowel analysis showed that mean F_0 values for the African-American and European-American speakers were not significantly different (123.2 Hz vs. 124.7 Hz, respectively). In addition, F_0 standard deviations and range values were also observed not to be significantly different.
- In a comparison of aerodynamic and acoustic characteristics of voice in adult African-American and adult Caucasian speakers, Sapienza (1997) observed no significant differences in mean fundamental frequency obtained from sustained vowels as a function of either race or gender. Sapienza (1997) concluded that "for vowel production there are more similarities than differences in the vocal function between African American and White speakers" (p. 415). Any differences in the voice characteristics of African-Americans compared with Caucasians were attributed more to linguistic and cultural difference rather than to laryngeal anatomical ones.
- Awan and Mueller (1996) examined speaking F_0 characteristics of Caucasian, African-American, and Hispanic kindergartners. Results showed mean speaking F_0 to be significantly lower in African-American versus Hispanic children (236.4 Hz vs. 248.5 Hz) but not different from Caucasian children

(236.4 Hz vs. 241.7 Hz). Pitch sigma was similar among all three groups, and ranged from a mean of 4.38 semitones in Caucasian males to a mean of 5.59 semitones in Caucasian females.

Although previous studies have been ambiguous in terms of the effects of race of speaking F_0, caution should be exercised when applying the normative speaking F_0 data collected solely from one racial group to decisions regarding the speaking F_0s of other racial groups. Regardless of whether possible anatomical differences in the speech/voice mechanisms of different races exist or not, there may be significant linguistic and societal differences (e.g., differences in pragmatic and interaction styles) between racial and/or dialect groups that may affect speaking F_0 and/or F_0 variability.

Aging Characteristics of Voice

Infancy and Preadolescence

Kent (1976) has reviewed the research on developmental changes in fundamental frequency from birth to adulthood. The fundamental frequency drops slightly during the first 3 weeks of life, then rises until about the fourth month, and then stabilizes for approximately 5 months. When the child is 1 year old, the fundamental frequency lowers rapidly until he or she is about 3 years old. The pitch and F_0 level then gradually lower to the point of onset of puberty. Fundamental frequency levels begin to be distinguishable by sex at about 11 years of age and certainly by 13 years of age. In females, the fundamental frequency lowers little more than an octave from birth to adulthood; in males, fundamental frequency lowers approximately 2 octaves. The age periods of most rapid change in fundamental frequency levels are: the first 4 months, 1 to 3 years, and 13 to 17 years. Because girls mature faster than boys, they may approach adolescence with slightly lower SFF (Perkins, 1985).

In terms of pitch and F_0 variability, data from Eguchi and Hirsh (1969, as cited in Kent, 1976) indicate that variability decreases with age from infancy through 10 to 12 years of age. Pitch variability in the infant voice may reflect a low level of neuromuscular coordination and limited ability to control the tension of the vocal folds (Colton & Casper, 1996).

The pitch range (both in continuous speech and in total phonational range) varies considerably with age. Although the physiological range of the voice (i.e., the range encompassing all possible vocal pitches and including vegetative and emotional voice use as in crying, screaming, etc.) may be relatively stable across the life span (Aronson, 1990a; Van Oordt & Drost, 1963), the actual useable or musical range (Damste, 1970) of the voice appears to be restricted somewhat during childhood. It has been reported that children should be capable of varying pitch for a number of intonational forms (e.g., request, question) and gestures by the first year (Tonkova-Yampol'skaya, 1968 cited in Kent, 1976). As males and females move through puberty and into adulthood, the range of useable vocal pitches will extend to approximately 2 to 3 octaves.

Adolescence

During puberty there is normally a change in the speaking frequency of the voice because of growth changes in the larynx (mutation). The male pitch lowers approximately one octave, and the female pitch 3 to 4 semitones (Perkins, 1985). According to Aronson (1990a), complete mutation of voice takes place within 3 to 6 months, during which time the neck lengthens and the larynx descends and grows in size. In addition to changes in the laryngeal mechanism itself, the drastic vocal F_0 changes observed in the male going through puberty are also reflective of the development of secondary sex characteristics. Pedersen et al. (1986) examined F_0 measures in relation to pubertal development in 48 normal males in three groups (8.7 to 12.9 years, 13 to 15.9 years, and 16 to 19.5 years). Mean speaking F_0 dropped considerably (as expected) among the three groups (273 Hz vs. 184 Hz vs. 125 Hz). In addition, speaking F_0 correlated quite strongly with height ($r = -0.82$), pubic hair stage ($r = -0.87$), testis volume ($r = -0.78$), and total testosterone ($r = -0.73$). The authors concluded that speaking F_0s greater than 200 Hz and low levels of serum testosterone probably represent values for a boy in puberty. A study by Boltezar, Burger, and Zargi (1997) indicated that one of the main characteristics of the adolescent voice was pitch instability/variability. These authors examined voice characteristics of 51 adolescent boys and girls (22 males; 29 females) between the ages of 10 and 17 years. These authors observed a mean F_0 for males of 199.56 Hz (SD = 57.3 Hz) and 261.66 Hz for females (SD = 60.96 Hz). In addition, Boltezar et al. (1997) reported that the coefficient of F_0 variation (i.e., the relative standard deviation of F_0) from sustained vowel /ɑ/ productions was greater in both adolescent males and females than normal expectations (1.10%). This was particularly true for the male adolescent voice, with the adolescent female voice being somewhat more stable. The authors attribute this instability to differential development between nervous control and peripheral speech mechanism growth (gradual vs. rapid development).

The Elderly Voice

Age-related changes in the speech mechanism may include increased stiffness of respiratory and laryngeal structures, muscle and nervous system degeneration, reduced speed of neural transmission, and reduction in vocal tract mucous glands (Kahane, 1990). However, the magnitude of aging effects varies from person to person (Morris & Brown, 1994b) and appears to be related to overall physical condition rather than chronological age as an absolute (Ramig & Ringel, 1983).

As the female approaches and then goes through menopause, it has been observed that the pitch of the voice may lower (Awan & Mueller, 1992; Perkins, 1985). This lowering has been associated with factors such as hormonal changes and edema (Gilbert & Weismer, 1974; Honjo & Isshiki, 1980). Figure 2–4 shows the possible effects of aging on the speaking F_0 of the female voice across various age groups (five age groups with 10 subjects per group) as reported by Awan and Ziminsky-Ammon (1996). Mean speaking F_0 results showed that the 18- to 30-year-old group produced significantly higher mean speaking F_0s than all the other age groups. No significant difference in mean speaking F_0 was observed between the 40- to 49- and 50- to 59-year-old groups and the 60- to 69- and 70- to 79-year-old groups. In addition, a significant inverse correlation ($r = -0.69$, $p < .001$) was observed between mean speaking F_0 and age. In Figure 2–5, the mean speaking F_0 of the young adult group (18 to 30 years of age) minus 2 SD was used as a value to judge voice change for the older subjects (i.e., Z-scores were calculated for each subject using the mean and standard deviation of the young adult female group as the control group). Results show increasing percentages of each aging group with subjects producing mean speaking F_0s substantially lower than the mean speaking F_0 of the young adult group.

The possible pitch and F_0 changes reported in the aging female voice are not definitive; there is a tremendous amount of variability in voice change as a result of aging (Awan & Mueller, 1992), with many elderly women able to maintain appropriate pitch and overall voice function throughout the life span.

In contrast to the female, the male vocal pitch and F_0 appear to remain relatively stable throughout adulthood. However, there have been studies (Hollien & Shipp, 1972; Honjo & Isshiki, 1980; Shipp, Qi, Huntley, & Hollien, 1992) that indicate that some men may experience a rise in the pitch and F_0 of the voice during senescence. It has been hypothesized that pitch and frequency elevation in the elderly male voice may be due to changes in vocal fold tissue mass and/or an imbalance between cricothyroid and thyroarytenoid muscle forces (Shipp et al., 1992). Again, substantial variation in pitch effects with aging should be expected. However, it is interesting to speculate that, just as we begin life with similar pitch voices, men and women may also end life with similar vocal pitch.

Evidence exists that the variability of vocal pitch during continuous speech may be affected by advanced age. This variability may be observed in terms of (1) changes in intonation patterns and (2) pitch instability. It has been specu-

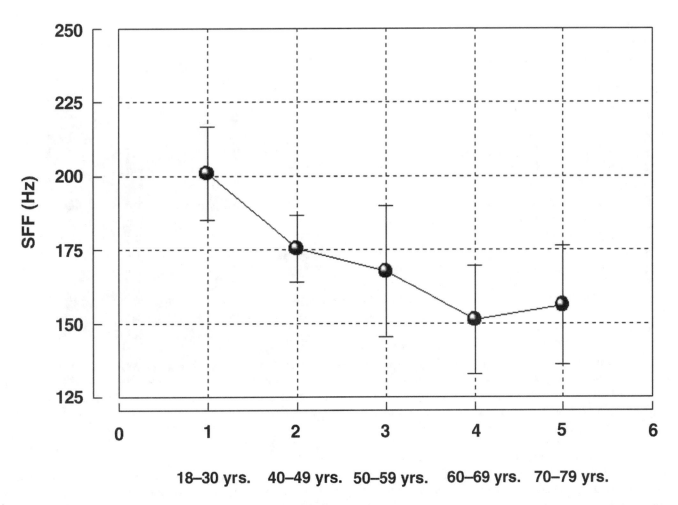

Figure 2–4 Mean SFF of Aging Women. Mean speaking fundamental frequency (SFF) and standard deviations across aging groups. (Correlation between aging and SFF: $r = -0.69$, $p < .001$)

lated that as we age, decrements in motor/sensory control of the speech mechanism may occur. These decrements may reflect neurochemical changes in the basal ganglia (Liss, Weismer, & Rosenbek, 1990), decrements in sensory feedback, decreased speed and accuracy of motor control, and structural and physiological changes in the laryngeal mechanism (Kahane, 1990). The results of the age-related changes may be observed as an increased pitch range used for intonation purposes in continuous speech (Awan & Mueller, 1992). This characteristic was also observed by Morris and Brown (1994b), who speculate that F_0 variability may be a cohort effect of older people being accustomed to using greater voice inflections. In addition, increased pitch variability resulting in a "shaky" or even tremulous voice production has been reported (Caruso, Mueller, & Xue, 1994; Mueller, 1998). Results reported by Awan and

Ziminsky-Ammon (1996) (see Figure 2–6) indicated that elderly females (60- to 69- and 70- to 79-year-old groups) produced significantly higher pitch sigma (F_0 standard deviation converted to semitones) than younger female groups (18- to 30-, 40- to 49-, and 50- to 59-year-old women) during continuous speech productions. In addition, a significant correlation ($r = 0.61$, $p < .001$) was observed between mean pitch sigma and age. In Figure 2–7, Z-scores were calculated for each subject using the mean and standard deviation of the young adult female group as the control group. Results show 40% to 50% of the 60- to 69- and 70- to 79-year-old subjects produced mean pitch sigma substantially higher than the mean pitch sigma of the young adult group. Increased F_0 standard deviations have also been reported in elderly versus young men during sustained vowel productions by Orlikoff (1990).

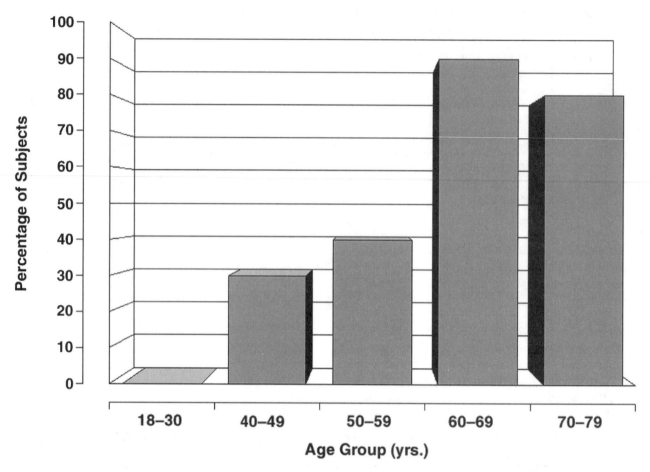

Figure 2–5 Mean SFF of Aging Women. Percentage of subjects per aging group with mean speaking F_0s <=2 standard deviations below the mean speaking F_0 of the young adult female group. (Percentage of Subjects with Z-Scores $\leq$–2.0 Re: Young Adult Comparisons [18–30 yrs.])

Declinations in pitch/frequency range in elderly subjects have also been observed. Ptacek et al. (1966) examined the performance of young adult (less than 40 years of age) and older adult (greater than 65 years of age) subjects on various measures of phonatory performance, including maximum frequency range. Results indicated that geriatric subjects had significant reductions in their total frequency ranges compared with young adults. Frequency range differences between groups averaged approximately 4 tones, mainly due to the higher frequencies that younger subjects were able to phonate. These findings concurred with those reported by Kaplan (1960), who stated that "there is a decrease in the range of the voice, particularly for the high frequencies" as the process of "calcification proceeds, and the cartilages and muscles become less elastic" (p. 145). The frequency

ranges of geriatric men and women were observed to be slightly greater than 2 octaves/24 semitones (26.5 and 25.1 semitones, respectively). In contrast, frequency range measurements averaged slightly below 3 octaves/36 semitones for young adults (34.5 for men; 32.8 for women), with similar frequency ranges observed between genders. Linville (1987) conducted a study to provide information on the maximum phonational frequency range (MPFR) capabilities during three distinct stages of physiological aging; 25 to 35 years of age ($n = 24$), 45 to 55 years ($n = 20$), and 70 to 80 years ($n = 23$). Results indicated that elderly women had significantly smaller F_0 ranges (mean = 28.96 semitones) than did middle-aged or young women (34.00 and 33.13 semitones, respectively). Results also indicated that changes occur at both ends of the MPFR as women age and that these

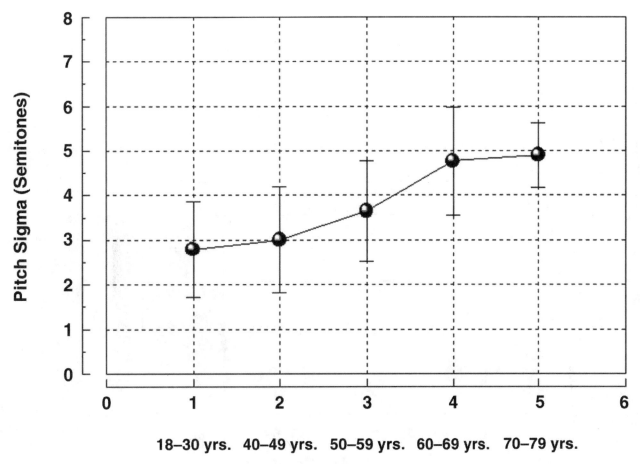

Figure 2–6 Mean Pitch Sigma of Aging Women. Mean pitch sigma (in semitones) and standard deviations across aging groups. (Correlation between aging and pitch sigma: $r = 0.61$, $p < .001$.)

changes occur during different stages of adult life. The 45- to 55- and 70- to 80-year-old subjects demonstrated the ability to produce lower frequencies than the 25- to 35-year-old subjects.

The "Super" Normal Voice: Effects of Vocal Training

It is important for the speech/voice clinician to realize that vocal training may expand "normal" voice expectations and capabilities. Several researchers have hypothesized other mechanisms of frequency control that may be exercised to great advantage by male and female subjects with vocal training. At a sublaryngeal level, several researchers (Gould, 1977; Gould & Okamura, 1974; Large, 1971) have found that trained singers have an increased respiratory capacity compared with untrained singers or the normal population. This increased respiratory capacity primarily lies in an in-

creased vital capacity and a decreased residual volume. Hixon and Hoffman (1978) have also observed that singers use different respiratory postures than do untrained singers. Singers may extend their abdomens beyond their relaxed positions to take advantage of maximum expiratory force. Although it has been noted earlier that an increase of sub-glottic pressure of 1 cm H_2O increases the frequency of phonation by only 2 to 4 Hz (Hixon et al., 1971), a considerable rise in subglottic pressure would result in a substantial increase in fundamental frequency range. In this manner, trained singers may be able to use their greater respiratory capacity and different respiratory postures to produce higher F_0s than untrained singers in the normal population, and thereby increase their F_0 ranges.

Subjects with vocal training have been observed to use different mechanisms of laryngeal control than the normal untrained population that may affect their capacity to gen-

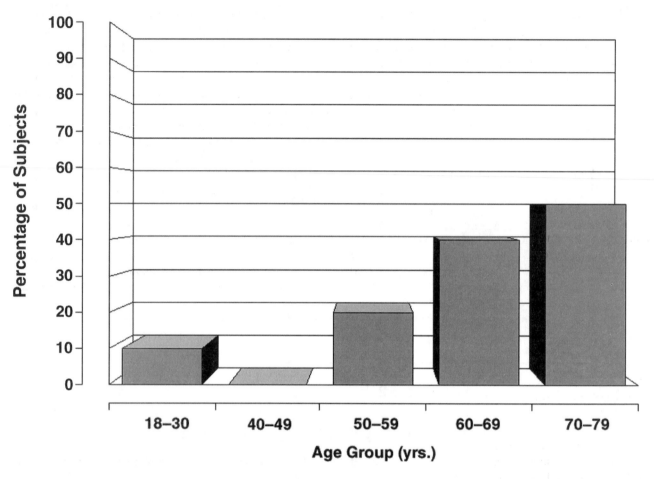

Figure 2–7 Pitch Sigma. Percentage of subjects per aging female group with mean pitch sigma ≥ 2 SD above the mean pitch sigma of the young adult female group. (Percentage of subjects with Z-scores ≥ 2.0 re: young adult comparisons [18–30 yrs.])

erate increased F_0 ranges. Pressman (1942) described a mode of vocal fold vibration used by trained singers at high frequencies in which the vocal folds are adjusted to allow only the anterior two-thirds to vibrate. Gould (1977) has described this mode of vibration as analogous to the results obtained when a stringed instrument is fingered to shorten one of the strings, resulting in the production of a higher tone. It has also been speculated that trained singers may use isometric contractions of the laryngeal musculature to produce wide ranges of acoustic output (Titze, 1989). In isometric contraction, the shape of the muscle (length, thickness, etc.) does not appreciably change, and only the tension varies. Greater tension in the folds would result in an increased fundamental frequency. This increase in fundamental frequency would be independent of the mechanism of

vocal fold lengthening, which primarily controls vocal fold tension in untrained subjects. In light of the aforementioned differences between trained and untrained subjects in terms of frequency control mechanisms, it has been speculated that trained subjects would have a greater fundamental frequency (F_0) range and would be able to produce higher F_0s than the normal or untrained population (Troup, 1981).

It has been speculated by several researchers (Coleman & Mott, 1978; Van Oordt & Drost, 1963) that trained singers are able to use the limits of their vocal capacity and yet maintain an acceptable degree of quality and control during singing. In effect, the "musical" range of phonation for a trained singer is quite similar to his or her "physiological" range. In contrast, the normal population of untrained singers has a "musical" range of controlled phonation that is highly distinct from the "physiological range." In the normal untrained population, the "physiological range" may be used in activities such as screaming, crying, shouting, etc. These are all activities in which no constraints are placed on quality, pitch, or duration of phonation (Fairbanks, 1960).

Tables 2–1, 2–2, and 2–3 present examples of speaking F_0, F_0 standard deviation/pitch sigma, and total phonational frequency range data for normal voice subjects.

WHAT TO EXPECT: ABNORMAL VOICE

If the mass, length, and tension characteristics of the vocal folds are affected in a voice disorder, then the vibratory characteristic of frequency (as well as perceived pitch) may be affected. So, in a very simple view, we may expect that a disorder that involves an additive lesion to the vocal fold(s) (e.g., vocal polyp) would increase the mass of the fold(s) and, therefore, decrease the frequency of vibration. Unfortunately, the effects on vocal pitch and F_0 are not always as simple as we might expect. We must remember that there is a complex interaction between the mass, length, and tension characteristics we have mentioned. In this example of a vocal fold lesion, the polyp may very well lead to an increase in mass but may also result in an increase in stiffness of the vocal fold tissue and cause the patient to compensate for the voice difficulties with increased muscular tension. Now the actual effect of the additive lesion on vocal frequency is very much in question; vocal frequency may remain at the patient's habitual level or even increase. The point being made is that the interaction of the physical determinants of vocal frequency is a complex one that is also influenced by the patient's own reaction to the voice disorder. In the diagnostic process, the clinician must apply his or her knowledge of anatomy, physiology, and acoustics to arrive at the best diagnostic interpretation of how a particular voice disorder may be revealing itself in the patient's voice characteristics. The possibility of highly variable effects on vocal F_0 should be kept in mind as we look at some of the possible effects of various disordered states.

Puberphonia/Mutational Falsetto

As males move from childhood to adulthood, a substantial lowering of the pitch and F_0 of the voice is generally observed. This lowering is observed during the period of puberty. Although voice change often occurs without any residual voice problem, disturbed mutation can occur. In some cases, the male subject retains a childlike, higher pitched voice after puberty, resulting in a voice versus age mismatch and pitch abnormality. Luchsinger and Arnold (1965) classified disturbed mutation in boys into three clinical forms: (1) delayed mutation, (2) prolonged mutation,

and (3) incomplete mutation. In all three forms, the voice is characterized by high pitch, chronic hoarseness, and pitch breaks. The continued use of the high pitch level of childhood is called *mutational falsetto* or *puberphonia* (Colton & Casper, 1996). Aronson (1990a) has described the mechanical cause of mutational falsetto as the overcontraction of the cricothyroid muscles, accompanied by a pronounced elevation of the entire larynx during phonation.

One may speculate on a number of possible reasons why the retention of the child pitch level may occur in cases of puberphonia (Aronson, 1990a; Colton & Casper, 1996; Morrison & Rammage, 1993) as shown below.

- The patient may have experienced an embarrassing pitch break (i.e., rapid, noticeable, uncontrolled shift in the pitch of the voice). As a consequence, the patient continues to use the child pitch level (which may be falsetto in register) because he may believe it is more "stable" than the new, adult pitch level.
- The adult pitch level may be unstable because of some underlying weakness in the phonatory mechanism that was only revealed during the period of voice change.
- Endocrine disorders may delay laryngeal development.
- Severe hearing loss may affect perception and control of the voice during adolescent voice change.

Cases of puberphonia are often confirmed by the criteria below.

- Presence of secondary sex characteristics (Pedersen et al., 1986) and age level at which voice change would be expected.
- An otherwise normal speech/vocal mechanism.
- Capability to produce the expected lower pitch level. This is the key area where the speech/voice pathologist's skills come into play, because we must somehow elicit this voice. Some patients may be able to produce other voices (i.e., an authoritative voice, a shouted voice, an imitated voice) that are produced at the expected natural pitch level. Other patients may produce more natural pitch levels during vegetative voice productions (e.g., cough, sigh, grunt, etc.).

Although puberphonia/mutational falsetto is most commonly reported for male patients, the condition may also affect women. The woman with puberphonia also maintains a childlike voice after puberty. However, the pitch abnormality may be less noticeable compared with the male condition, because the female voice does not undergo as drastic a shift in pitch level as the male voice.

Table 2–1 Speaking Fundamental Frequency (in Hz)

Author	Gender	No. of Subjects	Age (yr.)	Mean & SD	Range
Fitch & Holbrook (1970)	M	100	$\bar{x}$ = 19:6	116.65 (1.05 T)	85.0–155.0
	F	100	$\bar{x}$ = 19:5	217.00 (0.85 T)	165.0–255.0
Hollien & Jackson (1973)[a]	M	157	17:9–25:8 ($\bar{x}$ = 20:3)	123.3 Hz	90.5–165.2
Hollien & Shipp (1972)	M	25	20–29	119.5	N/A
	M	25	30–39	112.2	N/A
	M	25	40–49	107.1	N/A
	M	25	50–59	118.4	N/A
	M	25	60–69	112.2	N/A
	M	25	70–79	132.1	N/A
	M	25	80–89	146.3	N/A
McGlone & McGlone (1972)	F	10	7:6–8:6	275.8 (0.6 T)	N/A
Horii (1975)	M	65	26–79 ($\bar{x}$ = 54.1)	112.5 (17.3)	84–151
Honjo & Isshiki (1980)	M	20	69–85	162.0 (30.7)	N/A
	F	20	69–85	165.0 (32.5)	N/A
Hudson & Holbrook (1981)[b]	M_B	100	18–29	110.15 (16.21)	81.95–158.50
	F_B	100	18–29	193.10 (18.58)	139.05–266.10
Murry & Doherty (1980)	M	5	55–71 ($\bar{x}$ = 63.8)	122.9	104.0–137.7
Stoicheff (1981)	F	21	20–29 ($\bar{x}$ = 24.6)	224.3	192.2–275.4
	F	18	30–39 ($\bar{x}$ = 35.4)	213.3	181.0–240.6
	F	21	40–49 ($\bar{x}$ = 46.4)	220.8	189.8–272.9
	F	17	50–59 ($\bar{x}$ = 54.4)	199.3	176.4–241.2
	F	15	60–69 ($\bar{x}$ = 65.8)	199.7	142.8–234.9
	F	19	70+ ($\bar{x}$ = 75.4)	202.2	170.0–248.6
Bennett (1983)[c]	M	15	$\bar{x}$ = 8:2	234.0 (19.76)	204.0–270.0
	F	10	$\bar{x}$ = 8:2	235.0 (12.31)	221.0–258.0
	M	15	$\bar{x}$ = 9:2	226.0 (16.42)	198.0–263.0
	F	10	$\bar{x}$ = 9:2	222.0 (8.25)	209.0–236.0
	M	15	$\bar{x}$ = 10:2	224.0 (14.68)	208.0–259.0
	F	10	$\bar{x}$ = 10:2	228.0 (9.37)	215.0–239.0
	M	15	$\bar{x}$ = 11:2	216.0 (15.04)	195.0–259.0
	F	10	$\bar{x}$ = 11:2	221.0 (13.43)	200.0–244.0
Ramig & Ringel (1983)[d]	$M_{Y,G}$	8	26–35 ($\bar{x}$ = 29.5)	121.93 (1.91 ST)	N/A
	$M_{Y,P}$	8	25–38 ($\bar{x}$ = 32.3)	127.30 (2.61 ST)	N/A
	$M_{M,G}$	8	46–56 ($\bar{x}$ = 53.0)	118.36 (3.02 ST)	N/A
	$M_{M,P}$	8	42–59 ($\bar{x}$ = 52.6)	122.85 (2.17 ST)	N/A
	$M_{O,G}$	8	62–75 ($\bar{x}$ = 67.5)	125.98 (2.96 ST)	N/A
	$M_{O,P}$	8	64–74 ($\bar{x}$ = 69.1)	132.89 (2.43 ST)	N/A
Horii (1983)	M	18	10–12	226.5 (20.5)	192.1–268.5
	F	18	10–12	237.5 (15.9)	198.1–271.1
Moran & Gilbert (1984)	M	2	24–29	152.0	137.0–167.0
	F	3	24–29	244.0	220.0–278.0
Pedersen et al. (1986)	M	19	8.7–12.9	273.0	N/A
	M	15	13.0–15.9	184.0	N/A
	M	14	16.0–19.5	125.0	N/A

continues

Table 2–1 continued

Author	Gender	No. of Subjects	Age (yr.)	Mean & SD	Range
Kent et al. (1992)	F	19	65–80 ($\bar{x}$ =71.8)	194.0 (6.0)	N/A
Shipp et al. (1992)[e]	M_Y	10	21–35 ($\bar{x}$ = 25.3)	120.67 (10.87)	103.54–139.08
	M_M	10	46–71 ($\bar{x}$ = 57.7)	106.22 (2.27)	91.0–131.24
	M_O	10	77–90 ($\bar{x}$ = 83.7)	149.23 (19.97)	116.39–187.57
Awan & Mueller (1992)[f]	F_Y	9	$\bar{x}$ = 21.18 (1.06)	207.67 (16.38)	186.0–230.0
	F_E	9	$\bar{x}$ = 101.7 (2.40)	176.92 (22.61)	135.35–210.33
Awan (1993)[g]	M	10	18–30	123.00 (12.54)	102.0–137.0
	F	10	18–30	206.60 (14.99)	186.0–230.0
Morris et al. (1995)[h]	M	18	20–35	125.8 (11.1)	N/A
	M	14	40–55	117.2 (9.4)	N/A
	M	18	>65	130.1 (16.7)	N/A
Murry et al. (1995)[i]	M_Y	9	20–35	137.0 (0.9 ST)	N/A
	M_O	6	59–73	139.0 (6.9 ST)	N/A
	F_Y	10	20–35	195.0 (1.2 ST)	N/A
	F_O	7	59–73	170.0 (2.3 ST)	N/A
Awan & Mueller (1996)[j]	M_W	15	5:1–6:3	240.07 (15.89)	211.89–263.06
	F_W	20	5:1–6:1	243.35 (22.17)	195.20–291.10
	M_B	18	5:0–6:0	241.31 (18.05)	204.94–274.35
	F_B	17	5:1–6:0	231.48 (14.99)	208.08–261.73
	M_H	16	5:1–6:0	248.99 (20.18)	219.16–287.51
	F_H	19	5:1–5:11	248.04 (14.45)	217.56–274.03
Awan & Ziminsky-Ammon (1996)	F	10	18–30 ($\bar{x}$ = 23.80)	200.85 (15.70)	N/A
	F	10	40–49 ($\bar{x}$ = 43.40)	175.37 (11.18)	N/A
	F	10	50–59 ($\bar{x}$ = 54.80)	167.66 (22.23)	N/A
	F	10	60–69 ($\bar{x}$ = 65.20)	151.16 (18.30)	N/A
	F	10	70–79 ($\bar{x}$ = 72.30)	156.08 (20.19)	N/A
Morris (1997)[k]	M_W	15	$\bar{x}$ = 8.4 (0.4)	213.0 (15.0)	N/A
		15	$\bar{x}$ = 9.4 (0.3)	219.0 (18.0)	N/A
		15	$\bar{x}$ = 10.5 (0.2)	220.0 (21.0)	N/A
	M_B	15	$\bar{x}$ = 8.3 (0.4)	230.0 (22.0)	N/A
		15	$\bar{x}$ = 9.5 (0.2)	217.0 (39.0)	N/A
		15	$\bar{x}$ = 10.6 (0.2)	204.0 (37.0)	N/A
Author	M	51	18–30 ($\bar{x}$ = 24.03)	124.54 (17.72)	86.90–169.28
	M	14	40–80 ($\bar{x}$ = 52.75)	126.86 (25.67)	103.98–207.00
	F	205	18–30 ($\bar{x}$ = 22.85)	207.52 (15.68)	176.56–274.46
	F	17	31–45 ($\bar{x}$ = 37.69)	201.78 (11.68)	182.15–218.00
	F	20	46–80 ($\bar{x}$ = 55.06)	190.74 (16.40)	168.32–225.70

M = male; F = female; $\bar{x}$ = mean; ST = semitones; T = tones; N/A = not available.

[a] Data from extemporaneous speech only.

[b] Data from black ($_B$) subjects.

[c] Longitudinal study—same male and female subjects studied over a 3-year period.

[d] Young ($_Y$), middle age ($_M$), and old age ($_O$) subjects in good ($_G$) and poor ($_P$) condition. Data from reading of a standard passage.

[e] Young ($_Y$), middle-aged ($_M$), and old ($_O$) subjects.

[f] Young ($_Y$) versus elderly ($_E$) female subjects.

[g] Data from nonsingers only

[h] Data from nonsingers only.

[i] Young ($_Y$) and older ($_O$) subjects. Data from a standard reading passage averaged over three times daily on three different days.

[j] Data from white ($_W$), black ($_B$), and Hispanic ($_H$) children.

[k] Data from white (M_W) and black (M_B) subjects (spontaneous speech data only).

Muscle Tension Dysphonias (MTDs)/Hyperfunctional Voice

Increased tension within the vocal musculature may be of functional or organic origin. In functional cases, the increased tension may occur as a result of factors such as emotional stress, use of inappropriate pitch level, or retained compensatory activity after some previous organic disturbance (e.g., laryngitis). Excessive muscular tension may also be due to underlying neurological disturbance, as in spasticity (Darley et al., 1975).

When excessive muscular activity occurs in those muscles that increase the lengthening and tensing aspects of vocal fold function, the result may be an increase in pitch and F_0 level. We have all experienced this at times of emotional stress. Imitation of someone who is trying to speak when he or she is about to cry will characteristically result in tension in the laryngeal region and increased pitch level. Excessive muscular tension may also occur as a compensation during periods of vocal fatigue. This effect was observed by Stemple, Stanley, and Lee (1995), who examined acoustic, aerodynamic, and videostroboscopic characteristics associated with laryngeal fatigue resulting from prolonged voice use. Subjects were 10 adult women (mean age = 25.3 years). Analyses were made before and 2 hours after reading at a sound pressure level of 75 to 80 dB. Results indicated

Table 2–2 Fundamental Frequency Standard Deviation and Pitch Sigma

Author	Gender	No. of Subjects	Age (yr.)	Mean & SD	Range
Hollien & Jackson (1973)[a]	M	157	17:9–25:8 ($\bar{x}$ = 20:3)	1.6 T	0.5–2.5
Horii (1975)	M	65	26–79 ($\bar{x}$ =54.1)	2.41 ST (0.48)	1.46–3.54
Murry & Doherty (1980)[b]	M	5	55–71 ($\bar{x}$ = 63.8)	1.88 ST	1.0–3.2
Stoicheff (1981)	F	21	20–29 ($\bar{x}$ = 24.6)	3.78 ST	N/A
	F	18	30–39 ($\bar{x}$ = 35.4)	3.92 ST	N/A
	F	21	40–49 ($\bar{x}$ = 46.4)	4.00 ST	N/A
	F	17	50–59 ($\bar{x}$ = 54.4)	4.33 ST	N/A
	F	15	60–69 ($\bar{x}$ = 65.8)	4.25 ST	N/A
	F	19	70+ ($\bar{x}$ = 75.4)	4.70 ST	N/A
Horii (1985)[c]	M	12	24–40	0.27 ST (0.09)	0.14–0.47
Linville & Fisher (1985)V	F	25	25–35	1.47 Hz (0.39)	0.84–2.39
		25	45–55	1.68 Hz (0.43)	1.08–2.69
		25	70–80	2.52 Hz (1.49)	1.06–8.05
Linville (1988)V[d]	F	22	18–22 ($\bar{x}$ = 20.32)	0.11 ST (0.04)	0.05–0.33
Linville, Skarin, & Fornatto (1989)V	F	20	67–86 ($\bar{x}$ = 76.09)	0.34 ST (0.19)	0.10–0.74
Orlikoff (1990)[e]	M_Y	6	26–33 ($\bar{x}$ = 30.0)	1.06 Hz (0.65)	0.69–2.37
	M_E	6	68–80 ($\bar{x}$ = 73.3)	2.63 Hz (0.75)	1.32–3.44
Shipp et al. (1992)[f]	M_Y	10	21–35 ($\bar{x}$ = 25.3)	1.76 ST (0.26)	1.34–2.30
	M_M	10	46–71 ($\bar{x}$ = 57.7)	2.25 ST (0.45)	1.61–3.08
	M_O	10	77–90 ($\bar{x}$ = 83.7)	2.60 ST (0.60)	2.08–3.85
Wolfe, Fitch, & Cornell (1995)	M&F	20	18–30	1.86 (1.89)	0.33–7.52

continues

Table 2–2 continues

Author	Gender	No. of Subjects	Age (yr.)	Mean & SD	Range
Awan & Mueller (1996)[g]	M$_W$	15	5:1–6:3	4.38 ST (1.78)	2.18–9.36
	F$_W$	20	5:1–6:1	5.59 ST (1.81)	2.92–8.98
	M$_B$	18	5:0–6:0	5.26 ST (1.44)	2.85–8.28
	F$_B$	17	5:1–6:0	5.03 ST (2.04)	2.64–10.71
	M$_H$	16	5:1–6:0	5.39 ST (2.59)	2.75–11.08
	F$_H$	19	5:1–5:11	4.64 ST (1.67)	2.53–9.64
Morris (1997)[h]	M$_W$	15	$\overline{x}$ = 8.4 (0.4)	2.5 ST (0.9)	N/A
		15	$\overline{x}$ = 9.4 (0.3)	1.9 ST (0.7)	N/A
		15	$\overline{x}$ = 10.5 (0.2)	2.3 ST (0.8)	N/A
	M$_B$	15	$\overline{x}$ = 8.3 (0.4)	2.1 ST (0.7)	N/A
		15	$\overline{x}$ = 9.5 (0.2)	2.5 ST (0.9)	N/A
		15	$\overline{x}$ = 10.6 (0.2)	3.2 ST (0.7)	N/A
Awan & Ziminsky-Ammon (1996)[i]	F	10	18–30 ($\overline{x}$ = 23.80)	2.79 ST (1.07)	N/A
	F	10	40–49 ($\overline{x}$ = 43.40)	3.00 ST (1.19)	N/A
	F	10	50–59 ($\overline{x}$ = 54.80)	3.65 ST (1.13)	N/A
	F	10	60–69 ($\overline{x}$ = 65.20)	4.77 ST (1.21)	N/A
	F	10	70–79 ($\overline{x}$ = 72.30)	4.90 ST (0.72)	N/A
Author[j]V	M	20	18–30	0.29 ST (0.09)	0.17–0.54
	F	20	18–30	0.22 ST (0.07)	0.13–0.45
	M&F	10	5–6	0.29 ST (0.06)	0.20–0.37

M = male; F = female; V = vowel production; $\overline{x}$ = mean; ST = semitones; T = tones; N/A = not available.

[a] Data from extemporaneous speech only.

[b] Speech—converted from tones.

[c] Vowel—data reported from modal register phonations and reported in semitones.

[d] Data from the vowel /ɑ/ only.

[e] Vowel—data from healthy young men (M$_Y$) and healthy elderly men (M$_E$). F$_0$ SD represents 0.96% vs. 2.12% of the reported sustained vowel F$_0$, respectively.

[f] Speech—young ($_Y$), middle-aged ($_M$), and old ($_O$) subjects.

[g] Data from white ($_W$), black ($_B$), and Hispanic ($_H$) children.

[h] Speech—data from white (M$_W$) and black (M$_B$) subjects (spontaneous speech data only).

[i] Speech.

[j] Data for the vowel /ɑ/ only.

increased speaking F$_0$ after fatigue (mean F$_0$ = 223 Hz [SD = 25 Hz] versus 204 Hz [SD = 20 Hz]).

Although increased pitch is most commonly associated with excessive tension, decreased pitch may also be observed in this condition. A number of studies (Awan, 1999; Blood, 1994; Morrison & Rammage, 1993) have reported that methods to relieve excessive muscular tension and hyperfunction may result in decreases in pitch and F$_0$ level. Why would increased muscular tension result in decreased pitch and F$_0$? It may be hypothesized that (1) increased tension may be localized to the thyroarytenoid/vocalis muscle(s), resulting in shorter, more massive folds (when not in conjunction with antagonistic cricothyroid constric-tion), and/or (2) anterior-posterior squeezing of the larynx, which often accompanies stress and tension, may result in a shortening of the vocal folds and lower pitch (Morrison & Rammage, 1993).

Psychological Disorders

The previous discussion of MTDs indicated that the emotional state of the speaker may be clearly reflected in the characteristics of the voice. The same appears to be true for certain psychological states. Cases of psychosis, schizophrenia, and clinical depression may be characterized in part by changes to the pitch and F$_0$ of the voice. In particular,

Table 2–3 Total Phonational Frequency Range

Author	Gender	No. of Subjects	Age (yr.)	Mean & SD	Range
Hollien & Jackson (1973)	M	157	17:9–25:8 ($\bar{x}$ = 20:3)	19.4 T	14.5–27.0
Ramig & Ringel (1983)[a]	$M_{Y,G}$	8	26–35 ($\bar{x}$ = 29.5)	32.20 ST (8.77)	N/A
	$M_{Y,P}$	8	25–38 ($\bar{x}$ = 32.3)	26.65 ST (7.10)	N/A
	$M_{M,G}$	8	46–56 ($\bar{x}$ = 53.0)	28.29 ST (8.74)	N/A
	$M_{M,P}$	8	42–59 ($\bar{x}$ = 52.6)	26.84 ST (3.57)	N/A
	$M_{O,G}$	8	62–75 ($\bar{x}$ = 67.5)	31.37 ST (4.38)	N/A
	$M_{O,P}$	8	64–74 ($\bar{x}$ = 69.1)	24.30 ST (7.12)	N/A
Pedersen et al. (1986)	M	19	8.7–12.9	34.4 ST	N/A
	M	15	13.0–15.9	37.5 ST	N/A
	M	14	16.0–19.5	41.4 ST	N/A
Linville (1987)	F	24	25–35	33.13 ST (3.43)	28–40
	F	20	45–55	34.00 ST (3.22)	27–38
	F	23	70–80	28.96 ST (4.13)	19–35
Linville et al. (1989)	F	20	67–86 ($\bar{x}$ = 76.0)	36.4 ST (4.1)	29.0–44.0
Awan (1991)[b]	M	10	18–30	29.10 ST (5.02)	N/A
	F	10	18–30	25.80 ST (4.87)	N/A
Morris et al. (1995)[c]	M	18	20–35	36.6 ST (4.2)	N/A
	M	14	40–55	36.9 ST (5.0)	N/A
	M	18	>65	29.7 ST (5.2)	N/A

M = male; F = female; $\bar{x}$ = mean; ST = semitones; T = tones; N/A = not available.

[a] Young (Y), middle age (M), and old age (O) subjects in good (G) and poor (P) condition. Data from sustained vowel /ɑ/.

[b] Data from nonsingers only—musical range was evaluated rather than physiological range.

[c] Data from nonsingers only.

pitch variability appears to be substantially reduced in cases of both schizophrenia and severe clinical depression, resulting in monotone/monopitch voice consistent with flat affect (Andrews, 1995; Leff & Abberton, 1981).

Neurological Disturbance

Damage to the neuromotor system as a result of disease or trauma may result in dysarthrias. Descriptions of the five major groups of dysarthria are provided below (mixed dysarthrias caused by damage in multiple components of the motor system are also possible) (Colton & Casper, 1996; Darley et al., 1975; Dworkin, 1991).

Pyramidal/upper motor neuron (UMN) disorders: The upper motor neurons are the direct motor pathways linking the cortex with the other motor centers and, in particular, the lower motor neuron system

(originating at the "bulb"—the pons and the medulla). UMN damage releases inhibition over lower centers, resulting in spasticity. Spasticity is primarily characterized by hypertonia, muscle weakness, limited range of movement, and hyperreflexes. In spasticity, motor disruption may be unilateral or bilateral, although most prominent characteristics result from damage to the UMNs bilaterally. Dysfunction generally affects all aspects of the speech mechanism (to varying degrees), as well as the extremities.

Extrapyramidal disorders (hypokinetic dysarthrias): Hypokinesia is associated with damage or dysfunction to the extrapyramidal motor system, basal ganglia, and the substantia nigra. The extrapyramidal system is responsible for maintaining a foundation of basic muscle tone, posture, and readiness on which voluntary activities take place. Normal function of this system depends on a balance between neurotransmitters produced in portions of the basal ganglia and the substantia nigra (acetylcholine and dopamine, respectively). Hypokinesia is associated with a relative deficiency of dopamine, resulting in slowness, limited range of motion, and rigidity. Resting tremor may also be observed. Parkinson's disease is a characteristic example of hypokinesia.

Hyperkinetic disorders: Hyperkinesias are also associated with extrapyramidal system damage and neurotransmitter imbalance (in this case, a relative deficiency of acetylcholine). These disorders are characterized by the presence of uncontrolled movements, some quick (uncontrolled movements sustained less than 1 second in duration, such as jerks, tics, chorea) and some slow (uncontrolled movements sustained more than 1 second in duration, such as athetosis, dyskinesias, dystonias). Tremors such as organic or essential tremor have also been characterized as hyperkinetic in nature.

Ataxia: The cerebellum is responsible for "finetuning" movements by regulating the force, speed, timing, range, and direction of movements. Cerebellar damage results in ataxia, characterized by inaccurate, incoordinated movements, slowness, and hypotonia.

Lower motor neuron (LMN) disruptions: Disruptions of the lower motor neurons affect the final common pathways through which all movements (voluntary and involuntary) must pass before muscle contraction. A LMN and the muscle fibers supplied by it are referred to as the *motor unit* and are composed of the cranial nerve cell bodies (within the "bulb"), the nerve axons, the myoneural junction, and the muscle itself (Darley et al., 1975). Damage within the motor unit results in flaccidity, characterized by hypotonia, weakness, limited range of motion, and hyporeflexes. Unlike UMN damage, LMN disorders may be isolated to particular muscles or muscle groups. Therefore, it is possible for an individual to have isolated laryngeal dysfunction in combination with adequate function in other components of the speech mechanism.

Dysarthric effects on voice production have been described by a number of sources (Andrews, 1995; Boone & McFarlane, 1988; Canter, 1963; Colton & Casper, 1996; Darley et al., 1975; Dworkin, 1991; Haynes et al., 1992). Habitual pitch and F_0 may be affected by hypotonic (e.g., flaccidity) versus hypertonic (e.g., spasticity; Parkinsonism) states (lowered vs. raised, respectively). In addition, pitch range and variability are also often affected by dysarthric states. Monopitch and restricted pitch range have been observed in Parkinson's disease (Canter, 1963; Darley et al., 1975; Dromey, Ramig, & Johnson, 1995), superior laryngeal

nerve disruption (Aronson, 1990a; Luchsinger & Arnold, 1965), and vocal fold paralysis (Boone & McFarlane, 1988). In contrast, excessive pitch variability has been reported in spastic, ataxic, and hyperkinetic states (i.e., conditions in which hypertonicity occurs, lack of coordination of muscular activity occurs, or in which sudden, uncontrolled muscular contractions may occur). Vocal tremor, often associated with motor disruption, but for which a specific site of lesion is unclear (Aronson, 1990a), is an example of noticeable rhythmic variation in pitch. Spasmodic dysphonia (often acknowledged as a type of focal dystonia and hyperkinetic state) may also be observed to have elevated habitual pitch levels.

Examples of studies that have reported on the effects of neurological disease on pitch and F_0 characteristics can be found below.

- Canter (1963) reported on the speaking F_0 characteristics of patients with Parkinson's disease as compared with a group of age-matched controls. A substantially higher mean speaking F_0 was observed in the Parkinson's group versus the controls (mean SFF = 129 Hz vs. 106 Hz, respectively).

- Kent and Rosenbek (1982) observed monopitch and flattened F_0 contour as key characteristics of patients with various neurological lesions (ataxic, right hemisphere, and Parkinson's patients). These authors reported that the reduction in intonation patterns associated with motor speech disorders contributed to decreased acoustic contrasts and distortion in the speech signal. The overall result may be a reduction in intelligibility.

- Zwirner, Murry, and Woodson (1991) examined the phonatory characteristics of three dysarthric groups (Parkinson's disease, Huntington's disease, and cerebellar ataxia) versus a group of normal controls. Results for mean speaking F_0 showed no significant differences between groups. However, F_0 standard deviation (described as reflecting long-term phonatory instability) was observed to be significantly greater in the Huntington's and cerebellar ataxic groups versus the normal controls.

- Kent et al. (1992) described sustained vowel F_0 characteristics in a group of 10 amyotrophic lateral sclerosis (ALS) patients. Results showed that ALS patients exhibited abnormal F_0 values compared with a group of normal controls. However, no statistical difference was observed between the two groups because of the highly variable nature of F_0 in the ALS patients, with some deviant ALS F_0 values substantially lower than normal controls and some substantially higher.

- Dromey et al. (1995) described changes in speaking F_0 characteristics in a single Parkinson's disease patient before and after therapy by use of the Lee Silverman Voice Treatment approach (in this approach, the patient is encouraged to increase vocal intensity by increasing phonatory effort, vocal fold adduction, and respiratory support). Results indicated that mean speaking F_0 increased 15 to 20 Hz from before to after treatment. In addition, the speaking F_0 standard deviation was also observed to increase, reflective of increased intonation variations in connected speech. The authors speculated that improved F_0 characteristics after treatment were a result of improved compensation for laryngeal and respiratory rigidity characteristic of Parkinson's disease.

- Countryman, Hicks, Ramig, and Smith (1997) reported a case study of a 60-year-old man with idiopathic Parkinson's disease. Countryman et al. (1997) documented both decreased speaking F_0 and decreased F_0 standard deviation before therapy.

Mass Lesions and Distributed Tissue Change

Lesions (e.g., nodules, polyps, tumors) or added mass (e.g,. edema) that develop on or within the vocal fold tissue may have several variable effects on the pitch and frequency of the voice.

- Habitual pitch may be lowered because of the increased mass of the vocal folds, as in cases of edema, benign growths, and erythema (Boone & McFarlane, 1988; Dworkin & Meleca, 1997). Andrews (1995) reports lower than normal F_0 in cases of Reinke's edema, laryngeal granuloma, and contact ulcers.
- Habitual pitch may be increased because of increased stiffness of the fold(s) and compensatory increased laryngeal tension.
- Habitual pitch and mean SFF may not be significantly affected at all by the presence of laryngeal tissue changes (Baken, 1987).
- Pitch variability may occur (e.g., diplophonia, pitch breaks) because of altered vibratory characteristics (Haynes et al., 1992).
- Monopitch and decreased pitch ranges (Boone & McFarlane, 1988) may be observed because of restricted range of lengthening/tensing motion within the vocal folds. Andrews (1995) reports decreased speaking F_0 variability (reflective of reduced intonation) may be observed in cases of increased mass and stiffness of the vocal folds or swollen vocal folds.

The studies below exemplify the variable effects of lesions on vocal F_0 characteristics.

- Murry (1978) observed no significant difference in mean speaking F_0, F_0 standard deviation, or speaking F_0 range in cases of benign mass and laryngeal cancer as compared to normals. The author concluded that speaking F_0 should not be expected to necessarily lower in cases of organically based voice disorders.
- Hufnagle and Hufnagle (1984) examined the relationship between speaking F_0 and vocal quality in a group of eight dysphonic women diagnosed with vocal nodules. Results showed that the mean speaking F_0 of these patients was similar to published norms for normal young adult women. In addition, no significant changes in speaking F_0 or F_0 standard deviation occurred between before therapy and after therapy. These authors suggested that "there is no difference between SFF in normal speakers and those with vocal cord pathologies" (p. 98).
- Hirano, Tanaka, Fujita, and Terasawa (1991) described the F_0 characteristics of 1563 voice patients compared with a group of normal controls. Several observations were: (1) The effects of laryngeal carcinoma were variable, with abnormally low habitual F_0s observed in female patients, but abnormally high results observed in male patients. It was speculated that carcinoma may reduce the ability to stretch and thin the vocal fold (resulting in low F_0) or increase the stiffness of the vocal fold cover (resulting in high F_0). (2) Habitual F_0 was observed to be decreased in cases of acute laryngitis and Reinke's edema in men. It was speculated that this result was due to increased mass and a decreased stiffness in the cover of the vocal fold. (3) F_0 range was observed to be decreased in almost all disease groups. Overall, the authors concluded that measures of F_0 are recommended to assess aspects of vocal function and possible effects of treatment in dysphonic patients.

Effects of Smoking

Because smoking is associated with the development of additive mass conditions such as Reinke's edema, precancerous conditions such as leukoplakia, and laryngeal carcinomas (Colton & Casper, 1996), it is important to discuss the possible effects of smoking on voice. In addition, smoking is a significant irritant of the vocal fold mucosa and is associated with the development of chronic edema, laryngitis, and erythema. Studies of the general effects of cigarette smoking on the voice are limited. However, several studies have specifically attempted to investigate the effects of smoking on various frequency characteristics of the voice as shown below.

- Gilbert and Weismer (1974) measured the speaking F_0s of 15 smokers and 15 nonsmokers, and found that the F_0s of adult female smokers were significantly lower than those of the nonsmoker group on an oral reading task but not in spontaneous speech. The authors concluded that a thickening of the vocal folds and the connective tissue as a result of smoking caused the lowering of the F_0 on the oral reading task.

- Sorensen and Horii (1982) studied the effects of long-term smoking on fundamental frequency in both male and female subjects. A significant difference between the F_0 values was found for the male smokers and nonsmokers in the spontaneous speech and oral reading tasks. Although nonsignificant, similar trends were observed for the female smokers and nonsmokers on these same tasks. The difference in F_0 values for sustained vowel phonation was not significant for both smokers and nonsmokers, regardless of sex. Although there was a lack of statistical significance in all measures taken, the authors emphasized that the prepathological changes in acoustic measures of the voice signal need to be studied to understand how disease affects the larynx.
- Murphy and Doyle (1987) found that smoking cessation for as few as 40 hours resulted in an increase in fundamental frequency. Speech and sustained vowel samples of two subjects were collected before, during, and after a 40-hour period of smoking cessation. The F_0s of the two subjects returned to baseline once they began smoking again.
- Awan and Coy (1992) compared the voice characteristics of 15 young adult female smokers and 15 female nonsmokers (mean ages of 24.7 years and 24.4 years, respectively). Results showed the mean speaking fundamental frequency, as well as the maximum fundamental frequency of the smoking group, to be significantly lower than that of the nonsmoking group. The difference between minimum F_0s of the two groups was not significant. Furthermore, the mean speaking range of the smokers was significantly less than the mean speaking range of the nonsmokers.
- Hewlett, Topham, and McMullen (1996) investigated whether average speaking fundamental frequency is lower in smokers than in nonsmokers. The subjects were a young group (18 to 24 years of age) consisting of 20 nonsmokers and 14 smokers versus a middle-aged group (43 to 60 years old) consisting of 11 nonsmokers and 13 smokers. Although nonsignificant, results revealed a trend for lower mean speaking F_0s for both age groups within the smokers group compared with the nonsmokers group.
- Hewlett et al. (1996) also compared fundamental frequency ranges of 20 female smokers and 20 female nonsmokers. Although the lower limits of the frequency scale of smokers appeared to be similar to those of the nonsmokers, the upper end of the frequency scale was substantially restricted, thereby narrowing the total frequency range.
- Awan and Knych (2000) observed significantly greater pitch sigma in groups of smoking and nonsmoking young adults in both continuous speech and sustained vowel productions. No significant differences were observed in terms of mean speaking F_0. The observed increases in pitch sigma were felt to reflect possible reduced phonatory control over vocal F_0, possibly due to (1) tissue changes in the vocal fold mucosa, and/or (2) possible effects of smoking on nervous system control of phonatory behavior.

Deafness/Hearing Impairment

The control of various parameters of phonation, including pitch and frequency, occurs in part by means of the hearing mechanism. Patients with congenital or early childhood hearing losses of a severe nature have been observed to have variable effects on speaking F_0 and F_0 variability as used for intonation purposes as shown below.

- Monsen (1979) reported on the F_0 characteristics of syllabic production in 24 hearing-impaired children versus a group of normal controls. Although no differences were observed in mean F_0, the type of intonation contour used by the hearing-impaired subjects appeared to be a key characteristic in differentiating hearing-impaired from normal subjects and in differentiating the better from poor deaf speakers. Compared with normal subjects, many hearing-impaired subjects showed differences in the duration of F_0 contour and the variability of contour (some subjects producing flat intonation patterns and others producing highly variable contours). Monsen (1979) indicated that the deviant intonation contours observed may be due to poor control over respiratory supply and vocal fold tension.
- Horii (1982b) reported on the F_0 characteristics of 12 hard-of-hearing women (mean hearing loss of 91.2 dB secondary to congenital or early childhood losses) and 12 normal age-matched controls. Oral reading and spontaneous speech utterances were analyzed. Results indicated increased mean speaking F_0 and decreased F_0 standard deviation of the hard-of-hearing group in all conditions.

PITCH AND FREQUENCY: TUTORIAL

In this section, the reader will listen to voice characteristics and review the analyses of several voice samples that will illustrate (1) both normal vocal pitch and a number of the commonly observed voice pitch deviations and (2) methods of quantitatively analyzing the frequency capabilities of the voice. All of the voice samples discussed in this section can be found in the C:\VDP directory.

Continuous Speech Sample: Child Voice (Female)

Using the Windows Explorer program, double-click on the C:\VDP folder to find the file to be discussed. In this step, we will be analyzing the file P&F1.WAV. If you click on the file name using the L. mouse button, you will hear a 5-year-old female repeating the second sentence of "The Rainbow Passage." In listening to the pitch of this subject's voice, the clinician must primarily determine whether it would be normal for the patient's age, gender, etc. The pitch characteristics heard in this sample would seem appropriate for a kindergarten-aged child (not too high or too low). In addition, her pitch variations (intonation patterns) appear to be acceptable for the sentence that is being read—she does not have monopitch, nor does she have any excessive variations in pitch during her speech sample.

To quantify the pitch characteristics of this subject's voice, the clinician could compute measures of fundamental frequency (F_0). As we have previously learned, the F_0 is a measure of the number of cycles of vocal fold vibration per second. The examples that will be presented in this tutorial have been analyzed using the EZVoicePlus voice analysis software (VoiceTek Enterprises, Nescopeck, PA). However, the principles to be discussed will be applicable to most any voice analysis program the clinician may choose to use. Computation of the F_0 contour and associated statistics are shown in Figure 2–8.

The various measures of vocal F_0 confirm that this is a voice with appropriate frequency and pitch characteristics. The mean F_0 value of 250.782 Hz is well within the expected range for a young, school-aged child. The F_0 standard deviation is a measure of the average variability of the voice and is often observed to be approximately 10% of the mean speaking F_0. In this sample, the F_0 standard deviation appears a little low, as is her pitch sigma (F_0 standard deviation converted to semitones), although within normal limits. In addition, because her pitch variability and intonation were considered perceptually normal, the slightly low F_0 SD and pitch sigma would be considered clinically insignificant.

Continuous Speech Sample: Child Voice (Male)

Male and female voices are very similar in terms of mean speaking F_0 before puberty. As an example of this, a speech sample from a 5-year-old male is also provided for analysis.

Using the Windows Explorer program, double-click on the C:\VDP folder to find the file to be discussed. In this step, we will be analyzing the file P&F2.WAV. If you click on the file name using the L. mouse button, you will hear a 5-year-old male repeating the second sentence of "The Rainbow Passage." The pitch of this male's voice is very similar to the 5-year-old female voice previously analyzed (in fact, if you listen closely, it is actually a little higher pitched than the female child sample). The speech pattern of this child is a little halting (probably because of some hesitancy during the reading of the passage). However, his intonation patterns should be perceived as appropriate for the sample he is reading.

Computation of the F_0 contour and associated statistics are shown in Figure 2–9.

The main screen of the EZVoicePlus program shows the F_0 contour/trace for this child's continuous speech sample. The F_0 trace graphically depicts the varying F_0 of the voice during speech, corresponding to the pitch fluctuations used in normal intonation patterns. The F_0 analysis shows a slightly higher, although relatively similar, mean speaking F_0 in this male subject compared with the previously analyzed female child voice (278.377 Hz vs. 250.782 Hz). This child's F_0 standard deviation closely approximates the expected 10% of mean speaking F_0 (pitch sigma [3.63 semitones] is also within normal expectations). This child uses more pitch variability in his speech than the previous example—this is reflected in the greater F_0 SD, greater pitch sigma, and greater overall speaking range (i.e., lowest to highest F_0) during speech compared with the female child. Note that the EZVoicePlus program has been set to compute range in semitones (STs). The range in Hz would be 129.938 Hz.

Continuous Speech Sample: Adult Voices (Female and Male)

As children mature through puberty into adolescence, both genders will experience a lowering of vocal pitch and corresponding lowering in mean speaking F_0. However, the lowering of pitch and F_0 in the postpubertal male voice is substantially lower than that of the female. These characteristics are observed in the next samples to be discussed.

Using the Windows Explorer program, double-click on the C:\VDP folder to find the file to be discussed. In this step, we will be analyzing the file P&F3.WAV. If you click on the file name using the L. mouse button, you will hear a young adult female (24 years old) repeating the second sentence of "The Rainbow Passage." The pitch of this adult female's voice is clearly lower than the previous examples heard for male and female child voices. Again, intonation patterns should be perceived as being appropriate.

Computation of the F_0 contour and associated statistics are shown in Figure 2–10.

This example of an adult female speaking voice shows a mean speaking F_0 of 196.786 Hz, well within expectations

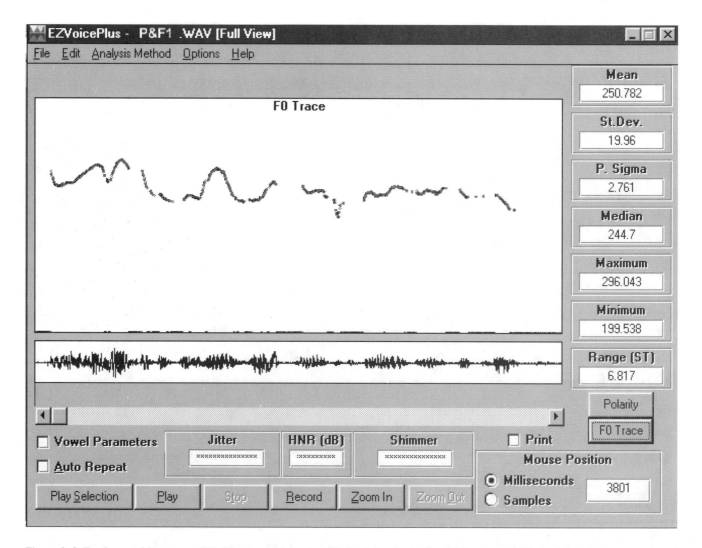

Figure 2–8 Fundamental Frequency (F_0) Contour and Associated F_0 Statistics for the Second Sentence of "The Rainbow Passage" Produced by a 5-Year-Old Female

for normal women. Again, measures of F_0 standard deviation and pitch sigma are also within expected limits, consistent with the perception of normal intonation.

✎ We will next analyze an example of a normal adult male voice. If you click on the file P&F4.WAV using the L. mouse button, you will hear a young adult man (25 years old) repeating the second sentence of "The Rainbow Passage." As expected, the pitch of the speaking voice is again lower than the previous example (adult woman). In addition, listen for short periods of vocal fry phonation (i.e., the lowest vocal register) at the ends of several unstressed words in this sentence (particularly the word "light"). Occasional episodes of vocal fry would be considered normal. Again, intonation patterns should be perceived as being appropriate.

Computation of the F_0 contour and associated statistics are shown in Figure 2–11.

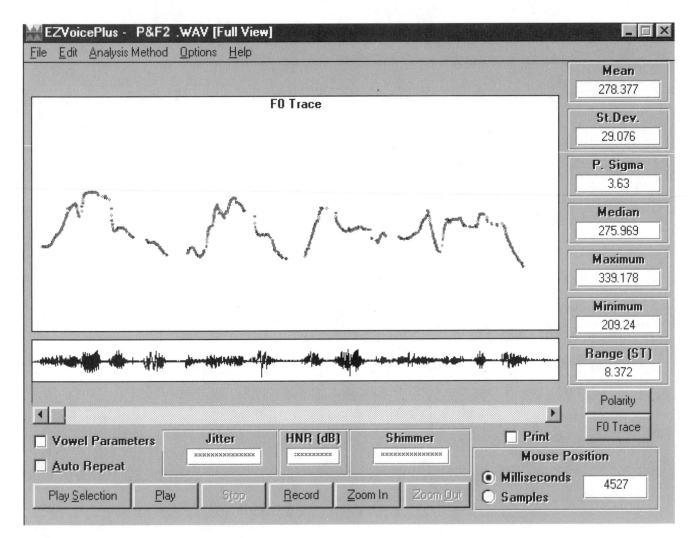

Figure 2–9 Fundamental Frequency (F₀) Contour and Associated F₀ Statistics for the Second Sentence of "The Rainbow Passage" Produced by a 5-Year-Old Male Subject

A mean speaking F_0 of 128.191 Hz is observed for this example of an adult male speaking voice, well within expectations for normal men. Again, the perception of normal intonation corresponds with F_0 standard deviation and pitch sigma levels within expected limits. This subject's occasional periods of vocal fry at the ends of several of the words in the sentence are produced at a substantially lower frequency than his average frequency level and correspond to the minimum frequency measurement of 104.549 Hz.

Disordered Samples: Continuous Speech

Effects of Roughness on Speaking Pitch and Frequency

It has been mentioned that voice quality deviations may affect the accuracy of our perceptions of vocal pitch. This is demonstrated in the next example of an adult man, who was characterized as having mild-to-moderate roughness as the primary voice quality deviation. The rough quality in the voice was secondary to a unilateral vocal polyp.

☙ If you click on the file P&F5.WAV using the L. mouse button, you will hear an adult man (60 years old) repeating the second sentence of "The Rainbow Passage." This patient had complained of a "low, rumbling sound" in his voice. Initial perceptual impressions of the vocal pitch corroborated the presence of roughness in the voice and an accompanying low pitch.

Computation of the F_0 contour and associated statistics are shown in Figure 2–12.

Although this patient was perceived as having a low pitch voice, the results of F_0 analysis show that this patient actually has a mean speaking F_0 of 150.522 Hz, which would be considered high normal/borderline abnormal. This is an example where the perception of pitch was adversely affected by the presence of roughness in the voice. In this case, initial perceptions did not match with the results of objective analysis. When this occurs, the clinician must read-

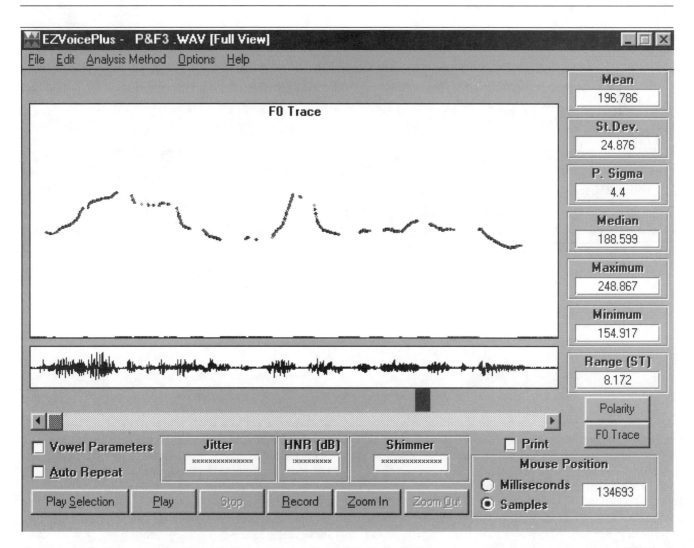

Figure 2–10 Fundamental Frequency (F_0) Contour and Associated F_0 Statistics for the Second Sentence of "The Rainbow Passage" Produced by a 24-Year-Old Female Subject

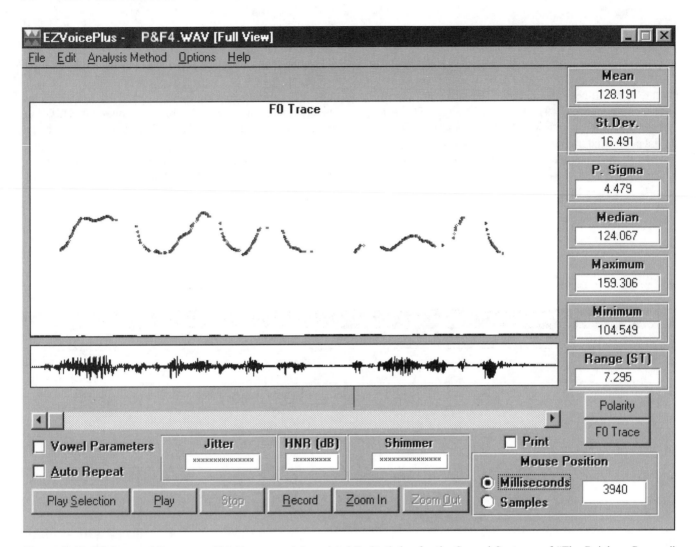

Figure 2–11 Fundamental Frequency (F_0) Contour and Associated F_0 Statistics for the Second Sentence of "The Rainbow Passage" Produced by a 25-Year-Old Male Subject

dress and, if necessary, revise the initial clinical hypotheses regarding the patient's voice problem(s). It was suspected that compensatory muscle tension may have caused the increased speaking frequency observed and may also have been contributing to his rough quality.

Reduced Pitch and Frequency Variability in Vocal Hypofunction

🐚 In this next example, click on the file P&F6.WAV using the L. mouse button. You will hear a speech sample from an adult woman (41 years old) who had been diagnosed with a unilateral vocal fold weakness. This patient's voice had been characterized as having a moderate degree of breathiness. The key pitch characteristic to notice in this example is the presence of relatively "flat" intonation throughout the sentence, resulting in an inanimate sounding voice.

Computation of the F_0 contour and associated statistics are shown in Figure 2–13.

The measures of F_0 standard deviation and pitch sigma confirm the perception of reduced pitch variability. The

F_0 SD of 7.443 Hz and pitch sigma of 1.162 Hz are both considerably below expectations, meaning that the average frequency variability of this patient's voice was quite limited. The overall speaking range of only 2.83 semitones also confirms the restricted intonation.

Analysis of Total Phonational Range

In the previous examples, we have concentrated on characteristics of the speaking voice (mean F_0, etc.). In these next examples, we will look at some other methods of frequency analysis that are often used to quantify vocal pitch and frequency characteristics and possible changes in the voice

as a result of a voice disorder. First we shall look at the method for computing total phonation range (i.e., the total F_0 range from lowest frequency in modal register to the highest in falsetto).

✎ In this next example, click on the file P&F7.WAV using the L. mouse button. You will hear a 38-year-old male patient's lowest and highest phonations combined into a single sound file. In obtaining the patient's total phonational range, the subject was first asked to phonate down to his lowest note/pitch level in modal register. The instructions to the subject were, "Using the vowel /ɑ/, I want you to start at a

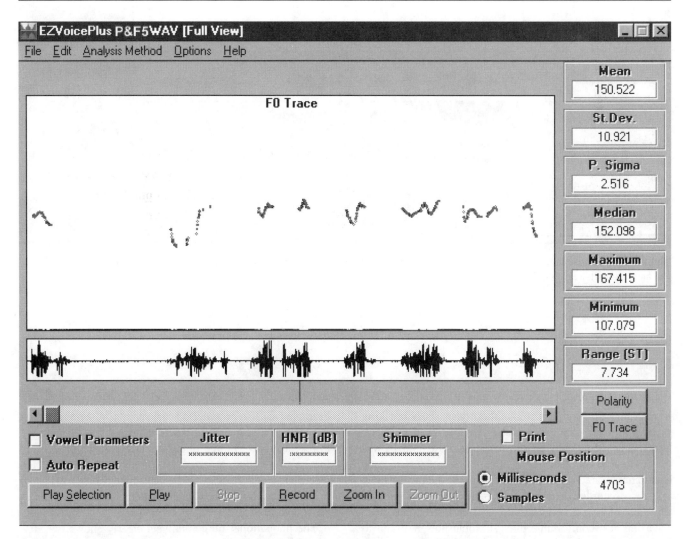

Figure 2–12 Fundamental Frequency (F_0) Contour and Associated F_0 Statistics for the Second Sentence of "The Rainbow Passage" Produced by a 60-Year-Old Male Patient (Unilateral Vocal Polyp)

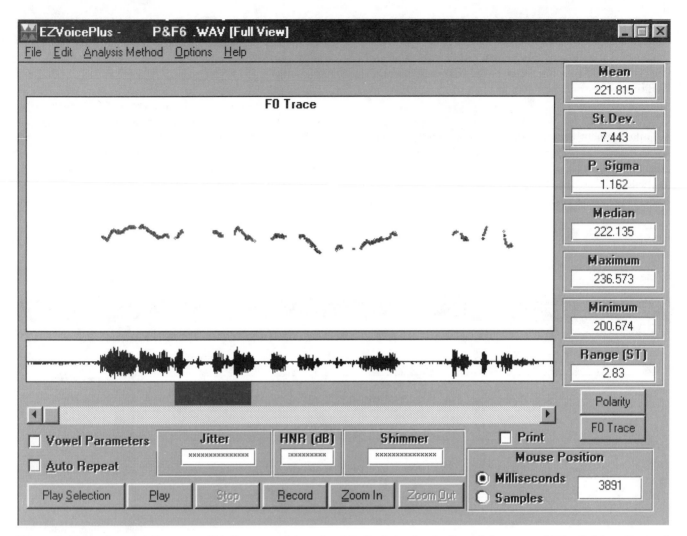

Figure 2–13 Fundamental Frequency (F₀) Contour and Associated F_0 Statistics for the Second Sentence of "The Rainbow Passage" Produced by a 41-Year-Old Female Patient (Unilateral Vocal Fold Paresis)

comfortable pitch and go down in steps until you reach the lowest note that you can hold without your voice breaking or cracking." An example was also provided for the patient. When the patient got to the lowest note he could hold, he was encouraged to repeat it two to three times and sustain each production for 2 to 3 seconds. A sample of the lowest pitch was then recorded. The patient was next asked to phonate up to his highest note in falsetto register. Instructions were "Starting at a comfortable pitch, I would now like you to go up in steps until you reach the highest note that you can produce without your voice breaking or cracking, including

falsetto register—falsetto is a thin, reedy type of voice." An example was also provided for the subject. When the patient got to the highest note he could hold, he was encouraged to repeat it two to three times and sustain each production for 2 to 3 seconds. A sample of the highest pitch was then recorded.

Computation of the F_0 contour and associated statistics are shown in Figure 2–14.

The phonational range analysis clearly shows two distinctive F_0 traces/contours for the lowest versus highest frequency phonations. In addition, the total phonational range is automatically calculated in semitones (26.272 STs). This range would be considered within normal expectations for a person without vocal training. In this example, the mean F_0 is simply the average between the low- versus high-frequency phonations and does not have any significance.

Example of a Pitch Glide

Pitch glides are often incorporated into the voice diagnostic to examine (1) the ability of the patient to lengthen and tense the vocal folds in a continuous manner and (2) to assess the patient's ability to produce continuous phonation during this stressful task. In addition, Stemple (1993) includes pitch glides as a key component of his vocal function exercises to "stretch" the vocal folds.

✎ In this next example, click on the file P&F8.WAV using the L. mouse button. You will hear a 38-year-old male patient (the same patient as in the previous example) carrying out a pitch glide. The patient was asked to glide (i.e., change his pitch continuously from lowest to highest pitches) from his very lowest note to his very highest (including falsetto) using the vowel /ɑ/. An example was provided for the patient by the clinician. When perceptually judging the pitch glide, it is important to assess (1) the range of pitches produced and

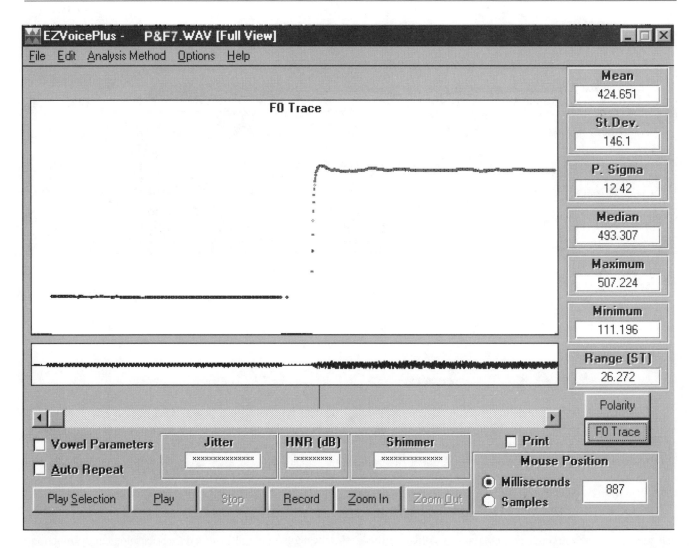

Figure 2–14 Measurement of the Total Phonational Range. The patient's lowest and highest frequency productions have been combined into one sound file for analysis.

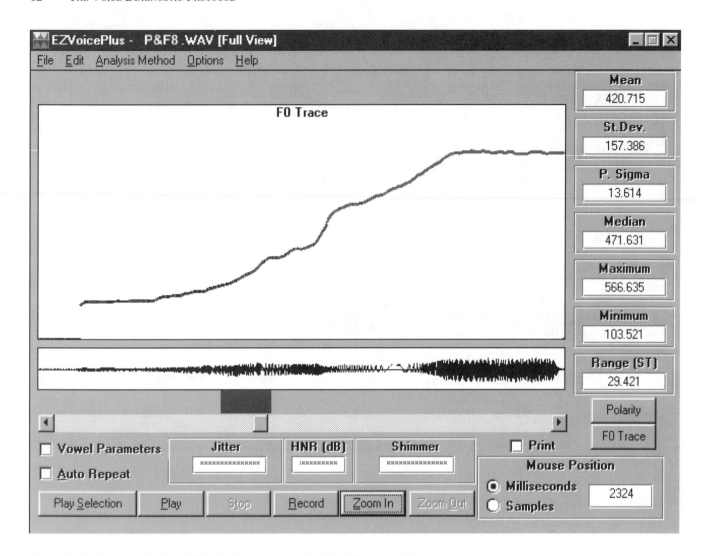

Figure 2–15 Analysis of a Pitch Glide for Measurement of the Total Phonational Range

(2) the ability to control phonation without any noticeable phonation or pitch breaks. Some slight vocal instability may be observed during the period of register transition (modal to falsetto).

Computation of the F_0 contour and associated statistics are shown in Figure 2–15.

This example shows a relatively steady frequency change as the patient produces the pitch glide. The patient has then held out his highest frequency phonation, resulting in the plateau at the end of the F_0 trace/contour. The slight variability in the contour of the glide corresponds with the change into falsetto register. This patient has produced a phonational range of 29.421 semitones (more than adequate for a patient without vocal training).

Variability of Vocal F_0 in Sustained Vowels: Vocal Tremor

In vocal tremor, we observe a rhythmic variation in pitch and/or loudness of the voice. Tremors are often considered to be signs of possible underlying neurological dysfunction. However, it should also be remembered that there are normal tremors that occur as a result of factors such as fatigue or anxiety/stress. In addition, many people (particularly those with singing experience) will add a purposeful tremor referred to as *vibrato* to sustained phonations. In the next two examples, we will hear and analyze samples of both normal and abnormal tremor.

✎ In this next example, click on the file P&F9.WAV using the L. mouse button. You will hear an adult female subject sustaining the vowel /ɑ/. A rhythmic variation in pitch can be heard in this sample, which may be perceived by some as unsteady, "wobbly," or quavering (Colton & Casper, 1996).

Computation of the F_0 contour and associated statistics are shown in Figure 2–16.

The F_0 contour/trace clearly shows evidence of a vocal tremor in this particular sample. Rather than a relatively flat contour (which would be expected in a normal voice), a rhythmic fluctuation in vocal F_0 is shown by the presence of repetitive "hills and valleys" in the contour. In this particular example, it was determined that the tremor was due to the use of vibrato, a purposeful tremor commonly used by trained singers.

✎ In the next example, we will hear and analyze a sample of abnormal tremor. Click on the file P&F10.WAV using the L. mouse button. You will hear a sustained vowel /ɑ/ produced by an adult female subject who had been diagnosed with

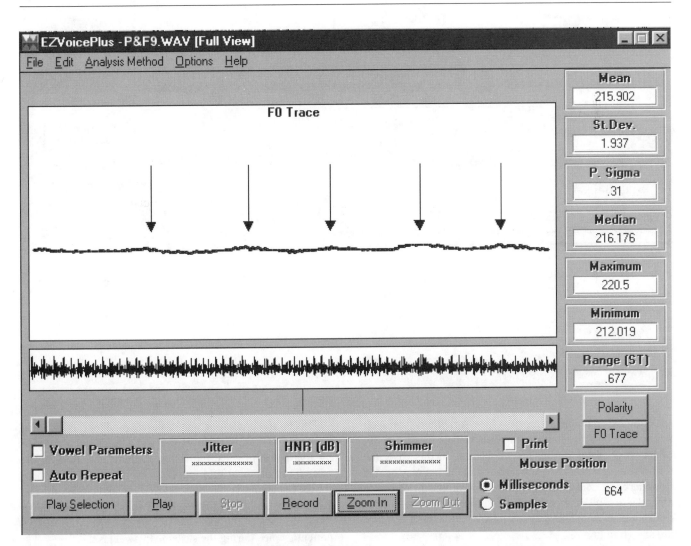

Figure 2–16 An Example of a "Normal" Tremor (Vibrato). The arrows indicate the periods of rhythmic frequency variations during the sustained vowel production.

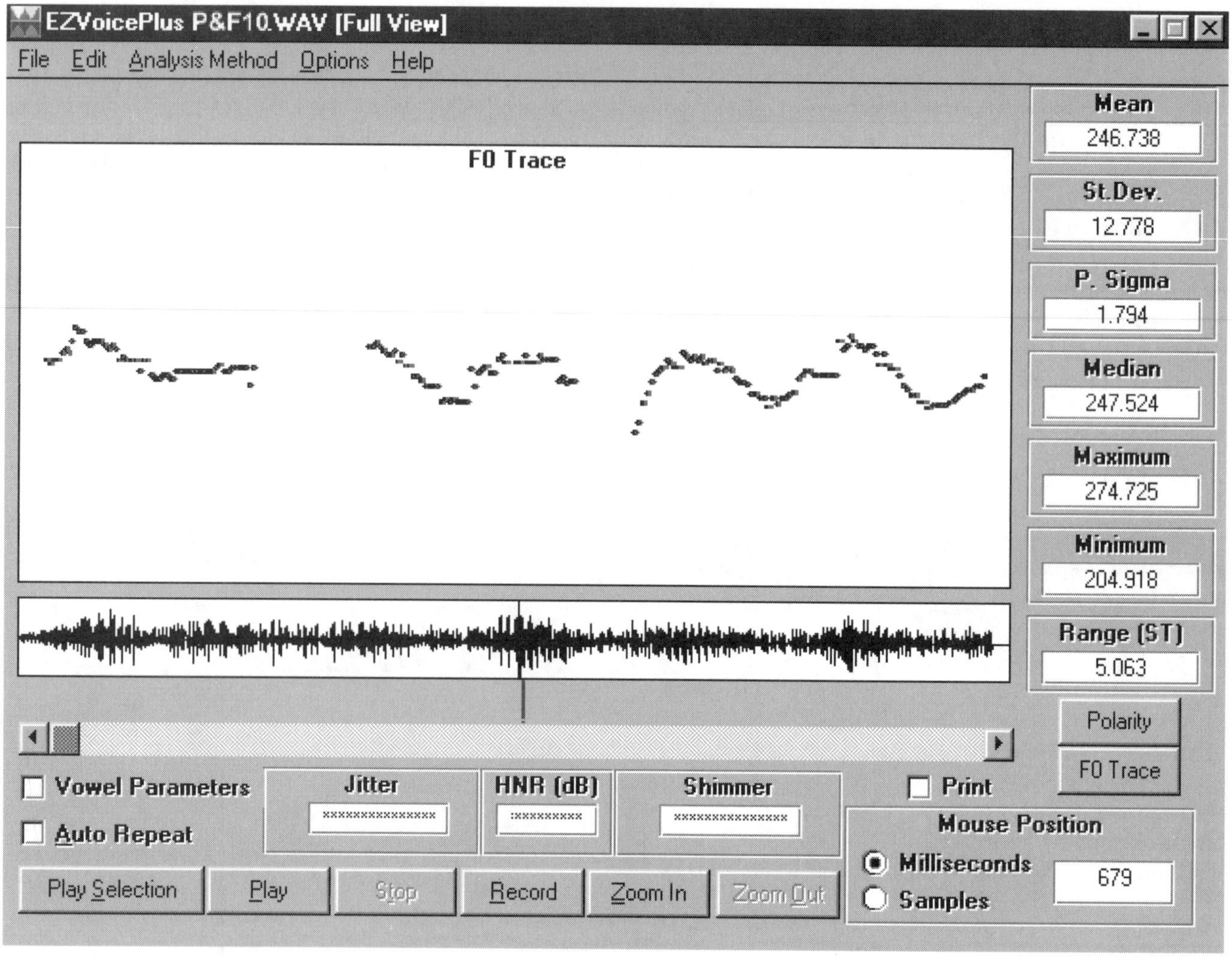

Figure 2–17 An Example of an Abnormal Tremor Observed during Sustained Vowel Production by a Patient Diagnosed with Spasmodic Dysphonia (Adductory Type)

spasmodic dysphonia (adductory type). A rhythmic variation in pitch can be heard in this sample, as well as spasm activity of the vocal folds during her phonation. In this case, the tremor and spasm activity are not purposeful but may be due to underlying neurological dysfunction similar in nature to dystonia (a type of hyperkinesis) or essential tremor.

Computation of the F_0 contour and associated statistics are shown in Figure 2–17.

The F_0 trace/contour again shows evidence of a vocal tremor, with each spasm of the vocal folds accompanied by a variation in vocal frequency. Extreme variations in the periodicity of vocal fold vibration may also be responsible for the blank areas ("drop-outs") in the F_0 trace/contour. The F_0 standard deviation (in Hz), pitch sigma (STs), and range (STs) document the extreme frequency variability of this patient's voice during the sustained vowel task.

CHAPTER 3

Evaluation of Vocal Loudness/Intensity

DEFINITION

Sound is the perception of pressure changes in air (Baken, 1987). In an oscillogram, the magnitude of these pressure changes is reflected in the *amplitude* of the wave. The human ear is sensitive to a vast range of pressure changes (from a minimum of .0002 dynes/cm^2 (for *most* people, not all) to >600 dynes/cm^2). The *intensity level* of a signal refers to the power of the signal (proportional to the square of the pressure) and is commonly reported in decibels (dB). Intensity represents a comparison of the sound pressure level (SPL) of an observed signal to a reference sound pressure. In contrast to the objective measure of intensity, *loudness* is the perceptual attribute that corresponds to the magnitude of the pressure changes (Baken, 1987).

Although an often somewhat overlooked phenomenon, loudness/intensity evaluation is also an important component of the voice diagnostic protocol. Bless and Hicks (1996) state that loudness relates not only to the degree of respiratory force but also to the amplitude of vocal fold vibration. In addition, Colton and Casper (1996) indicate that vocal loudness is affected by (1) glottal resistance to the expiratory airstream and (2) the rate of airflow change at the moment of closure. It appears that loudness/intensity evaluation is an essential component of our evaluation because it provides us with information about the coordination between phonatory and respiratory mechanisms.

CONTROL OF VOCAL LOUDNESS/INTENSITY

Vocal loudness/intensity depends on an interaction of subglottal air pressure, adjustments at the level of the vocal folds, and the configuration of the supraglottal vocal tract (Baken, 1987). Because phonation at different intensities assesses the sublaryngeal, laryngeal, and supralaryngeal limits of the phonational system (Gauffin & Sundberg, 1980; Gramming & Sundberg, 1988), intensity range would seem to be a potentially important measure in the assessment of vocal function and performance (Michel & Wendahl, 1971).

In his seminal study on vocal intensity, Isshiki (1964) investigated the relationship between voice intensity (SPL), subglottic air pressure, airflow rate, and glottal resistance. His results indicated that at very low frequencies, airflow rate remained almost unchanged or even slightly decreased with increases in vocal intensity. The glottal resistance increased with vocal intensity. In contrast to this, the flow rate in high-frequency phonation was found to increase greatly with intensity, but glottal resistance remained constant. Isshiki (1964) concluded that the glottal resistance was dominant in controlling intensity at very low pitches (i.e., laryngeal control). Glottal resistance became less dominant as the frequency was increased, until at extremely high frequencies the intensity was controlled almost entirely by the flow rate (expiratory muscle control). Isshiki (1964) suggested that voice intensity at the level of the larynx may be controlled by three factors: flow rate (expiratory effort), glottal resistance (glottal closure), and efficiency (duration of the open phase controlled by physiological laryngeal forces). It has been estimated that a decrease in the open quotient (OQ) (the ratio of the duration of the open period of the vocal folds to the total period of the cycle) from 1.0 to 0.5 may lead to an increase in intensity of 7 dB (Flanagan, 1958). In addition, the decrease in OQ may result in the accentuation of the high-frequency component of the glottal sound (Flanagan, 1958; Fletcher, 1950). This spectral change may also contribute to the increase in intensity because the resonant frequencies of the vocal tract (formants) are generally situated at higher frequencies.

In a further study of vocal intensity and flow rate, Isshiki (1965) states that the intensity of a normal laryngeal voice generally is controlled by two variables: (1) the contraction of the laryngeal adductor muscles (encompassing the factors of glottal resistance and efficiency) and (2) the expiratory force (encompassing the factors of subglottal air pressure and flow rate). To augment vocal intensity, both variables synergistically increase in varying degrees, depending on the frequency level. The results of Isshiki's (1965) study confirmed the results of his earlier (1964) study, which indicated that glottal resistance was observed to play a more important role in varying the intensity at low frequencies, and expiratory force was considered the dominant factor at high frequencies. Isshiki's (1964, 1965) results were further supported by the EMG data of Hirano, Ohala, and Vennard (1969), in which increased activity in the vocalis and lateral cricoarytenoid muscles was observed during intensity changes at low pitches, but not at high pitches.

In contrast to studies detailing the interaction of respiratory and laryngeal control for vocal intensity, Faaborg-Andersen (1957) found no relation between changes in loudness and activity levels in the vocalis and cricothyroid muscles. In support of this view, Sawashima (1974) described vocal intensity as being primarily controlled by respiratory factors. Folkins and Kuehn (1982) have tentatively concluded that if laryngeal adjustments in loudness change do exist, they are probably less systematic than adjustments for pitch control.

The aforementioned factors dealing with intensity control are based on respiratory and laryngeal adjustments. However, Stevens and House (1961) discuss the fact that different vowels produced with the same vocal effort have different overall intensity levels. The range of overall intensity levels for the vowels of American English is approximately 4 to 5 dB, with /i/ and /u/ (with small anterior vocal tract openings) having the lowest intensity levels and /ae/, /ɑ/, and /ɔ/ (with relatively large anterior vocal tract openings) the highest intensity levels (Stevens & House, 1961). These observations would appear to support those of Fairbanks (1960), who reported that vowel intensities were correlated with the size of the anterior opening of the vocal tract. Stevens and House (1955) and Fant (1970) showed that the overall intensity of a vowel is determined largely by the frequency of the first vowel resonance (first formant), with higher first formant frequencies resulting in higher relative intensities. Lindblom and Sundberg (1971) have reported similar relationships between intensity, mouth opening, and first formant frequency.

Gauffin and Sundberg (1980) have observed that vowel intensity at soft levels mainly depends on the amplitude of the voice source fundamental. Thus, the vowel intensity reflects primarily the respiratory and laryngeal facets of intensity control. However, in loud phonation, voice-source overtones (often the second partial/harmonic) strongly determine the intensity value (Gauffin & Sundberg, 1980; Gramming & Sundberg, 1988). It appears evident that vowel intensity may reflect not only respiratory and laryngeal function but also the resonant qualities of the supralaryngeal vocal tract. It has also been noted by Gramming and Sundberg (1988) that the intensity level of a vowel will decrease if the frequency of the fundamental is higher than that of the first formant of a vowel.

The following conclusions may be made about the control of intensity:

- Intensity of voice is affected by the total speech production system.
- At low fundamental frequencies, glottal resistance (laryngeal control) may be dominant in controlling intensity.
- At higher frequencies, intensity is controlled almost exclusively by respiratory factors.
- Although laryngeal adjustments for intensity control exist, they are not as systematic as laryngeal adjustments for frequency changes.
- Low-intensity SPL is primarily indicative of respiratory and laryngeal facets of intensity control, whereas voice-source and vocal tract resonance interactions also affect loud intensity control.

Interaction of Frequency and Intensity Control

Although Hixon et al. (1971) have indicated that changes in subglottal air pressure do not effect significant changes in fundamental frequency, the opposite effect may not be true. Given the interaction of air pressure and laryngeal status, it is not surprising that vocal intensity changes with increases in F_0 (Baken, 1987). Stone and Ferch (1982); Komiyama, Watanabe, and Ryu (1984); and Awan (1991) have confirmed the effect of increases in F_0 on SPL and have observed that the intensity increase with F_0 is roughly linear, with the rate of intensity increase affected by intended loudness level (maximum, minimum, or comfortable).

- Awan (1991) observed that SPL increased with increasing frequency at a rate of approximately 1.0 dB for each 10% increase in frequency along the total phonational range when producing maximum intensity levels (correlation between dB SPL and frequency level: $r = 0.89$, $p < .001$). Trained singers showed a rate of SPL increase of approximately 2.3 dB per 10% increase in phonational range (correlation between dB SPL and frequency level: $r = 0.88$, $p < .001$).
- SPL increased with increasing frequency at a rate of approximately 1.4 dB for each 10% increase in phonational range when producing minimum intensity levels (correlation between dB SPL and frequency level: $r = 0.98$, $p < .001$). Trained singers showed a rate of SPL increase of approximately 2.7 dB per 10% increase in phonational range (correlation between dB SPL and frequency level: $r = 0.99$, $p < .001$) (Awan, 1991). In an earlier study, Stone and Ferch (1982) had also observed that the increase in intensity with F_0 is roughly linear at a rate of from 7.5 to 12 dB per octave.
- At comfortable loudness levels, SPL increased with increasing frequency at a rate of approximately 1.3 dB for each 10% increase in phonational range (correlation between dB SPL and frequency level: $r = 0.97$, $p <$

.001). Trained singers showed a rate of SPL increase of approximately 2.4 dB per 10% increase in phonational range (correlation between dB SPL and frequency level: $r = 0.96$, $p < .001$) (Awan, 1991).

The interaction between frequency and intensity may be explainable in the following manner. To increase fundamental frequency, increases in activity are mainly observed in cricothyroid and vocalis, but also in posterior cricoarytenoid and interarytenoids. These increases in the muscular contraction result in great increases in vocal fold tension. To overcome the high vocal fold tension, increases in subglottal air pressure and transglottal airflow rate may be necessary. The result is high-frequency phonation accompanied by high intensity. The fact that high-intensity phonation often accompanies high-frequency phonation does not imply that vocal intensity is controlled by laryngeal factors. Respiratory mechanisms work independently or in conjunction with laryngeal control mechanisms.

PERCEPTUAL ASSESSMENT OF LOUDNESS

The perceptual assessment of loudness generally focuses on the same three parameters that were used in pitch evaluation: (1) habitual loudness, (2) loudness variability, and (3) loudness range.

Habitual Loudness

Habitual loudness is analogous to the most commonly used loudness or average loudness level. No single loudness level would be considered normal. Instead, the habitual loudness level should be appropriate for the speaking situation (Boone & McFarlane, 1988; Case, 1996; Haynes et al., 1992; Murry, 1982; Prater & Swift, 1984; Stemple, 1993). Prater and Swift (1984) indicate that the habitual loudness level should be loud enough to be heard over background noise but not be so loud that it brings discomfort or distraction to the listener. Abnormal habitual loudness level is found in speakers who use vocal loudness/intensity levels conspicuously higher or lower than typical for a particular speaking situation (Weinberg, 1983).

Loudness Variability

Normal stress/intonation patterns require the use of loudness variability. A stressed word or syllable is generally produced with an increase in perceived loudness. Loudness variations are an important aspect of *prosody*, the physical attributes of speech that are used to alter or accentuate the linguistic nature of an utterance. When a patient speaks with little or no fluctuation in loudness, the result may be a "boring, colorless voice" (Prater & Swift, 1984, p. 50). This type of voice has been referred to as *monotone* (Prater

& Swift, 1984) or as displaying *monoloudness* (Colton & Casper, 1996).

In addition to loudness variations as applied to suprasegmentals, *loudness instability* is also an aspect of variability that must be attended to by the clinician. Abrupt changes in loudness may be observed in phonation breaks (Haynes et al., 1992). In vocal tremor, rhythmic variations in loudness (as well as pitch) are observed, particularly during the production of sustained vowels. In addition, vocal loudness should be controlled throughout an utterance and not decrease noticeably at the end of a sentence.

Loudness Range

The loudness range, from minimal to maximal levels, is also an important aspect of loudness evaluation (Haynes et al., 1992). The assessment of loudness range is believed to be an essential aspect of vocal evaluation because voice production at different loudness levels assesses the function and interaction of all components (respiratory, laryngeal, and supralaryngeal/articulatory) of the speech mechanism affecting phonation. It is generally considered that vocal dysfunction will reduce the available loudness/intensity range (Bless & Hicks, 1996). Andrews (1995) states that observations of voice characteristics such as the presence of voice/phonation breaks and quality changes at different levels should be noted during the evaluation of loudness range.

Methodological Considerations

Judgments of vocal loudness may have great relevance to the patient and be a standard by which vocal improvement will be judged after therapy. However, a difficulty with judgments of loudness is that loudness and intensity are not linearly related. It has been observed that the sensation of loudness increases more slowly than the actual increase in intensity (Borden, Harris, & Raphael, 1994). Therefore, it is possible that a patient may be using higher than normal levels of vocal intensity (possibly resulting in misuse or abuse of the vocal mechanism [Colton & Casper, 1996]) that will not be perceived by the clinician. As with all types of perceptual assessment methods, issues of training and experience of the listener must also be considered when assessing the accuracy of loudness judgments.

HOW TO DO IT: PERCEPTUAL ASSESSMENT OF LOUDNESS

Habitual Loudness

As in the case of pitch evaluation, perceptual assessment of vocal loudness may be easily reported using a multipoint scale. Ratings of habitual loudness may be applied to (1) a picture description/spontaneous speech sample and/or (2) "The Rainbow Passage" sample, which was obtained for the vocal ratings and analysis described in the previous chapter. The main difference in rating loudness is that it is necessary to evaluate the patient's habitual loudness level under various conditions. Prater and Swift (1984) suggest the following:

- Assessment of vocal loudness in conjunction with differing levels of background noise.

- Assessment of vocal loudness while standing close to the examiner (conversational distance) versus 10 to 15 feet away. This allows assessment of the ability to vary habitual loudness level as a function of proximity to other individuals (Prater & Swift, 1984).

Once a judgment is made regarding the patient's habitual loudness level, the result may be reported using a categorical/equal-appearing interval (EAI) rating scale in the following format:

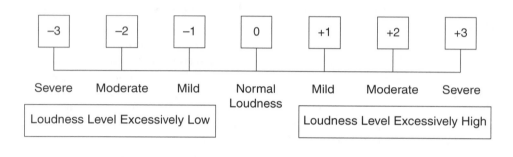

Note that the central point of the scale is zero (i.e., no substantial difference from normal expectations), with ratings of excessively loud voice (positive numbers) and ratings of excessively low vocal loudness (negative numbers) rated on either side of the normal expectation point. Definitions for mild, moderate, and severe are the same as those presented in Chapter 1.

Perceptual Assessment of Loudness Variability

Similar categorical/EAI scales as used for the rating of habitual loudness may be applied to the rating of loudness variability:

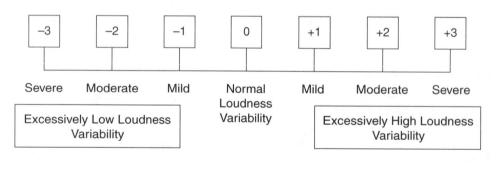

It is recommended that ratings of loudness variability/intonation be applied to continuous speech samples. Observation of vocal tremor and effects on vocal loudness are best carried out on a sustained vowel sample.

In addition, Prater and Swift (1984) and Andrews (1995) suggest the use of contrastive stress tasks in which the primary stress in a phrase or sentence is varied so as to create differences in meaning.

Perceptual Assessment of Loudness Range

To assess loudness range, Andrews (1995) has suggested having the patient read the numbers 1 through 9 (provided on a chart), with number 1 being a quietest/softest loudness level and the number 9 being the loudest level. The patient is asked to gradually change loudness level as he or she counts from smaller to larger numbers and to gradually reduce loudness level when counting backwards. The size of the numerals is varied to represent the expected change in loudness.

QUANTITATIVE EVALUATION OF INTENSITY

Methodology

The measurement of vocal intensity is generally conducted using a *sound level meter* (SLM; see Figure 3–1). A basic SLM consists of a microphone, an amplifier, a frequency weighting circuit, and a meter (analog or digital) calibrated in decibels (re: 0.0002 dynes/cm^2) (Nicolosi et al., 1989).

When the SLM detects a sound disturbance, the intensity of the sound wave is shown on the SLM meter. The mouth-to-microphone distance substantially affects the intensity of the sound being measured and must be kept as constant as possible if accurate readings of vocal intensity are to be made. A mouth-to-microphone distance of 30 cm (approximately 12 inches) has been suggested (Schutte & Seidner, 1983). Two commonly used frequency weighting circuits are A-weighting and C-weighting. Schutte and Seidner (1983)

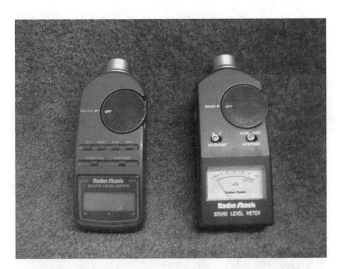

Figure 3–1 Digital (left, Radio Shack Cat. No. 33-2055) and Analog (right, Radio Shack Cat. No. 33-2050) Sound Level Meters. *Source:* Reproduced with written permission of RadioShack Corporation.

suggested use of A-weighting during vocal intensity measurements, presumably because it reduces the influence of low-frequency ambient noise. However, Gramming and Sundberg (1988) showed that the use of an A-weighted circuit resulted in substantially reduced intensity measurements for low-frequency and low-intensity vowel productions compared with a linear weighting circuit (i.e., C-weighting). This was expected because A-weighting attenuates the low-frequency range (i.e., < 500 Hz) where the fundamental frequency of the voice is found for most phonations (particularly modal register phonations). Therefore, it can be argued that C-weighting would be preferred for measures of vocal intensity because it (1) measures uniformly over the frequency range (up to approximately 10 kHz) and (2) will not discriminate against low frequencies such as those often found in the F_0s of speech and most singing.

With the aforementioned methodological considerations in mind, we are now ready to carry out measures of intensity, which correspond to the perceptual measures of loudness we have previously described.

Habitual Intensity Level

Low-cost sound level meters (e.g., Radio Shack Cat. No. 33-2055 and 33-2050) can provide real-time (i.e., almost "instantaneous") estimates of vocal intensity but generally do not provide the user with an average level. Using the SLM itself, the best we can do is estimate a *modal intensity level* (i.e., the most commonly or frequently occurring intensity). To obtain the modal intensity level, the following steps should be used.

Method 1

1. Have your patient seated. Although for many conditions, standing would be optimal, the patient will have a greater tendency to move and therefore disrupt the mouth-to-microphone distance. Ideally, attach your SLM to a tripod or some other stand so that it is located 30 cm (approximately 1 ft.) directly in front of the patient's mouth (0-degree angle of incidence).

2. Turn on the SLM and set the range selector to 70 dB. Also, select C-weighting and slow response. The meter may look something like Figure 3–2 on an analog SLM. When the range selector is set for 70 dB, the meter will respond to intensity levels between 60 and 76 dB (70 dB is indicated when the meter needle points to 0). The 70-dB setting is suggested because conversational speech levels generally range from 65 to 75 dB (1 ft. mouth-to-microphone distance).

3. Ask your patient to read "The Rainbow Passage": "I would like you to read this passage in your normal

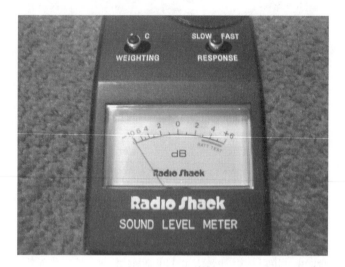

Figure 3–2 Close-up View of the Analog Meter on the Radio Shack Cat. No. 33-2050 Sound Level Meter. Zero (0) dB Corresponds to the User Selected Setting on the Range Selector. *Source:* Reproduced with written permission of RadioShack Corporation.

speaking voice. Please try not to move too much as you are speaking."

4. As the patient is reading, closely watch the decibel meter for the most frequently occurring intensity level. The meter will be in a constant state of fluctuation. However, the use of the slow-response setting should allow the meter to "linger" somewhat at the displayed intensity levels, making it easier to identify the most commonly/consistently occurring intensity value (i.e., the modal intensity level).

Method 2: Intensity-by-Count Method

As an alternative method by which an estimate of habitual intensity level may be obtained, see below.

1. Follow steps 1, 2, and 3 as described in Method 1.
2. Make and record observations of the intensity of speech approximately every 3 seconds during the reading of "The Rainbow Passage."
3. Your list of intensity observations can be reviewed for the modal intensity level or averaged to result in the mean intensity level. The clinician should be able to record approximately 9 to 10 intensity observations for a patient reading "The Rainbow Passage" at a normal speaking rate. In addition, an estimate of intensity range may also be computed.

Several newer models of SLM allow the user to capture the maximum and minimum intensity values within a signal. This will allow the clinician to compute an estimate of the intensity range for the utterance. Figure 3–3 shows a clinician monitoring a patient's vocal intensity using the intensity-by-count method.

Computer programs are also available by which measures of intensity may be made (e.g., Visi-Pitch; CSL). These programs are useful for visually depicting the intensity changes over time for a particular utterance or for measurements of the intensity range. However, they do not provide the user with a true measure of mean vocal intensity level because (1) it is unknown what the reference amplitude/pressure is for the reported intensity level, and (2) it is unknown under which conditions the unknown reference was recorded (e.g., mouth-to-microphone distance). Recall that in the calculation of intensity, the reference pressure/amplitude and its equivalent decibel value must be known (e.g., 0.0002 dynes/cm^2 = 0 dB). Therefore, if the program arbitrarily reports that the mean intensity for an utterance is 58 dB, the intensity level cannot be regarded as valid because we do not know the reference level used in the reported intensity.

It is clear that without a known reference, accurate measures of intensity will be invalid. However, a fairly simple procedure can be used that will result in a calibrated reference by which SPL measures may be accurately calculated by means of a strip chart recorder or (more feasibly) a computer algorithm. This procedure could be carried out with any voice analysis program that will provide a statistical average amplitude for the sound waveform being measured.

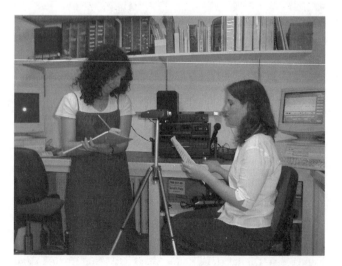

Figure 3–3 Clinician Monitoring Speaking Intensity Using the Intensity-by-Count Method. The sound level meter is attached to tripod with a mouth-to-microphone distance of 12 inches (30 cm).

One of the most common methods for estimating the effective level of a sound waveform is the root mean squared (RMS) amplitude. To calculate mean speaking intensity, the steps below should be followed.

1. Place some type of tone generator approximately 30 cm from your SLM at a 0-degree angle of incidence (i.e., directly in line with the SLM microphone). The actual frequency of the tone does not appear to be crucial, with various calibration tone frequencies used (Awan, 1991; Sapienza & Dutka, 1996; Winholtz & Titze, 1997). I have a preference for relatively low frequency (200 to 300 Hz) complex waves (i.e., a wave containing more than one frequency) such as could be played by an electronic keyboard. This tone will be your calibration tone.

2. As the tone is being generated, record the tone with your computer program or record the tone with an alternative recording device (high-quality tape recorder, MD, DAT, etc.). If using some alternative recording device, set your recording level so that the calibration tone "peaks" at –6 volume units (VU); this will allow for your patient's voice to fluctuate at least 6 dB above the calibration tone without becoming distorted. As the tone is being recorded, read the intensity of the tone from your SLM (use C-weighting; adjust the range selector as appropriate). Ideally, your tone should be in the vicinity of 70 dB, because average speaking intensity from 30 cm is generally observed to be in the range of 70 dB. Keep this information because later we will need to know the intensity level (in dB) that is equivalent to the RMS amplitude of the calibration tone.

3. You are now ready to record your patient's speech. ***DO NOT ADJUST ANY OF YOUR GAIN SETTINGS OR RECORDING LEVELS AND DO NOT CHANGE THE MOUTH-TO-MICROPHONE DISTANCE.*** It is essential that all recording conditions be the same when recording your patient's speech as they were for recording the calibration tone.

4. After your recording, use a voice analysis software package to calculate the RMS amplitude of the calibration tone and the speech sample. When analyzing sustained vowel samples, the RMS amplitude of the entire sample can be used. However, continuous speech presents difficulties because of the possible presence of pauses/silences within the utterance. These pauses/silences cannot be included in the statistical analysis of the intensity of the continuous speech sample because they will tend to lower the average intensity level. It is sug-

gested that you isolate each continuous portion of the speech sample and calculate a RMS amplitude for each portion. These individual portions would then be averaged using a weighted average formula (Awan & Mueller, 1992; see Chapter 2).

5. When you have calculated the RMS amplitude for your speech sample and the calibration tone, incorporate your results into the following formula (Sapienza & Dutka, 1996):

$$dB\ SPL\ (speech\ sample) = dB\ SPL\ (calibration\ tone) + 20 \times LOG(\frac{RMS(Speech\ Sample)}{RMS(Calibration\ Tone)})$$

One of the difficulties with recording accurate intensity levels is the maintenance of a standard mouth-to-microphone distance. In an attempt to avoid significant patient movement problems, Winholtz and Titze (1997) described a method in which a headset microphone is placed on the patient and used to record a calibration tone (produced by a small tone generator unit attached to the patient at a similar distance from the headset microphone as the patient's mouth) while a SLM simultaneously records the tone from a standard distance (e.g., 30 cm). In this manner, the speech signal amplitude may be related to a known SPL (i.e., a reference is established). After the calibration procedure, the patient's voice recording (obtained using the headset microphone) may then be compared with the calibration signal (in terms of RMS amplitude) and converted to SPL at a later time. Although this procedure does help in maintaining a steady mouth-to-microphone distance, two microphones (headset microphone and the SLM microphone) are now required for the intensity measurement rather than one.

Total Intensity Range: The Phonetogram

In the phonetogram, the phonatory capabilities of the voice with respect to F_0 and sound intensity are plotted on a frequency (Hz)-by-intensity (SPL) graph. The phonetogram (see Figure 3–4) displays fundamental frequency range and intensity range, as well as the area of interaction between these two measures.

In deriving a phonetogram, minimal instrumentation can be a simple SLM and a tone generator (pure tone oscillator, pitch pipe, tuned musical instrument) (Schutte & Seidner, 1983). The subject is asked to sustain a vowel at given frequencies (either at 10% intervals of the fundamental frequency range or at the range of whole musical tones that fit within the frequency range) at two vocal intensities (Baken, 1987):

Pianissimo: A vowel sustained as quietly as possible without whispering

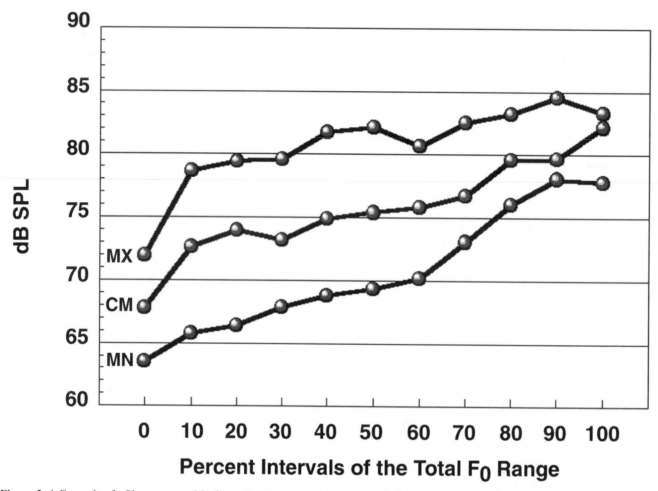

Figure 3–4 Example of a Phonetogram. Maximum (MX), comfortable (CM), and minimum (MN) intensity phonations are elicited at 10% intervals of the total phonational F_0 range.

Fortissimo: A vowel sustained as loudly as possible without pitch breaks

Various recommendations for conducting the phonetogram have been presented by the Union of European Phoniatricians (UEP) (Schutte & Seidner, 1983). Among these recommendations is that a mouth-to-microphone distance of 30 cm be used in conjunction with the A-weighting scale on SLMs (although, as previously discussed, C-weighting may be better suited to voice analysis). At this distance, an omnidirectional microphone is capable of measuring low-intensity productions despite the commonly present surrounding noise. Background noise is recommended not to exceed 40 dB. It has been suggested that the vowel /ɑ/ be used because it has a high first formant frequency that will not interact with the F_0 for most male F_0 ranges and a large part of the female F_0 range. Gramming and Sundberg (1988) observed that using vowels with low first formant frequencies (e.g., /i/) may cause a reduction in SPL, especially when a vocal F_0 becomes higher than the first formant.

It is evident from this description that the phonetogram can be successfully derived with a minimum amount of equipment. This greatly increases the cost-effectiveness of this method in comparison with many other acoustic and nonacoustic methods of vocal assessment. Also, this noninvasive technique yields a plot of frequency and intensity data that result from adjustments of the whole speech mechanism.

HOW TO DO IT: THE PHONETOGRAM

1. Obtain the patient's total phonational range (as previously described in Chapter 2).
2. Compute the 10% intervals of the frequency range. If you intend on obtaining a complete phonetogram, you will test your patient at 11 frequency levels (0%, 10%, 20%…100%). Note that the complete phonetogram can be a time-consuming task. Therefore, Bless and Hicks (1996) suggest a shorter version of the phonetogram. Phonations are elicited at 10%, 50%, and 80% levels of the frequency range. I also suggest the addition of the 30% level (for minimum intensity productions) and 40% level (for maximum intensity productions) to this shortened phonetogram because (1) the 30% to 40% level is often the last frequency in modal register before register transition into falsetto, and (2) these levels often elicit the greatest dynamic range of the voice.
3. The target frequency that the patient has to match can be presented by means of a frequency/tone generator or, perhaps more reasonably, by means of a tuned musical instrument (e.g., electronic keyboard). If using a musical instrument, convert the target frequencies to the nearest musical note using the chart provided in Chapter 2 (Exhibit 2–1). If the patient requires the tone to be played continuously, present it through a headphone.
4. Have your patient positioned 30 cm from the microphone of your SLM (C-weighting, slow response, range selector adjusted as necessary). Seating will keep the patient most steady; however, many patients may prefer standing, particularly for maximum intensity phonations. Most studies have asked their patients to produce only maximum and minimum intensity level phonations at the test frequencies. However, Awan (1991) and Bless and Hicks (1996) suggest the inclusion of comfortable intensity levels. At each semitone level to be tested, provide the patient with the following instructions (Awan, 1991):
   - For comfortable intensity: "Using the vowel /ɑ/, I would like you to hold this note (as presented by means of a speaker or headphone) at whatever loudness is most natural and comfortable for you."
   - For maximum intensity: "Using the vowel /ɑ/, I would like you to hold this note (as presented by means of a speaker or headphone) as loudly as possible without shouting or screaming."
   - For minimum intensity: "Using the vowel /ɑ/, I would like you to hold this note (as presented by means of a speaker or headphone) as softly as possible without whispering."
5. It is suggested that phonations should be at least 2 to 3 seconds in duration with no excessive breathiness or other quality deviation.
6. Coleman (1993) suggests starting at low-frequency/semitone levels and progressing upward. Maximum, comfortable, and minimum intensity levels are sampled at each target frequency/semitone level.
7. The results can be plotted by use of a standard spreadsheet program and/or graphics program.

The reader is encouraged to refer to Coleman (1993) for a detailed discussion of the sources of variation in phonetograms and for alternative testing procedures.

Pros and Cons of the Phonetogram

Bless and Hicks (1996) note two key advantages to the use of the phonetogram as shown below.

- The phonetogram may be considered a good means of tracking changes in organic conditions, with improved voice function reflected in expansion of the phonetogram area.
- The phonetogram does not need to be a complicated or expensive procedure.

Bless and Hicks (1996) have also described possible disadvantages of the phonetogram as shown below.

- The complete phonetogram can be a time-consuming test.
- Interpretation of the phonetogram has not been well defined.
- Variables such as singing training experience and elicitation procedures may affect test outcome.

The Phonetogram Versus the Audiogram

The graphic display of vocal performance at various frequency and intensity levels is similar in nature to the clinical assessment of hearing performance, resulting in the audiogram. Many similarities between the phonetogram and the audiogram may be made:

- The hearing thresholds recorded on the audiogram are not absolute (i.e., they do not remain constant, but tend to fluctuate somewhat as a function of the subject's physical, emotional, and mental state) (Newby, 1979). In a similar fashion, recordings of minimum and maximum frequency and intensity range may fluctuate. However, the fluctuations of performance in both audiograms and phonetograms are often nonsignificant (Gelfer, 1986; Stone & Ferch, 1982) and, at a given moment, can be established with a high degree of precision.

- Both audiograms and phonetograms may be used to aid in the diagnosis of impairment. Both tests are not meant to be all-inclusive but must be supplemented by other diagnostic information (i.e., medical examination, case history). However, just as it is often possible to make generalizations regarding hearing impairment from an audiogram appearance alone, it would seem likely that generalizations about the diagnosis of vocal impairment could be made from the appearance of the phonetogram. Examples of representative phonetograms for vocally disordered patients have been presented by Gramming (1988); Pabon and Plomp (1988); Sulter, Wit, Schutte, and Miller (1994); and Heylen, Wuyts, Mertens, De Bodt, Pattyn, Croux, and Van de Heyning (1998).

- Both audiograms and phonetograms may be useful in determining (1) the need for rehabilitative measures, (2) the type of rehabilitation necessary, and (3) the results of rehabilitative measures over time.

- Although the data recorded on the audiogram are not elicited from actual communication situations (i.e., pure tones are used to elicit hearing threshold responses), estimates of the effect of hearing loss on speech can be made from pure tone audiograms. In estimating the effect on speech of a particular hearing loss, two things are important: the amount of loss through the speech frequencies (.5, 1, and 2 kHz), and the configuration of the audiogram curve (Newby, 1979). In a similar manner, the phonetogram may be used to estimate the effects of voice disruption on speech/singing capabilities. Voice disruption may be gauged in terms of (1) reductions in intensity and/or frequency range and (2) the shape of the phonetogram contours and the area between them.

HIGH FREQUENCY–LOW INTENSITY SINGING ("HIGH-QUIET")

In the event that a phonetogram cannot be conducted, it may still be valuable to assess the patient's ability to produce high-pitched quiet phonation. The ability to produce low-intensity phonation at high frequencies may depend on the relatively healthy status of the vocal folds (Andrews, 1995; Bastian, Keidar, and Verdolini-Marston, 1990; Verdolini, 1994). Bastian et al. (1990) rated subjects (both normal

subjects and clinical patients) in terms of their phonatory characteristics during the production of high-pitch quiet singing ("Happy Birthday" was one of the tasks used). Patient performance was rated on a scale of 1 to 10, with 1 representing extremely delayed phonation, discontinuous phonation, and failure to phonate quietly. At the other extreme, a rating of 10 represented immediate phonatory onset, continuous phonation, and quiet phonation. In addition to perceptual ratings, subjects were also evaluated with videostroboscopic techniques and categorized in terms of normal, vocal fold mucosal swelling, muscle tension dysphonia, and vocal fold bowing. Results revealed that all subjects rated from 1 to 4 had some impairment of the membranous vocal folds (vocal fold swelling, inclusive of acute swelling, nodules, and polyps), with the larger the swelling, the worse the vocal performance. Subjects rated 8 to 10 were judged to have normal appearing vocal folds; those rated 5 to 7 had laryngeal abnormalities in some cases.

Verdolini (1994) speculates that the inability to produce high-quiet phonation may be due to (1) prevention of high-frequency phonation by the presence of mass lesions and (2) the requirement for increased subglottal pressure to put increased mass folds into vibration, thereby negating "quiet" phonation. The inability to produce quiet phonation may also be related to the necessity for increased phonation threshold pressure (PTP) in cases in which the vocal fold mucosal cover has been damaged or dehydrated. PTP is the minimum subglottal pressure required to initiate vocal fold vibration (Fisher & Swank, 1997). The reduction in dynamic range that is implied when subjects cannot achieve quiet singing has also been reported in studies dealing with phonetograms.

HOW TO DO IT: "HIGH-QUIET" SINGING

If the clinician has already completed a phonetogram, the necessity for another task assessing the ability to carry out high pitch, quiet phonation may be unnecessary. However, if the phonetogram has not been completed, Verdolini (1994) provides instructions for the assessment of the high-frequency/low-intensity singing task consistent with those carried out in the Bastian et al. (1990) study as shown below.

1. Ask the patient to sing the first two phrases of "Happy Birthday" at a high pitch, as quietly as possible. Verdolini (1994) suggests that the target pitch should be the musical note E4 for adult men (approximately 330 Hz) and musical note A4 for adult women and prepubescent males (approximately 440 Hz). The target pitch may be presented using either a pitch pipe or keyboard.

2. A SLM is to be placed approximately 3 ft. from the patient's mouth, with the target intensity in the 50- to 55-dB range.
3. During the singing task, the clinician should note the occurrence of delayed phonatory onset, discontinuous phonation (i.e., phonation breaks), and relatively louder phonation (i.e., greater than the target intensity range). Verdolini (1994) recommends rating the productions on the same 1 to 10 scale as defined in the Bastian et al. (1990) study, in which 1 = extremely delayed phonatory onset, discontinuous phonation, relatively loud phonation, and 10 = immediate onset, continuous phonation, and relatively quiet phonation.

It is expected that subjects with relatively normal vocal folds will generally be rated in the 8 to 10 range. Patients with membranous vocal fold abnormalities are often rated in the 1 to 4 range.

WHAT TO EXPECT: NORMAL VOICE

As was seen with vocal pitch/frequency, the age, gender, and body stature of the subject may have a substantial effect on the loudness/intensity of the voice. The normal vocal loudness/intensity should be adequate enough that the voice may be heard over background noise and should have adequate range and variability to allow the speaker to be heard in various situations.

The review of norms for mean speaking intensity can be problematic because different mouth-to-microphone distances study to study have resulted in a wide range of mean intensity observations. However, if we use the suggested distance of an approximately 1 ft. (30 cm) mouth-to-microphone distance, the intensity of continuous speech is generally observed to be in the range of 65 to 70 dB (Baken, 1987). The following studies confirm this observation:

1. In a study of the intensity characteristics of adult males (ages 40 to 80 years old), Ryan (1972) observed that mean reading intensity ranged from 69.2 to 71.3 dB. Similar results were observed for conversational speech intensity levels (68.1 to 70.7 dB).
2. Awan (1993) observed mean speaking intensity to range from 67.1 to 72.3 dB in groups of men and women with and without vocal training.
3. Morris and Brown (1994a) observed a mean speaking intensity of approximately 69 dB in groups of young versus elderly female speakers.

Table 3–1 presents a range of examples of speaking intensity values obtained from normal speakers.

Gender

Because of the greater enlargement of the thorax in the male, Aronson (1985) has reported a prominent increase in vital capacity as compared with females. This increase in vital capacity has also been related to gender differences in mean airflow rate (Baken, 1987; Koike & Hirano, 1968). Brown and McGlone (1974) have shown that airflow values and vocal intensity are strongly correlated. Koike and Hirano (1968) examined airflow rate in 21 male and 21 female adults, who were asked to sustain the vowel /ɑ/ for as long as possible at a constant pitch and loudness. Dividing the total air volume used by the duration of phonation resulted in mean airflow. Results indicated that men produced greater mean airflow rates than women (112.4 ml/s vs. 93.7 ml/s).

In addition to the increased respiratory capacity of men, differences in vocal tract length have also been observed between genders. According to Nordstrom (1977), the average oral cavity length of a female adult is about 85% of that of the average male adult, whereas the female pharynx length is only 77% of the corresponding male value. These differences in vocal tract length are significant for formant frequencies. Sundberg (1987) has shown that for most vowels, the average male formant frequencies are lower than the average female formant frequencies. Because men have a generally lower fundamental frequency than women, these fundamental frequencies may tend to interact with their lower formant frequencies, resulting in a general increase in vocal intensity at relatively lower frequencies than females (Sundberg, 1987). In contrast, the higher fundamental frequencies of women would interact with their formant frequencies at relatively higher frequency levels. It can be seen that, depending on the frequency of phonation, gender differences may or may not be observed in vocal intensity as a result of vocal tract differences.

On the basis of the aforementioned reasons, it would appear that men should have the capacity to produce greater vocal intensities than women. To a degree, this expected gender effect has been observed in studies by Awan (1989, 1993). In a study of the intensity and frequency characteristics of trained versus untrained singers, Awan (1993) observed that men used significantly greater intensity levels in speech regardless of vocal training or type of intensity measure (i.e., mean speaking intensity, maximum speaking intensity, or minimum speaking intensity). In contrast to the intensity of the speaking voice, Awan (1989) observed greater vocal intensities for male subjects only at particular levels of the total phonational frequency range. Awan's (1989) findings can be summarized as follows:

- No significant difference between men and women (without vocal training/experience) in mean minimum SPL as a function of frequency level. Stone, Bell, and

Table 3–1 Speaking Intensity (in dB)

Author	Gender	No. of Subjects	Age (yr.)	Mean & SD	Range
Ryan (1972)[a]	M	20	40–49	68.1 (2.3)	N/A
	M	20	50–59	68.7 (2.1)	N/A
	M	20	60–69	68.6 (1.6)	N/A
	M	20	70–79	70.7 (2.4)	N/A
Linville et al. (1989)[b]	F	20	67–86 ($\bar{x}$ = 76.0)	71.8 (4.0)	64.0–81.6
Awan et al. (1991)[c]	M&F$_H$	17	5–6	61.39 (2.76)	N/A
	M&F$_B$	17	5–6	61.20 (3.07)	N/A
	M&F$_W$	17	5–6	61.77 (3.12)	N/A
Awan (1993)[d]	M	10	18–30	71.36 (2.72)	65.29–75.06
	F	10	18–30	67.14 (2.05)	61.80–69.45
Morris & Brown (1994a)[e]	F$_Y$	25	20–35 ($\bar{x}$ = 27.2)	69.30 (5.57)	56.1–79.7
	F$_O$	25	70–90 ($\bar{x}$ = 79.4)	70.83 (5.46)	59.8–81.2
Morris et al. (1995)[f]	M	18	20–35	72.8 (4.7)	N/A
	M	14	40–55	70.1 (7.1)	N/A
	M	18	>65	72.4 (4.4)	N/A
Author[g]	M	29	18–30 ($\bar{x}$ = 24.24)	68.93 (2.60)	64.83–73.50
	M	12	44–58 ($\bar{x}$ = 51.69)	69.25 (2.80)	65.00–74.33
	F	85	18–30 ($\bar{x}$ = 22.57)	68.37 (2.17)	65.50–71.93
	F	9	36–41 ($\bar{x}$ = 38.99)	68.06 (1.78)	65.33–71.00
	F	13	46–80 ($\bar{x}$ = 57.71)	67.42 (2.93)	65.60–71.60

M = male; F = female; $\bar{x}$ = mean; N/A = not available.
[a] Data from impromptu speaking task only (12-in. mouth-to-microphone distance).
[b] Data from sentence reading (6-in. mouth-to-microphone distance).
[c] Data for Hispanic ($_H$), black ($_B$), and white ($_W$) kindergarten-age children (9-in. mouth-to-microphone distance).
[d] Data for untrained male and female adults only ($\approx$12-in. (30-cm) mouth-to-microphone distance).
[e] Data from young ($_Y$) and old-aged ($_O$) subjects in conversational speech (28.3-cm ($\approx$ 11-in.) mouth-to-microphone distance).
[f] Data from nonsingers only (25.4-cm (10-in.) mouth-to-microphone distance).
[g] Data from oral reading (12-in. mouth-to-microphone distance).

Clack (1978) had also observed this finding in a study of minimal intensity variations over the F_0 range.

- Men produced significantly greater mean comfortable SPLs at low frequency levels (0% and 10% of the total phonational frequency range) than women (without vocal training).
- Men produced significantly greater maximum SPL at the 40% frequency level (often the last frequency in modal register and the point of greatest dynamic range) than women (without vocal training). A previous study by Ptacek et al. (1966) had observed similar maximum vocal intensities observed between genders.

Effects of Aging on Vocal Loudness/Intensity

Infancy and Preadolescence

Because of their smaller respiratory capacities, it may be expected that the vocal intensity level of the childhood voice would be somewhat lower than that observed in adulthood. Although data in speaking intensity levels in children are scarce, Awan, Mueller, Larson, and Summers (1991) did observe substantially lower mean conversational speaking intensity levels in 5-year-old children (approximately 61 dB: mouth-to-microphone distance = 9 in.) compared with generally observed mean speaking intensity levels observed in adult speakers. Also, Sapienza and Stathopoulos (1994) observed that children had to expend more respiratory effort to achieve the same perceptual effect of increased loudness as adults.

In terms of overall dynamic range, Bohme and Stuchlik (1995) observed that maximum and minimum intensity levels were relatively consistent from ages 7 through 10 years for both males and females. In contrast, Komiyama et al. (1984) observed increases in dynamic range and associated phonetographic area between the ages of 8 and 9 years in both males and females.

Adolescence

During adolescence, both phonational frequency range and dynamic range increase, with dynamic range increases primarily caused by increased respiratory capacity. The result is an increase in phonetographic area (i.e., the space enclosed by the phonetogram). Pedersen, Moller, and Bennett (1990) observed that the phonetographic area correlated well with the development of secondary sex characteristics in females ages 8 to 19 years. In a study of 139 male and female subjects between the ages of 6 and 30 years, Komiyama et al. (1984) observed rapid increases in maximum intensity levels between 10 and 14 years and further increases in phonetographic area between 15 and 16 years. Komiyama et al. (1984) attributed these improvements in maximum intensity level and overall dynamic range to a generally larger physical constitution and vital capacity, particularly in male subjects.

The Elderly Voice

A review of research studies dealing with the effects of advanced age on loudness/intensity of the voice is somewhat ambiguous. Mueller (1997) reports that overall vocal loudness may be reduced in the elderly subject, although studies that have directly measured mean vocal intensity have not reported this finding (see below).

- Ryan (1972) measured vocal intensity in four groups of males ranging in age from 40 to 80 years. Mean reading intensity ranged from 69.2 to 71.3 dB (12-in. mouth-to-microphone distance) in reading and 68.1 to 70.7 dB in conversational speech, with the 70- to 79-year-old group producing significantly higher intensity levels than all other groups in both conditions (approximately 2 dB higher than the younger comparison groups). The author speculated that changes in sensory feedback with aging may have caused the elderly subjects to increase vocal effort during speech and, therefore, increase vocal intensity.
- Morris and Brown (1994a) examined vocal intensity in reading and sustained vowel production in young (25 to 35 years old) versus elderly (≥ 75 years old) women. No significant difference was observed in reading intensity (69.49 dB vs. 69.20 dB: mouth-to-microphone distance = 28.3 cm), and the authors concluded that speech intensity does not appear to be a significant variable in the perception of age in conversational speech. However, total dynamic range was observed to be restricted in the elderly subjects. The authors speculate that possible decrements in respiratory force and/or laryngeal valving may affect the total dynamic range in the elderly voice.
- Sapienza and Dutka (1996) investigated airflow and acoustic characteristics of the voice in healthy women between the ages of 20 and 75 years. Vocal intensity was measured from a central portion of a long duration sustained vowel /ɑ/ elicited at a comfortable effort level. Results showed no significant differences between aging groups in terms of mean intensity (mean dB SPL ranged from 78.88 dB to 81.45 dB across aging groups: mouth-to-microphone distance = 15 cm). In addition, no significant difference was observed in intensity variability across trials. The authors concluded that laryngeal senescence in healthy women may not be significant enough to affect the magnitude of phonatory function parameters such as vocal intensity.

The possible effects of advanced aging on vocal intensity may be similar in nature to those described for vocal pitch/frequency. The magnitude of aging effects on vocal intensity probably varies from person to person and appears to be related to overall physical condition rather than chronological age (Morris & Brown, 1994a; Ramig & Ringel, 1983).

Race

The possible effects of race, dialect, or cultural/linguistic background on vocal intensity have not been studied extensively. Awan et al. (1991) examined speaking intensity characteristics of Caucasian, African-American, and Hispanic kindergartners. Although no significant difference was observed in mean speaking intensity level, Caucasian subjects were observed to produce greater speaking intensity ranges than their African-American or Hispanic counterparts. Awan et al. (1991) speculated that the observed reductions in speaking intensity range in the non-Caucasian subjects may have been indicative of social conditioning. This finding appears to concur with the comment of Prater and Swift (1984) that cultural attitudes may be reflected in the use of decreased loudness levels in speech.

The "Super" Normal Voice: Effects of Vocal Training

Trained subjects have been observed to use novel mechanisms of vocal control that would enable them to produce a wider range of phonational intensities than the normal untrained population. In terms of respiratory capacity, Large (1971), Gould and Okamura (1974), and Gould (1977) have reported that the vital capacity of trained subjects is expanded at the expense of residual volume. Watson and Hixon (1985) have also reported that higher lung and rib cage volumes separated trained from untrained subjects. Along with this ability to store a greater vital capacity, trained subjects have been observed to use different respiratory postures than untrained subjects (Hixon & Hoffman, 1978). These authors suggest that trained subjects extend their abdomens out beyond the relaxed position to take advantage of maximum expiratory forces. The abdominal wall has been shown to actively contribute to changes in subglottic pressure (Sundberg & Leanderson, 1987). Overall, it would appear that trained subjects have the capacity to use a greater storage of air (vital capacity) in conjunction with a greater expiratory force than untrained subjects. This interaction would imply the capacity to produce greater phonational intensities and intensity ranges.

Bouhuys, Proctor, and Mead (1966) and Proctor (1974) have reported that in trained subjects, the rate of airflow decreases with increases in SPL, whereas in the untrained subject, production of the same tone at a lower SPL requires a comparatively high rate of airflow. These findings imply a more efficient respiratory mechanism in trained subjects, because trained subjects may use less of their capacity in producing a similar intensity tone as untrained subjects. In turn, the trained subject would have a greater amount of inspiratory reserve with which to produce greater subglottal pressures and greater overall intensities.

At the laryngeal level, differences between trained and untrained subjects have been observed that would also appear to give trained subjects an advantage in producing increased maximum intensity phonations and greater intensity ranges. Studies by the Bell Telephone Laboratories (1940) have shown vocal fold closure time to be greater for trained singers. This increased closure time results in a more efficient conversion of airflow to acoustic energy, especially in the higher harmonics (Large, Baird, & Jenkins, 1980). As was previously noted, it has been estimated that decrease in the OQ may result in increases in vocal intensity (Flanagan, 1958). The Bell Telephone Laboratories (1940) studies have also indicated that the displacement or amplitude of vocal fold vibration is smaller than for the untrained voice in the production of a sound of similar intensity. These studies concluded that it was this ability to better control the flow of air that would enable the trained voice to radiate a greater amount of sound power than the untrained voice or to radiate a similar amount of sound power with a lower airflow.

Trained subjects have also been observed to use the supralaryngeal mechanism to produce high-intensity vocal output. In an x-ray investigation of female singers, Johansson, Sundberg, and Willbrand (1983) noted that as soon as the first formant frequency of a chosen vowel was lower than the fundamental frequency, the first formant was changed and tuned to a frequency near that of the fundamental. This "tuning" was controlled by adjusting the jaw opening in accordance with phonation frequency. If the phonation frequency was changed, the jaw opening was also changed accordingly. Sundberg (1987) notes that the gain from this simple principle of adjusting the jaw opening in accordance with phonation frequency can be considerable, with gains of 30 dB possible. The gain arises as soon as the first formant joins the frequency of phonation. This tuning must be

extremely precise because Gramming and Sundberg (1988) have observed that the intensity level of a vowel will decrease if the frequency of the fundamental is higher than that of the first formant of a vowel.

Troup (1981) has summarized the advantages of vocal training in the following statements:

- The lungs and the thoracic and abdominal musculature come under better control; the efficiency of operation increases; and a physical enlargement of the lungs and chest can result, as well as an increase in vital capacity.
- The vocal folds become more efficient, and the valving action either in or below the larynx also changes in such a way as to increase the efficiency of the source (longer, complete closure phase for the folds, ability to radiate a higher sound level for the same airflow).
- The vowel formants used in speech serve quite well to describe sung vowels, except when the fundamental pitch rises above the first formant; here, the jaw is dropped to raise the first formant toward the fundamental frequency.

In light of the aforementioned differences between trained and untrained subjects in terms of intensity control mechanisms, it has been speculated that trained subjects would be able to produce greater maximum intensities and intensity ranges than the normal or untrained population (Troup, 1981). Results from several studies shown below appear to support this speculation.

- Colton (1973) measured the SPLs of phonation produced at different vocal intensity and frequency levels in the modal and falsetto registers in eight trained male singers and eight male nonsingers. Results showed that trained singers tended to exhibit larger SPLs in both registers, although significant differences between the two groups occurred at only a few experimental conditions.
- Gramming, Sundberg, Ternstrom, Leanderson, and Perkins (1988) conducted a phonetographic study using trained and untrained groups. The results of their study indicated that trained and untrained subjects differed consistently only in that the untrained subjects had slightly lower maximum intensity levels at the higher frequencies.
- Awan (1991) observed substantial differences in dynamic range and overall phonetogram area in trained singers versus subjects with limited singing experience. In contrast to many previous studies of vocal range, this study attempted to elicit "musical range," in which substantial constraint (on vocal frequency, quality, and duration) was used. The author concluded that controlled phonation may be the key to revealing

the underlying differences in vocal capabilities (such as dynamic range) in seemingly different vocal groups.

In addition to effects on overall dynamic range, vocal training may also affect characteristics of the speaking voice. Awan (1993) examined speaking voice characteristics in addition to phonetograms for trained singers versus subjects with limited singing experience. Results indicated that trained female singers used significantly greater mean speaking intensity levels than untrained females (69.85 dB vs. 67.14 dB: 12 in. mouth-to-microphone distance), and trained singers used significantly greater intensity ranges in speech than the untrained group, regardless of gender (5.73 dB vs. 4.25 dB). In addition, overall intensity range correlated significantly ($r = 0.64$, $p < .05$) with speaking intensity range in the trained female singers, leading to the speculation that effects of vocal training for singing may carry over to everyday speaking situations.

WHAT TO EXPECT: ABNORMAL VOICE

Various disorders that affect the respiratory and/or laryngeal valving capability may adversely affect speaking intensity and/or dynamic range. In addition, abnormalities of vocal loudness/intensity may accompany psychological disorders and disruptions in other components of the speech mechanism.

Mass Lesions and Distributed Tissue Change

Several authors have stated that reduced speaking loudness/intensity and reduced dynamic range may accompany vocal fold lesions and associated laryngeal inefficiency:

- Speaking loudness/intensity levels may be reduced secondary to mass lesions of the vocal folds (Andrews, 1995; Boone & McFarlane, 1988; Prater & Swift, 1984). As an example, Hirano (1989) observed that size of glottic gap negatively correlated with maximum SPL level in polyp cases; in carcinoma cases, negative correlations between size of lesion and maximum SPL and SPL range were also observed. However, it should be noted that patients with vocal nodules, other lesions, or irregularities of the vocal fold margins may only be able to sustain phonation while using louder rather than softer voices, and thus may compensate for their disorder with hyperadduction and a louder voice (Andrews, 1995; Hirano, 1989). In addition, although the patient may have decreased loudness and hypofunction, many mass/additive lesions are a consequence of vocal abuse in which excessive loudness/excessive effort was the habitual speaking style of the patient

before the disorder developed (Haynes et al., 1992; Murry, 1982).

- In addition to changes in speaking loudness/intensity levels, inappropriate or limited loudness variation may also be observed (Andrews, 1995). Haynes et al. (1992) state that inappropriate loudness variability (e.g., loudness level "trailing off" at the end of a sentence) and phonation breaks may be associated with obstructive lesions. Bless and Hicks (1996) indicate that intensity range may be decreased in cases with Reinke's edema.

Neurological Disorders

Various neurologically based disorders may affect the ability to generate adequate respiratory force and/or build up subglottal pressure by means of laryngeal valving. The result may be disruptions in the ability to produce appropriate loudness/intensity levels.

Several authors have stated that speaking intensity/loudness levels may be reduced in neurological disorders such as parkinsonism and bulbar palsy (flaccidity) (Andrews, 1995; Darley et al., 1975; Murry, 1982; Prater & Swift, 1984). Countryman et al. (1997) reported decreased vocal loudness/intensity in a patient with Parkinson's disease and subsequent improvement in vocal loudness after voice therapy incorporating the Lee-Silverman Voice Treatment (LSVT). These authors attributed decreased vocal loudness to bowing of the vocal folds or other forms of glottal incompetence in combination with reduced expiratory volumes for speech (resulting from limited thoracic excursion and difficulty coordinating respiratory and laryngeal systems). In a study of 240 patients with unilateral vocal fold paralysis, Hirano, Mori, Tanaka, and Fujita (1995) observed mean speaking intensity to be abnormally low in approximately 70% of the subjects. These authors attributed their findings to glottic incompetence, poor neural control, and asymmetry of vocal fold vibration.

Certain neurological conditions may result in inappropriately high speaking intensity levels. Prater and Swift (1984) state that vocal loudness may be too high in neurological disorders resulting in respiratory and/or vocal hyperfunction. Haynes et al. (1992) state that dysarthric patients (particularly those with spasticity or dystonias) may present with a "booming" voice. Inappropriately loud voices have also been reported in patients with multiple sclerosis (Darley et al., 1975).

Neurological conditions may present with an inability to vary loudness/intensity for the normal production of intonation patterns. The result will be reduced loudness/intensity variability and overall dynamic range (Andrews, 1995; Darley et al., 1975; Haynes et al., 1992; Hirano et al., 1995; Prater & Swift, 1984). Reduced loudness variability is often referred to as *monoloudness* and was identified as one of the primary deviant speech dimensions in spastic, ataxic, and both hypokinetic and hyperkinetic dysarthrias by Darley et al. (1975). In contrast, the presence of hyperkinetic states (e.g., choreas, dystonias, vocal tremor) may produce excessive variations in loudness level (Andrews, 1995; Darley et al., 1975).

Psychologically Based Voice Disorders

Psychological disorders and personality disturbances may affect vocal loudness/intensity. Vocal loudness may be reduced in cases of inferiority complex and withdrawal (Boone & McFarlane, 1988; Murry, 1982; Prater & Swift, 1984). In addition, monoloudness presenting as a weak, "bland" voice may be observed in cases of depression (Andrews, 1995; Haynes et al., 1992; Murry, 1982; Prater & Swift, 1984).

Hearing Impairment/Deafness

Disruptions to the feedback mechanism(s) by which we control speech and voice production may also result in disruptions to vocal loudness. Several authors have indicated that hearing impairment may cause speaking loudness/intensity to be too high or too low, and overall loudness variability to be reduced (Andrews, 1995; Murry, 1982; Prater & Swift, 1984). Dworkin and Meleca (1997) state that sensorineural hearing loss may cause the patient to speak in an abnormally loud voice. On the other hand, a conductive loss may result in an abnormally soft voice. In the case of a conductive hearing loss, the patient may "hear" his or her own voice quite well (because of adequate bone conduction) and may believe that he or she is producing an adequately loud voice when it is, in fact, too quiet. In sensorineural losses, both air and bone conduction are detrimentally affected, causing the patient to increase vocal loudness as compensation.

Muscle Tension Dysphonias/Hyperfunctional Voice

The presence of excessive tension in the vocal musculature and/or excessive use of the voice may have variable effects on vocal loudness/intensity. Many hyperfunctional voices initially present with excessive loudness levels during speech (Boone & McFarlane, 1988; Haynes et al., 1992; Murry, 1982) followed by periods of reduced vocal intensity/loudness as a result of vocal fatigue. Vocal fatigue may lead to *myasthenia larynges* (vocal fold bowing secondary to continuous use) (Boone & McFarlane, 1988; Murry, 1982; Stemple, 1993). In addition to effects on habitual loudness/intensity level, loudness variability may be reduced in cases of excessive tension and elevated larynx (Andrews, 1995).

CHAPTER 4

Evaluation of Vocal Quality

PERCEPTUAL ASSESSMENT OF VOICE QUALITY

Definition

Characterization of voice *quality* is one of the key facets of perceptual assessment of the voice and an integral aspect of any voice evaluation. As stated previously, many clinicians and researchers believe that perceptual assessment is the basic foundation of voice evaluation and treatment because it presents (1) the comparative standard to which acoustic and physiological measures will be related and interpreted and (2) the essential gauge by which therapy recommendations will be made and evaluated.

The term *quality* may be defined simply as a distinguishing characteristic. Perhaps more specific to voice analysis, *quality* refers to the characteristic of a sound that distinguishes it from other sounds of similar pitch, loudness, and duration. Voice quality is one of the means by which we are able to distinguish between people of similar age and gender, even though they may be speaking with similar pitch and loudness. Quality is also one of the key parameters we will use to perceptually discriminate the normal from the disordered voice.

Various research methods provide insight as to what is meant by *normal* voice quality. It appears that most define what *normal* voice quality *is* by what it *is not*. Eskanazi, Childers, and Hicks (1990) defined normal voice "as a voice with no apparent pathology...and no unusual voice characteristics or habits" (p. 33). Karnell (1991) described normal voice quality as having no hoarseness. Awan and Mueller (1996) described their normal subjects as being "free of perceived voice disorders" (p. 574). Mendoza, Valencia, Munoz, and Trujillo (1996) determined that normal voices were "non-dysphonic" (p. 61).

Common Definitions for Dysphonic Quality

A wide variety of terminology has been applied to the description of the dysphonic voice qualities such as *creaky*, *tense*, *unstable*, *lax*, *guttural*, *strained*, and *husky*. It is, in fact, this wide diversity of terminology that may at times contribute to the difficulty with which voice quality judgments are made and communicated. Fortunately, review of the voice literature reveals several quality dimensions that have been consistently used to categorize dysphonic voice quality.

Breathy

The *breathy* voice is commonly perceived as a *whispery* or *airy* voice. Although we will discuss breathiness as a common attribute of disordered voices, a slight amount of breathy voice may be observed in the normal female voice (Klatt & Klatt, 1990) and may be a social marker of female gender emulated by others (Andrews & Schmidt, 1997).

In a physiological view, the term *breathiness* is associated with *hypoadduction* (i.e., lack of vocal fold adduction or closure) of the vocal folds and refers to the audible detection of airflow through the glottis during phonation. It is the combination of audible airflow with the quasiperiodic voice signal that results in the *airy* or *hazy* characteristic of the breathy voice. At its extreme, the breathy voice becomes similar to a whisper, in which the vocal folds cease to vibrate and only the aperiodic component of turbulent noise remains (i.e., *aphonia* caused by extreme hypoadduction).

Harshness

Unlike the breathy voice, the *harsh* voice appears to have no acceptable connotation under any circumstance. The harsh voice is commonly perceived as an unpleasant voice and associated with terms such as *coarse*, *strident*, *low-pitched noise*, and *rasping* (Askenfelt & Hammarberg, 1986; Fairbanks, 1960; Gelfer, 1993). In terms of underlying physiology, the harsh voice is associated with *hyperadduction* (i.e., excessive vocal fold adduction or closure) of the vocal folds and refers to the noise produced as a result of irregular vocal fold vibration (Askenfelt & Hammarberg, 1986; Eskanazi et al., 1990).

A term that has been used synonymously with harshness is *roughness* (Isshiki, Yanagihara, & Morimoto, 1966; Prater & Swift, 1984; Wolfe, Fitch, & Martin, 1997). Although both terms refer to irregularity of vocal fold vibration, the rough voice may be characterized by the presence of low-frequency noise components (Askenfelt & Hammarberg, 1986; de Krom, 1994; Eskanazi et al., 1990) versus a high-frequency noise found in the harsh voice (Askenfelt & Hammarberg, 1986). Current terminology in the perceptual assessment of voice appears to favor *roughness* over the term *harshness* (Wolfe et al., 1997).

Hoarseness

The term *hoarseness* is a hybrid descriptor that denotes a voice with both breathy and harsh/rough qualities simultaneously. Therefore, hoarseness originates from a combination of irregularity of vocal fold vibration and turbulent airflow through the glottis (Anders et al., 1988; Omori et al., 1997). This voice quality may arise, for example, in a patient who attempts to compensate for a breathy voice by using increased laryngeal tension and hyperadduction, thereby resulting in a harsh or rough component to the voice. In some cases, the harsh/rough component will predominate; in others, the breathy component will be most noticeable. In addition, the hoarse voice may also be characterized as *dry* versus *wet*, in which wet hoarseness is related to the presence of secretions at the vocal fold level (Andrews, 1995; Boone & McFarlane, 1988; Moore, 1971). A number of authors have concluded that hoarseness is probably the most common voice quality characteristic (Andrews, 1995; Boone & McFarlane, 1988).

HOW TO DO IT: PERCEPTUAL ASSESSMENT OF VOCAL QUALITY

The severity of a particular voice quality disruption (breathiness, hoarseness, roughness) may be rated on a 7-point categorical/equal-appearing interval rating scale ranging from 0 to 6. A 0 rather than a 1 is suggested as the lower anchor of the scale to represent the absence or minimal nature of the rated voice quality. The primary voice quality deviation observed is indicated with a check mark:

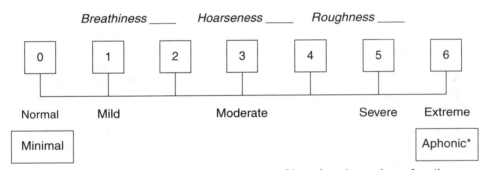

*Lack of phonation—may be due to extremes of hypofunction or hyperfunction.

In these rating scales, the severity terminology previously defined (mild, moderate, and severe) is used in conjunction with these primary voice quality terms/dimensions (e.g., mild breathiness, moderate hoarseness). Therefore, a mild breathiness would correspond to the audible airflow through the glottis during phonation that would most probably only be detected by a trained practitioner—the patient's ability to effectively communicate is not affected. Note that lack of phona-tion (aphonia) may be due to extremes of hypofunction *or* hyperfunction (Kinzl, Biebl, & Rauchegger, 1988).

In addition to the perception of the primary voice quality deviations, a number of alternative voice quality deviations may also be observed:

- **Instability:** This term refers to fluctuation in voice quality over time (de Krom, 1994; Orlikoff et al., 1999). As one moves through the previously described mild, moderate, and severe definitions, it can be seen that the ability to phonate changes from constant to intermittent to mainly absent. Therefore, instability of phonation is a deviation that is accounted for in these severity terms. The instability may be of two forms: (1) phonation intermittently or consistently ceased because of hypoadduction of the vocal folds or (2) phonation intermittently or consistently ceased because of hyperadduction of the vocal folds. In one of the few sources that attempts to provide definition to the mild, moderate, severe continuum, Andrews (1995) also refers to this factor of instability in describing tremor, which occurs intermittently on vowels and during sentences versus constant occurrences of the deviation.

- **Strain:** This is defined as the impression of vocal effort; a hyperfunctional state of phonation (de Krom, 1994; Hirano, 1981). The moderate and severe definitions provided here take into account the effortful characteristic consistent with both hypoadductive and hyperadductive states in which the speaker must use increased muscular force and tension in the attempt to produce phonation.
- **Diplophonia:** As previously described, diplophonia refers to irregularities in glottal vibration pattern in which alternating glottal periods are slightly different in period or shape (Monsen, 1979). Diplophonia was previously discussed as a pitch deviation. However, this characteristic often gives the impression of roughness in the voice.

Type of Sample Used in the Perceptual Assessment of Voice Quality

The literature dealing with perceptual assessment of voice quality generally focuses on use of sustained vowel productions (quite often the vowel /ɑ/ "*ah*"). de Krom (1994) has cited a number of reasons why sustained vowel productions are beneficial:

- Sustained vowel production is easily controlled and standardized (i.e., productions of similar vowels at consistent pitch, loudness, and duration may be consistently controlled). Connected speech samples may show great interspeaker variation in terms of articulatory aspects and dialectical influences that may affect the judgment of perceived voice quality.
- Sustained vowels may aid the listener in focusing more closely on the perceptual characteristics of the actual voice source signal.
- Perception of sustained vowel quality may relate better to many objective measures of voice quality (see *jitter*,

shimmer, and *HNR* in the next section) that generally yield valid and reliable measures only when applied to sustained vowel productions.

Although there are several practical reasons for using sustained vowels for perceptual assessment of voice quality, there may be issues of content validity that should be considered. Although sustained vowel production is convenient, it is not representative of conversational speech. A number of researchers have indicated that conversational speech samples may be more appropriate for perceptual voice quality evaluation for the following reasons:

- Conversational or continuous speech segments may allow for a more "adequate estimation of the voice status" (Askenfelt & Hammarberg, 1986, p. 51).
- Sustained vowel productions are unnatural/awkward for some speakers. This may result in uncharacteristic vocal behavior (de Krom, 1994).
- Connected speech involves increased physiological complexity (more complex and dynamic patterns of muscular activity) than sustained vowels, possibly resulting in more prominent voice quality deviations (Askenfelt & Hammarberg, 1986; Bassich & Ludlow, 1986; de Krom, 1994).

In an attempt to investigate the possible effect of sample type, de Krom (1994) examined the consistency and reliability of perceptual voice quality ratings from sustained vowels versus continuous speech samples. Results indicated that ratings of connected speech fragments were not necessarily more consistent or reliable than vowel segments. In addition, reliability of ratings on connected speech stimuli was lower than for vowel segments. These results were possibly caused by (1) distraction of the listener from nonvoice source information (e.g., dialect, rate) and/or (2) variability of voice quality within the connected speech segment. de Krom (1994) concluded that vowel segments appear to be acceptable for both acoustic and perceptual assessment.

Although de Krom's (1994) results support the use of sustained vowel productions in perceptual voice quality analysis procedures, it would appear that perceptual assessment of voice should include *both* sustained vowel segments and continuous speech samples (Fex, 1992). As stated previously, the inclusion of continuous speech samples appears to have strong face validity and may reveal voice aberrations not present during the sustained vowel sample. This book suggests that the identification and rating of voice quality be performed on three different samples:

- A sustained vowel /ɑ/ (at least 2 to 3 seconds in duration)
- A continuous and spontaneous speech sample (e.g.,

this sample may be obtained during the case history interview or from a picture description task).

- A reading sample (e.g., "The Rainbow Passage")

With these three samples, we have data on which perceptual assessment is applied, as well as data applicable to acoustic analysis methods. These three samples require the patient to produce voice under circumstances of differing vocal function while also providing us with an easily standardized method that can be repeated from patient to patient. In addition, these samples lend themselves well to comparisons to literature dealing with voice quality deviations.

QUANTITATIVE EVALUATION OF VOICE QUALITY

For a number of years, it has been a goal of voice clinicians and researchers to augment their perceptual assessment of voice quality with more "objective" methods. This is not to say that perceptual methods are imprecise—perceptual assessment of voice quality may be conducted in a valid and reliable fashion. However, as previously stated, factors of differential training, experience, and definition can make perceptual assessment problematic. In addition, we must face the fact that, even if definition and training were standardized across all voice clinicians, there would still be subpopulations of clinicians who possessed "finer" or more discriminating perceptual skills than other clinicians, which could result in differences in ratings of voice quality type and severity. These differences in the discriminatory capabilities of particular clinicians may be inherent characteristics that cannot be improved through academic or experiential factors. These interclinician variations in judging voice quality may represent the "artistic" aspects that combine with acquired training, experience, and definition to result in an accurate perceptual judgment.

So, we are in a situation in which even similarly trained clinicians may differ in their detection of the fine characteristics/nuances of the voice signal. This is, perhaps, where the addition of quantitative methods of voice quality evaluation may aid us the most. Theoretically, quantitative evaluation methods should reduce interjudge variability by reducing the subjective aspect of voice quality evaluation. In addition, because the methods we will discuss are based on computer algorithms, they have the following qualities:

1. The algorithms will always analyze voice signals in a similar manner every time. Therefore, there is no problem with the shifting of analysis definitions within a computer algorithm.
2. The results are provided in numerical format, allowing for built-in scaling and ease of communication.

By adding quantitative methods to our perceptual assessment techniques, perhaps we can achieve some degree of equality between clinicians in terms of their abilities to evaluate the qualitative aspects of the voice.

Vocal Quality and the Voice Waveform

Perkins (1985) stated that "the underlying premise for detection of laryngeal pathology is that a deviant condition will result in an acoustic 'signature' affecting fundamental frequency, intensity, or quality, singly or in combination" (p. 82). Haynes et al. (1992) have indicated that acoustic measures may be useful in the early detection of vocal pathological conditions, even though no visually detectable lesion or tissue change is present. In this next section, we will discuss some of the key acoustic parameters that are often affected by voice disorders and focus on the objective and quantifiable aspects of vocal quality.

The acoustic waveform is a time-by-amplitude waveform (i.e., an oscillogram). If we observe the waveforms of two different voices producing the same vowel (e.g., /ɑ/) at the same pitch and loudness, we will see similarities but also a key difference in the oscillograms (see Figure 4–1).

In terms of similarity, we will see that each waveform repeats itself over time. In particular, we will be able to measure the *period* of each waveform (i.e., the time it takes for the pattern of vibration to repeat itself; the time it takes for one complete cycle of vibration to complete) and see that they are identical. Of course, if we take the reciprocal of the period (1/p), we can compute the *frequency* of each wave. Frequency is the physical or measurable correlate of pitch. Therefore, if the frequency of each waveform is identical, we would generally perceive the waveforms to have similar pitch.

A second similarity between the two waveforms under scrutiny is that the *amplitude* (i.e., the "height" or vertical excursion) of each waveform is also quite similar, most notably at their *peaks* (i.e., the point of maximum vertical excursion). The amplitude is the physical or measurable correlate of loudness. Therefore, if the amplitudes of the two waveforms are identical, they would be perceived as having similar loudness.

The two waveforms are clearly similar in a number of ways, both measurable and perceptual. But what is the clear and obvious difference between the two waveforms? It is obviously the way each waveform looks (i.e., the visual appearance of each wave). The appearance or shape of a waveform is referred to as its *profile*. It is the profile of the wave that appears to relate to the perceived quality of a sound, because it is this aspect that differentiates our two waves of similar frequency/pitch and amplitude/loudness.

The reason that the waveform profiles of two different voice sources differ is that the spectral characteristics of the

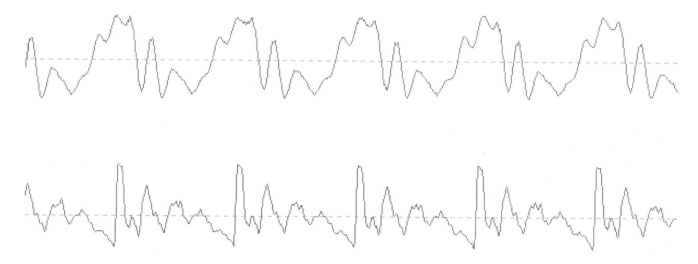

Figure 4–1 Two Waveforms Similar in Period/Frequency and Peak Amplitude, but Different in Profile

two waveforms are different. The term *spectral characteristic* refers to the concept that a single sound wave may be composed of many different frequencies, each with its own individual amplitude. In the case of a voice waveform, the *fundamental frequency* (i.e., the lowest or basic frequency of vibration as calculated from the waveform period) and its *harmonics* (i.e., integer multiples of the fundamental frequency) are blended together to produce a single, complex sound wave (i.e., a sound wave composed of more than one frequency). In an ideal periodic complex wave, we would observe the fundamental frequency and its harmonics as the *only* frequencies that have determined the waveform profile.

In particular, the profile of a sound wave is determined by two key factors:

1. The amplitudes of the individual frequency components of the complex voice wave. The voice is composed of a fundamental frequency and harmonics produced simultaneously. As the complex vibration produced by the vibratory source (vocal folds) moves through the supralaryngeal resonating cavities (e.g., the oral, pharyngeal, and/or nasal cavities), these various frequencies may have their amplitudes reinforced or diminished (i.e., *damped*). The effect of reinforcement or damping on the source spectrum is a function of the size and shape of the resonating cavities. Therefore, two different people produce different profile voice waveforms because there are anatomical variations from person to person that have differing resonatory effects on their voice sources.

2. The number of frequencies actually present in the complex sound wave. As waveforms become more complex (i.e., have more frequency components), we generally observe that the profile of the wave also becomes more complex. We observe more "peaks" and "valleys" in the profile of the wave (see Figure 4–2).

This second factor (the number of frequencies making up the waveform) is of particular importance in the consideration of voice quality. As we have discussed, the primary voice quality deviations (breathiness, harshness, and hoarseness) are all characterized by the presence of noise mixed in with the voice source signal (*additive noise*). In the case of breathiness, the excessive escape of air through the glottis during phonation adds turbulent noise (i.e., aperiodic vibration) to the periodic vibration of the vocal folds. In the case of the harsh/rough voice, irregularity of vocal fold vibration adds an aperiodic component to the vibratory behavior.

The addition of noise to the normal periodic (actually *quasiperiodic*) voice signal disturbs the repeating pattern of vibration in a number of key ways:

- The period (and thus, the frequency) of vibration is disrupted.
- The amplitude of vibration is disrupted.
- The profile of the waveform is disrupted.

In the last instance, the profile of the wave generally becomes increasingly complex and variable because the

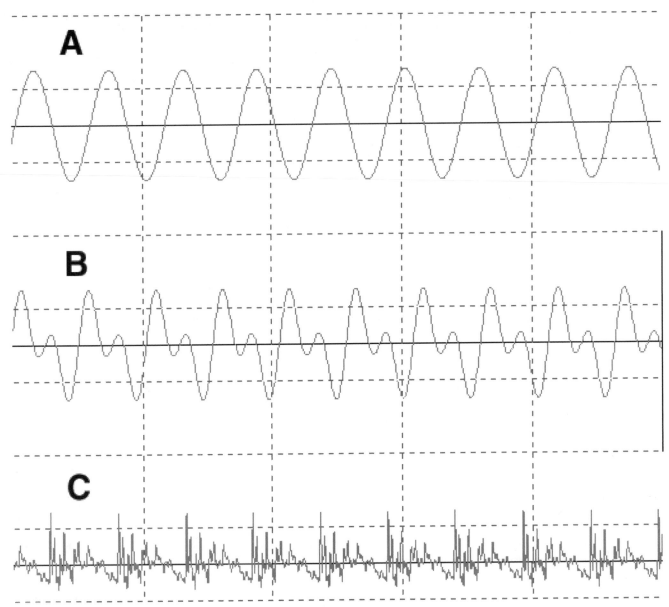

Figure 4–2 Waveforms Composed of One Frequency (A), Two Frequency (B), and Multifrequency Components (C). The complexity of the profile of each waveform increases with greater frequency content.

presence of additive noise has increased the number of frequencies present in the complex wave and, thus, increases its complexity. The reason that complexity is increased is that, theoretically, noise can have spectral components at *all* frequencies, not just at multiples of the fundamental frequency (Denes & Pinson, 1973). Therefore, the addition of aperiodic and periodic signals increases the complexity of the acoustic signal and its profile.

To summarize, quality of the voice is reflected in the profile (i.e., shape) of the voice waveform. Many voice disorders characteristically add noise to the quasiperiodic vibration of the voice. Additive noise disrupts the profile of the voice waveform by affecting the regularity of period and amplitude. In addition, the complexity of the wave is also increased (i.e., the profile becomes more detailed and variable cycle to cycle). The variations in frequency, amplitude, and profile are the characteristics we wish to quantify in voice quality evaluation. These variations are often referred to as *perturbations*, in which we observe random disturbances in periodic motion.

Methods of Quantifying Perturbations

Three particular methods have been used to quantify the voice signal perturbations that are characteristic of voice quality deviations. *Jitter* and *shimmer* are measures of *short-term instability* that quantify cycle-to-cycle variations in frequency and amplitude, respectively (Hartelius et al., 1997). In addition, *harmonics-to-noise ratio (HNR)* is also a method that detects cycle-to-cycle perturbations and was initially designed as a method for quantifying spectral noise.

Jitter

Jitter is a measure of the cycle-to-cycle perturbations in a vocal period (see Figure 4–3). Because the reciprocal of period is frequency, there are also methods of computing jitter that report results in Hz. Various methods have been proposed by which jitter may be calculated.

Mean Absolute Jitter

Mean absolute jitter is the mean absolute difference between sequential vocal periods. Although vocal period is computed in seconds, mean absolute jitter is generally reported in milliseconds (ms). In the following formula, we will (1) sum the cycle-to-cycle differences in period (in seconds); (2) divide the sum of differences by the number of differences (i.e., number of cycles –1); and (3) multiply the final result by 1000 to convert to milliseconds (ms):

$$\frac{1}{n-1}\left[\sum_{i=1}^{n-1}\left|P_i - P_{i+1}\right|\right] \times 1000$$

Jitter (%). Jitter (%) is also known as jitter factor. Mean cycle-to-cycle perturbation in frequency is reported in relation to the mean overall frequency of the voice signal. In this manner, the influence of F_0 is accounted for. In the following formula, we will (1) sum the cycle-to-cycle differences in frequency (in Hz); (2) divide the sum of differences by the number of differences (i.e., number of cycles –1); (3) divide the result by the mean frequency; and (4) multiply the final result by 100 to convert to a percentage (%):

$$\frac{\frac{1}{n-1}\left[\sum_{i=1}^{n-1}\left|F_i - F_{i+1}\right|\right]}{\frac{1}{n}\sum_{i=1}^{n}F_i} \times 100$$

Jitter (%) RAP. Jitter (%) RAP is similar to jitter factor but computed by use of relative average perturbation (RAP). This technique is used to remove relatively isolated and/or long-duration fluctuations in cycle-to-cycle perturbation. The calculation of jitter (RAP) is identical to that in jitter factor, with the exception that cycle-to-cycle differences are calculated by subtracting the frequency of the cycle under analysis from the average frequency of the current cycle plus two neighboring cycles. The result is a smoothed perturbation value:

$$\frac{\frac{1}{n-2}\left[\sum_{i=2}^{n-1}\left|\frac{F_{i-1}+F_i+F_{i+1}}{3} - F_i\right|\right]}{\frac{1}{n}\sum_{i=1}^{n}F_i} \times 100$$

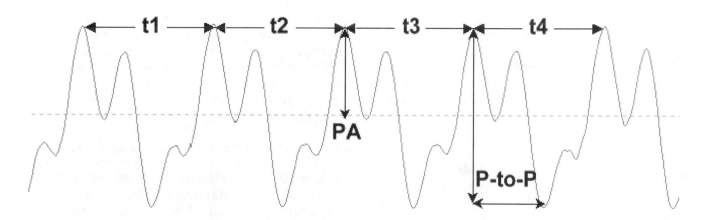

Figure 4–3 The Time (t1, t2, t3, t4...) It Takes to Complete Each Cycle of Vibration Is the *Period*. The reciprocal of period is *frequency*. Cycle-to-cycle variations in period or frequency are referred to as *jitter*. The amplitude of each cycle is often described as *peak amplitude* (PA) or *peak-to-peak amplitude* (P-to-P). Cycle-to-cycle variations in amplitude are referred to as *shimmer*.

Several studies have reported on the clinical usefulness of measures of jitter. Takahashi and Koike (1975) observed jitter to significantly correlate with ratings of roughness ($r = 0.55$), whereas Yumoto, Sasaki, and Okamura (1984) observed that jitter correlated significantly with perceived hoarseness ($r = 0.71$). In a study of children with vocal nodules, Kane and Wellen (1985) observed jitter to correlate significantly ($r = 0.68$) with perceptual ratings on a 7-point vocal severity scale. Wolfe and Steinfatt (1987) observed a correlation of 0.51 between vocal roughness and jitter obtained from sustained vowels /ɑ/ and /i/.

Shimmer

Shimmer is a measure of the cycle-to-cycle perturbations in amplitude. This measure has been commonly calculated from the *peak amplitude* (i.e., the value of the highest/greatest amplitude within each cycle—a decision is made before beginning analysis as to the use of positive or negative peaks), although others have calculated shimmer from peak-to-peak (Scherer, Vail, & Guo, 1995) and statistical average amplitudes (Hillenbrand, 1987) for each cycle under analysis (see Figure 4–3). In addition to various methods for actually defining amplitude, several methods for carrying out the calculation of shimmer have been proposed.

Shimmer (dB). Shimmer (dB) is an absolute measure of cycle-to-cycle variations in amplitude and expressed in decibels. In the following formula, we will (1) sum the cycle-to-cycle deviations in intensity (dB) and (2) divide the sum of differences by the number of differences (i.e., number of cycles –1):

$$\frac{1}{n-1}\left[\sum_{i=1}^{n-1}\left|20 \times LOG\left(\frac{A_i}{A_{i+1}}\right)\right|\right]$$

Shimmer (dB) RAP. Similar to shimmer (dB), shimmer (dB) RAP is computed by use of RAP. This technique is used to remove relatively isolated and/or long-duration fluctuations in cycle-to-cycle perturbation. The calculation of shimmer (RAP) is identical to absolute shimmer, with the exception that cycle-to-cycle deviations in intensity are smoothed by dividing the average amplitude of three successive cycles by the amplitude of the current cycle:

$$\frac{1}{n-2}\left[\sum_{i=2}^{n-1}\left|20 \times LOG\left(\frac{\frac{A_{i-1}+A_i+A_{i+1}}{3}}{A_i}\right)\right|\right]$$

Shimmer (%) RAP. In shimmer (%), the average cycle-to-cycle amplitude perturbation is divided by the average cycle amplitude. RAP removes relatively isolated and/or

long-duration fluctuations in cycle-to-cycle perturbation. In the following formula, we will (1) sum the cycle-to-cycle differences in amplitude by subtracting the amplitude of the cycle under analysis from the average amplitude of the current cycle plus two neighboring cycles; (2) divide the sum of differences by the number of differences (i.e., number of cycles –2); (3) divide the result by the mean amplitude; and (4) multiply the final result by 100 to convert to a percentage (%):

$$\frac{\frac{1}{n-2}\left[\sum_{i=2}^{n-1}\left|\frac{A_{i-1}+A_i+A_{i+1}}{3}-A_i\right|\right]}{\frac{1}{n}\sum_{i=1}^{n}A_i}\times 100$$

As with measures of pitch perturbation (jitter), several studies have reported on the clinical usefulness of measures of shimmer in the assessment of dysphonia. Takahashi and Koike (1975) observed ratings of both breathiness and roughness to correlate with shimmer ($r = 0.56$ and $r = 0.72$, respectively). Kane and Wellen (1985) reported a significant correlation of $r = 0.82$ between shimmer and rated vocal severity, whereas Wolfe et al. (1995) observed a significant correlation of $r = 0.54$ between shimmer and severity of dysphonia, and an $r = 0.56$ when shimmer was combined with measures of vocal F_0. A study by Wolfe et al. (1997) observed that measures of amplitude perturbation (shimmer) correlated strongly with perceived breathy/hoarse voice.

HNR

In the computation of HNR, a ratio comparing the estimated amplitude of the periodic portion of a sound wave to the estimated amplitude of the aperiodic component is achieved. A number of methods have been proposed by which HNR (a.k.a. SNR [signal-to-noise ratio] and NHR [noise-to-harmonics ratio]) may be computed (Kitajima, 1981; Kojima, Gould, Lambiase, & Isshiki, 1980). The most commonly used methods are based on work by Yumoto and colleagues (Yumoto, 1983; 1987; Yumoto, Gould, & Baer, 1982; Yumoto et al., 1984). As previously mentioned, the addition of aperiodic noise to the relatively periodic voice signal results in random perturbations/disturbances to the period (i.e., the "length" of each cycle as seen on an oscillogram) and amplitude (i.e., the "height" of each cycle) of a waveform, thus altering its profile. Yumoto et al. (1982) proposed that if a voice waveform could be "broken down" or separated into its individual cycles of vibration, an averaging of these cycles would essentially "remove" the random fluctuations in cycle profile. The resulting "average cycle" would represent the average periodic component of the voice signal (i.e., the "harmonic" or "signal" component). Yumoto et al. (1982) next proposed that if the average cycle were to be subtracted from each individual original cycle, the result/remainder would be an estimate of the noise (i.e., the random fluctuations in frequency and/or amplitude). Finally, statistical estimates of the power (Awan & Frenkel, 1994; Yumoto et al., 1982) or amplitude (Hillenbrand, 1987) of the periodic versus noise components are combined in ratio format (e.g., $20 \times$ LOG [H/N] for amplitude measures; $10 \times$ LOG [H/N] for power measures) to produce the HNR (expressed in dB).

A number of authors have indicated that HNR may be a more comprehensive measure of the voice signal (Awan & Frenkel, 1994; Eskanazi et al., 1990; Scherer et al., 1995) than jitter or shimmer. Two reasons for this are as follows:

1. HNR is able to detect all variations in waveform profile that occur as a result of the presence of additive noise, and, therefore, the measure is not restricted to variations that occur only in the vicinity of zero-crossings or peaks (Awan & Frenkel, 1994). Therefore, HNR examines not only period and amplitude but also waveshape (i.e., profile) measurements (Scherer et al., 1995).
2. By its nature, HNR takes into account the jitter and shimmer in a signal (Awan & Frenkel, 1994; Eskanazi et al., 1990).

Dworkin and Meleca (1997) state that there is generally a high correlation between HNR and perceptual ratings of voice disorders. A number of studies have supported the clinical usefulness of HNR in the assessment of dysphonic voice. Yumoto et al. (1982) observed a correlation of $r = 0.85$ between computed HNR and the spectrographic classification of degree of hoarseness in 41 dysphonic voice samples. In the same study, the difference in preoperative versus postoperative HNR had a correlation of $r = 0.944$ with a difference in preoperative versus postoperative spectrographic classification of hoarseness. Yumoto et al. (1984) observed that HNR correlated significantly ($r = 0.81$) with perceived degree of hoarseness in 87 voice samples ranging from normal to severely hoarse. Martin et al. (1995) used various acoustic measures to classify voice samples from 60 subjects diagnosed with unilateral vocal fold paralysis, vocal nodules, or functional dysphonia. Results indicated that dysphonic severity of rough voices was predicted most successfully by HNR. HNR also combined with jitter and shimmer to predict breathy voices (low HNR, increased shimmer, low jitter). In a similar study, Wolfe et al. (1997) examined various time-domain acoustic measures (i.e., measures obtained from the time $\times$ amplitude oscillogram) and their ability to predict perceptual severity in 51 dysphonic patients. Results indicated that NHR (similar in nature to HNR) was the most useful measure of dysphonic prediction across voice types (breathy, hoarse, and rough). NHR and jitter were most useful in discriminating vocal roughness. Wolfe et al.

(1997) concluded that measures that assess both harmonic and inharmonic components of the voice signal may predict perceptual severity better than those that focus solely on inharmonic components.

Methodological Considerations in Perturbation/Noise Measurement

Measures of jitter, shimmer, and HNR have generally all been conducted on the same type of voice sample: a sustained vowel production. A number of practical reasons for using this type of voice sample have been described (de Krom, 1994; Scherer et al., 1995) as follows:

- Sustained vowel production is easily controlled and standardized (de Krom, 1994). Scherer et al. (1995) state, "This task (sustained vowel production) is reasonable because it is essentially nonlinguistic, typically easily understood by the patient or subject, and can be imitated" (p. 1261).
- Valid and reliable measures of voice quality (as obtained by means of techniques such as jitter, shimmer, and HNR) may only be obtained from a steady-state vowel production (Baken, 1987; de Krom, 1994; Horii, 1979).

There are a number of important methodological issues that need to be taken into consideration when collecting sustained vowel samples from our patient.

Vowel Type

A number of studies have indicated that vowel type may affect measures of jitter. High vowels (i.e., high tongue position) such as /i/ and /u/ may have lower jitter values than a low vowel such as /ɑ/ (Deem, Manning, Knack, & Matesich, 1989; Sussman & Sapienza, 1994). Gelfer (1995) observed no vowel effect on jitter; however, analysis of the vowel /i/ was observed to result in lower shimmer than /ɑ/. Gelfer (1995) observed lower SNR on the vowel /ɑ/ compared with /i/ but only for low-frequency–low-intensity phonations.

Vowel Frequency

Several studies (Gelfer, 1995; Hollien, Michel, & Doherty, 1973; Horii, 1979) have observed that as the pitch (and therefore, frequency) of the voice increases, measures of jitter tend to lower. Titze (1991) indicates that jitter varies inversely with the firing rate of the motor units in the thyroarytenoid muscle (one of the muscles that influences the vibratory frequency of phonation). Therefore, higher fundamental frequencies are associated with increased motor-unit firing rates and, therefore, decreased jitter. Measures of absolute jitter (in ms) appear to be particularly frequency-dependent (Gelfer, 1995; Hollien et al., 1973; Horii, 1979), whereas the computation of percent jitter attempts to compensate for the influence of mean F_0 (Orlikoff, 1990).

Vowel type may influence the frequency of phonation. It has been speculated that the high tongue position for /i/ and /u/ may exert external tension on the larynx, resulting in a tilting of the thyroid cartilage (Honda, 1983; Sussman & Sapienza, 1994). The result of this external laryngeal tension is that the vowels /i/ and /u/ are often produced at a higher frequency than the vowel /ɑ/. As previously described, an increase in the frequency of the phonation may result in a decrease in measured jitter.

Vowel Length

Several studies have examined the length of vowel sample required to provide stable measures of jitter and shimmer. In this case, the length of sample is described in terms of number of phonatory cycles analyzed. In normal voice cases, as few as 20 to 40 cycles may be adequate to provide stable perturbation measures (Deem et al., 1989; Titze, Horii, & Scherer, 1987). However, disordered voice samples may require a larger number of consecutive cycles for analysis than nonpathological voices (Karnell, 1991), with greater than 100 cycles suggested as a minimum criterion (Karnell, 1991; Scherer et al., 1995).

Number of Vowel Repetitions

Scherer et al. (1995) have reported that the number of averaged vowel repetitions/tokens required to provide a stable measure increases the greater the voice perturbation of the patient. For patients of unknown voice characteristics, it is suggested that at least 15 repetitions/tokens should be sampled to establish a representative average for jitter and shimmer. Fewer tokens are required for stable measures of HNR. In contrast to Scherer et al.'s (1995) findings, most studies (1) use fewer samples that are then analyzed and averaged or (2) select a single sample for analysis that is "consistent," "representative," or "steady" (Walton & Orlikoff, 1994; Wolfe et al., 1995).

Vocal Intensity

Several studies have observed an inverse relationship between vocal intensity/loudness and perturbation (i.e., as intensity/loudness increases, perturbation decreases). Orlikoff and Kahane (1991) observed that jitter decreased significantly with increased vocal intensity; a similar trend was observed for shimmer. The authors speculate that less stable vibration of the vocal folds at low-intensity phonation may be responsible for their observations. Gelfer (1995) made similar observations in that low-intensity vowels consistently resulted in increases for both jitter and shimmer; however, SNR was observed to be a more stable measure of perturbation, with changes in intensity only affecting

SNR measures from the vowel /ɑ/. Gelfer (1995) speculates that low-frequency/low-intensity phonations may serve as an indicator of phonatory abnormality because this method of sampling phonation may be more sensitive to phonatory disruption.

Sampling Rate

When the voice signal is recorded for computer analysis, it must be converted into a data format that the computer can manipulate. This procedure is known as analog-to-digital (A-to-D) conversion. In this process, the sound wave is transformed into a series of numbers that represent the fluctuating amplitude of the signal over time.

When a sound is "sampled," we have a process analogous to taking a series of snapshots of some variable activity; the more snapshots or samples we have, the more accurate the reproduction of the activity being observed. For sound recordings and reproduction, many thousands of samples are required per second if we are to obtain an accurate reproduction of the observed sound wave (see Figure 4–4). Most computer sound cards are capable of recording the speech/voice wave at approximately 44,000 samples per second (44.1 kHz). This provides a high-quality recording of similar quality to the sound reproduced on most music compact discs.

A high sampling rate is particularly important for accurate measures of perturbation. The random fluctuations in the voice waveform profile may only be reproduced and measured if we have a high enough sampling rate to detect these variations. Titze et al. (1987) have suggested that sampling rates as high as 50 kHz to 100 kHz (for adult male and female voices, respectively) may be necessary. The accuracy of relatively low sampling rates may be improved by the use of *interpolation* techniques. Interpolation provides statistical estimates of waveform amplitudes that would be obtained in the event that a higher sampling rate had been used during the recording process.

Advantages in the Clinical Use of Perturbation Measures

1. Objective measures provide an unbiased aspect to the diagnostic process that lends an air of credibility to perceptual voice judgments (Fitch in Orlikoff et al., 1999).
2. Objective perturbation measures are relatively well defined (even though actual algorithms may vary) and easily communicated.
3. Perturbation measures may be able to identify small levels of aperiodicity that may be below the perceptual threshold of the listener. Therefore, the severity levels that may present the most difficulty in perceptual judgment (e.g., mild, mild-to-moder-

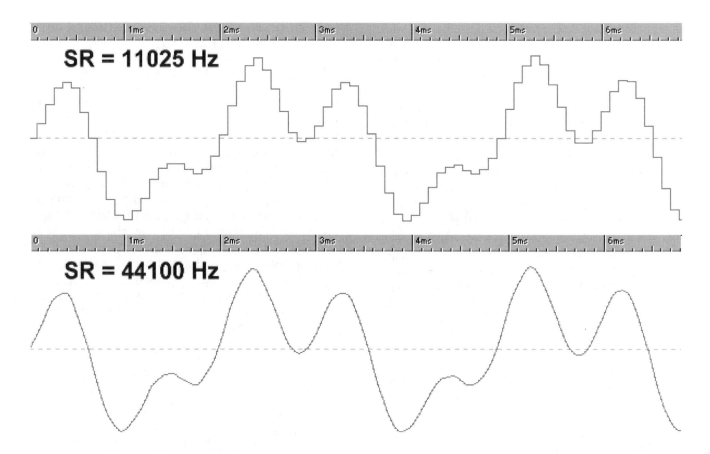

Figure 4–4 The Effect of Sampling Rate on Voice Recording. Two identical voice waveforms recorded at sampling rates (SR) of 11025 Hz (*top*) and 44100 Hz (*bottom*). The profile of the wave recorded with the higher sampling rate is a more accurate representation of the original analog signal than that recorded with the lower sampling rate.

ate) are those in which perturbation measures may be most helpful (Rabinov, Kreiman, Gerratt, & Bielamowicz, 1995).

4. Perturbation measures may direct the clinician to "listen with greater focus and to understand…a patient's variant and deviant vocal behaviors" (p. 101) (Haskell in Orlikoff et al., 1999).

5. Several studies have shown reasonably significant correlations between acoustic perturbation measures and voice quality categories (Kane & Wellen, 1985; Martin et al., 1995; Takahashi & Koike, 1975; Wolfe & Steinfatt, 1987; Wolfe et al., 1997; Yumoto et al., 1984).

In addition to the aforementioned advantages, Perkins (1985) believed that acoustic measures are preferable for assessing normal and abnormal phonatory performance because they are noninvasive, may be gathered and analyzed relatively quickly, permit calibration of the measuring instruments and quantification of the measured variable, and provide data for inferences and a wide range of interpretations of normal and abnormal laryngeal conditions and patterns of vocal fold vibration.

Cautionary Aspects of the Clinical Use of Perturbation Measures

1. Measures of perturbation are mainly applicable only with sustained vowel productions. However, measures from sustained vowels may not always relate to the perceptions of the quality of the voice made in continuous speech. Although studies have been conducted in which perturbation measures were applied to continuous speech samples (Hall & Yairi, 1992; Klingholz, 1990), traditional perturbation measures will be expected to show artificially

inflated noise levels (increases in jitter and shimmer, decreases in HNR) caused by possible interactions with unvoiced segments, intonation patterns, etc.

2. Interprogram reliability may be poor because of variation in computational algorithms for jitter, shimmer, and HNR. The normative data derived from one program/algorithm may not generalize to another.

3. Perturbation measures may be affected by various factors such as vowel phonatory frequency and intensity, vowel type, examination room noise level, microphone type, recording methods, etc. (although all these factors may also have substantial effects on perceptual judgments as well).

4. Variability in the relationship between acoustic measures of quality and (1) perceived vocal quality and (2) specific laryngeal behaviors responsible for perturbation has been observed. In contrast to the previously cited studies showing significant degrees of relationship between objective measures of quality and perceptual ratings, Wolfe et al. (1995) found no significant correlation between jitter and severity ratings of dysphonia. Bielamowicz, Kreiman, Gerratt, Dauer, and Berke (1996) have gone so far as to suggest "abandonment of jitter as a measure of pathological voice" (p. 134).

5. Perturbation measures depend on accurately identifying cycle boundaries (i.e., where a cycle of vibration begins/ends). Unfortunately, the presence of noise in the voice signal makes it more difficult to accurately identify where these cycle onsets/offsets are. The result is error in tracking the periodic vibration of the voice signal and, therefore, possible errors in measuring perturbation. Therefore, perturbation measures may become invalid, particularly with more severe voice disorders (Bielamowicz et al., 1996; Rabinov et al., 1995).

6. Ludlow, Bassich, Conner, Coulter, and Lee (1987) observed that "predictable changes do not occur in these measures (jitter and shimmer) with either morphological or tension changes in the vocal folds" (p. 505). Overall, Ludlow et al. (1987) believed that measures of jitter and shimmer were not adequate indices for the detection of laryngeal pathology.

It is clear that the clinician must balance the pros and cons of commonly used objective measures of vocal quality and interpret their results in an informed fashion. If the limitations in these measures are recognized and accounted for, they may still serve as important additions to our voice diagnostic procedures.

HOW TO DO IT: ELICITATION PROCEDURES FOR OBJECTIVE EVALUATION OF QUALITY

To apply our acoustic analysis techniques for the evaluation of vocal quality, we require our patient to provide a sustained vowel production. However, we would like this sustained vowel to have some reasonable similarity to the patient's voice characteristics during continuous speech performance. The method that this book proposes is the "1, 2, 3, 4" method of sustained vowel elicitation that has been previously discussed in Chapter 2. In this method, we obtain an estimate of the patient's speaking fundamental frequency level by having him or her "chant" a speech utterance (counting), followed by a sustained vowel /ɑ/ that approximates the chanted pitch/frequency. This method is similar to that described by Murry (1982), who described the patient counting and then sustaining the vowel /i/ from the word "three." The instructions below are given to the patient.

> "I want you to repeat the numbers "one, two, three, four." I would like you to chant them like this:"
>
> $\overrightarrow{\text{One}}, \overrightarrow{\text{two}}, \overrightarrow{\text{three}}, \overrightarrow{\text{four}}$
> (These words have a horizontal arrow over them to imply a flat intonation pattern.)
> ✎ "I want you to sustain the "or" of the number "four" and then match it with a vowel /ɑ/. You will sustain the vowel /ɑ/ for at least 2 to 3 seconds at a comfortable loudness level." (A sample file [1234.WAV] is provided on disk to demonstrate this method.)

Demonstrate the method above to the subject and have him or her repeat it once without recording to make sure that the patient understands what he or she is to do. If you are satisfied that the patient understands the procedure, have the patient repeat it again; when the patient begins sustaining the vowel /ɑ/, begin recording (use at least a 44-kHz sampling rate with 16 bits of resolution; if a recording time parameter is required, set for at least 3 seconds). Once your sample has been acquired, perform jitter, shimmer, and HNR analyses on the central 1 second of the vowel. Repeat the aforementioned steps two more times, and then average the perturbation measures.

Several benefits to using the aforementioned method for eliciting sustained vowel productions for vocal quality analyses are found below.

• This method of elicitation provides a pitch/frequency similar to that in continuous speech (we do not want an artificially high/low pitch level that may not correspond well with continuous speech characteristics). In addition, the use of a "comfortable loudness" level provides us with a loudness/intensity level that is habitual. Although it is recognized that frequency and intensity level may affect perturbation measures, we do not want our instructions to change the natural behavior of the patient. As an example, a hypofunctional patient may present with a low-intensity voice that also influences vocal perturbation. If we now ask the patient to produce a vowel at an intensity level that is higher than he or she habitually uses, we may cause the patient to produce a different quality voice with different levels of perturbation than would be found in the habitual voice.

- Use of the vowel /ɑ/ does not appear to raise the pitch of the voice (as with the vowels /i/ and /u/) and may be more beneficial in revealing vocal instability.
- Multiple repetitions allow for observation of possible variation in perturbation values but still at a manageable level (three repetitions) for clinical purposes and consistent with the method used in much of the clinical voice literature.
- The use of a relatively high sampling rate and bits of resolution will accurately capture most signals.
- The 2- to 3-second production provides us with a 100+ cycle sample for adequate analysis.
- The central vowel portion omits vowel onsets and offsets that may artificially inflate perturbation measures (however, the vowel onsets and offsets may be very valuable for perceptual analysis of vocal quality [de Krom, 1994]).

It is suggested that all recordings for objective voice analysis (particularly when conducting perturbation analyses on sustained vowel samples) be collected by means of direct digital recording into the computer. In particular, analysis from tape-recorded samples should be avoided whenever possible. Although Gelfer and Fendel (1995) showed that perturbation measures obtained from taped samples may still provide results within normal expectations, other research (Jiang, Lin, & Hanson, 1998; Titze et al., 1987) has indicated that distortions inherent in the tape format may elevate levels of perturbation and affect the validity of clinical judgments made in reference to measures of perturbation and noise.

A Note on F_0 Tracking Errors

When a computer algorithm makes pitch/F_0-tracking errors, the program has had difficulty in accurately identifying the cycle boundaries (i.e., beginning and ending points) for the waveform under analysis (see Figure 4–5). It must be understood that *all* frequency tracking algorithms will produce errors under certain circumstances (Papamichalis, 1987). These "errors" may reflect noise in the voice; in this case, they are really not errors because the periodic signal and its boundaries have been transformed into a new signal in which cycle boundaries have been randomly distorted/disturbed. However, other errors may reflect effects of factors such as (1) voluntary, rapid pitch changes as used in intonation/stress patterns, (2) coarticulatory effects, (3) a poorly recorded signal, (4) inappropriate setting of program parameters, and/or (5) a poor algorithm. Whatever the cause, the clinician must interpret the results of the analysis, because the presence of pitch/F_0-tracking errors may artificially elevate perturbation measures (or depress in the case of HNR) or at least make results increasingly variable (Rabinov et al., 1995). This interpretation requires that the clinician make a decision as to whether the F_0-tracking results are true reflections of the patient's voice signal or perhaps representative of error on the part of the clinician, patient, or instrumentation that was used. One aspect of this interpretation requires the clinician to match the visual/graphical and numerical results of the F_0-tracking and accompanying perturbation measures with their perceptions. If what you perceive and what you are measuring do not equate, reanalysis and reinterpretation are necessary.

F_0-tracking errors present a conundrum for the clinician and voice scientist. Generally, algorithms produce errors because of disturbances in the voice signal. In this case, "errors" are probably good (i.e., they are indication of the very thing we are trying to detect) and really shouldn't be considered errors at all. On the other hand, sometimes the magnitude of errors computed by the program may not correspond well with the perceived severity of the voice quality observed (in this case, perturbation may be artificially high). Therefore, we may be tempted to somehow correct or remove these errors from analysis (i.e., decrease measured perturbation) by changing various analysis parameters of the program being used. However, we may be removing the very aspects of voice measurement we want to observe and document. Obviously, this discussion emphasizes the key role the clinician/voice scientist has in not just carrying out the test but also in interpreting the results. Perhaps the suggestions listed below will aid in interpreting F_0 and perturbation measures.

- If you must adjust the program parameters to "correct" your analysis, correct as little as possible

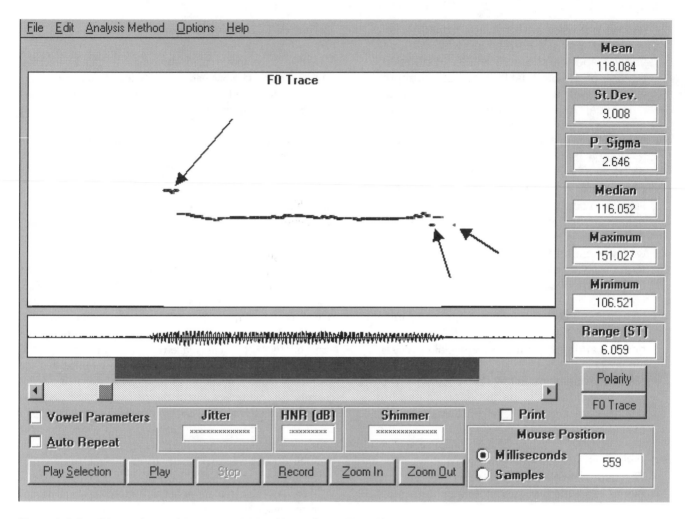

Figure 4–5 Possible Fundamental Frequency (F$_0$) Tracking Errors (Indicated by the Arrows) in a Sustained Vowel Analysis

before achieving a result that is, hopefully, consistent with perceptual judgments.

- Use the suggested program parameter settings for analysis with normal voices and accept any errors that occur as probably caused by voice dysfunction. Of course, make sure that you have carried out all elicitation tasks as accurately as possible and that you have obtained a high-quality recording.
- Whatever method you may choose to "improve" or "adjust" your analysis, remain consistent in your analysis procedures both intrapatient and interpatient. In this way, F$_0$ and perturbation measures that

you may carry out in the future will, hopefully, reflect voice change and not your method of analysis.

Software Analysis of Voice Signals

In the following pages, expectations for measures of vocal quality (both perceptual and quantitative) will be provided. In the discussion of methods of quantitative evaluation of vocal quality, expectations for normal and pathological voice will, in many cases, necessarily deal in generalities. This is because data obtained with different software programs are generally not directly comparable because of the use of different algorithms for the calculations (Bless & Hicks, 1996; Dworkin & Meleca, 1997). This problem is exemplified in two studies that have attempted to objectively evaluate commercially available software for voice analysis.

- Karnell, Hall, and Landahl (1995) analyzed sustained /ɑ/ phonations produced by 20 subjects being evaluated for potential voice disorders. Measures of F_0, jitter, and shimmer were obtained by three analysis systems, CSpeech, AUDED/SEG, and Kay 5500. Results indicated no significant differences and correlation coefficients ranging from .98 to 1.00 among measures of fundamental frequency. Comparisons of jitter measures, however, yielded significant differences between the AUDED/SEG and CSpeech results, but not between the AUDED/SEG and Kay 5500 measures. Agreement among the systems on measures of jitter was not as strong as for F_0 measures. Pearson correlation coefficients ranged from .29 to .64. Comparisons of shimmer measures obtained by means of the AUDED/SEG and Kay 5500 yielded a significant difference as did comparisons of AUDED/SEG and CSpeech. Pearson correlation coefficients ranged from .26 to .42. Results indicate that although there is strong agreement among measures of F_0 obtained using the three systems, measures of jitter and shimmer are not as highly correlated.
- Bielamowicz et al. (1996) compared F_0, jitter, and shimmer values obtained using CSpeech, CSL, and Sound-Scope computer software systems in addition to a hand-marking analysis system. Sustained vowels produced by 50 speakers with dysphonic voices ranging in severity from mild to severe were analyzed. The results below were described.

  1. Measures of mean F_0 among the systems were highly comparable, with the only significant difference occurring between values produced by the CSpeech and hand-marking systems. However, Spearman's rho correlations decreased significantly as severity of vocal pathology increased.
  2. Measures of jitter produced significantly different results between the CSpeech and CSL systems and between the CSL and SoundScope systems. Spearman's rho correlations ranged from .33 to .80. No relationship was found between degree of intersystem reliability and increases in dysphonia on measures of jitter.
  3. Significant differences were found between measures of percent shimmer obtained by CSpeech versus hand-marking system, SoundScope versus hand-marking, and CSpeech versus SoundScope. Correlations varied across severity levels (rho =

.66 to .95). Rank order correlations ranged from rho = .82 to .87 for values of mean shimmer in dB obtained from the CSL versus the hand-marking system.

Bielamowicz et al. (1996) conclude that even in slightly dysphonic voices, measures of jitter may not be reliable, citing errors in cycle matching or cycle boundary identification as possible explanations for the lack of intersystem reliability in obtaining these perturbation measures. The uses of different algorithms and different units of measure for jitter and shimmer were also offered as probable explanations for poor correlations among programs.

Although the results of the Bielamowicz et al. (1996) study appear somewhat discouraging, a multitude of studies have shown, and continue to show, that perturbation measures can be a valuable addition to a voice diagnostic protocol. A study by Hill, Meyers, and Scherer (1990) compared the success of obtaining information regarding laryngeal function from four techniques: videolaryngoscopy, videolaryngostroboscopy, electroglottography (EGG), and acoustic perturbation analysis. Voice evaluation was conducted with 28 subjects (2 normal, 26 disordered), with a technique judged to be successfully administered, "when recordings and data obtained appeared reliable and valid" (p. 201). Results showed that acoustic perturbation measures were successfully administered with 65% of the subjects. Unacceptable results were obtained with subjects who produced (1) highly aperiodic voice; (2) unacceptably short vowel prolongations; (3) extremely rough/fry-like voice; and/or (4) phonations containing transient disruptions or double excitations (e.g., double peaks). Although 35% of the subjects could not be acceptably analyzed by acoustic methods, 46% could not be evaluated by EGG, and 23% could not be successfully assessed by stroboscopic methods. The authors concluded that acoustic perturbation methods complemented the other techniques of voice evaluation and could be useful in a wide range of laryngeal abnormalities. The primary usefulness of perturbation methods appeared to be in the analysis of mild to moderate voice dysfunction.

WHAT TO EXPECT: NORMAL VOICE

Previous sections of this chapter have provided definitions of *normal* voice quality. In these definitions, it is clear that *normal* lies on a continuum that may range from excellent (i.e., one that appears to have professional training and good vocal tract excitement [Eskanazi et al., 1990]) to one that is adequate with no apparent pathology. A range of expectations may also be expected in terms of measures of perturbation and additive noise (jitter, shimmer, and HNR). As previously stated, it may not be valid to directly compare results taken from different software programs that may use very different algorithms in achieving their results. However, the following general guidelines for normal expectations for jitter, shimmer, and HNR have been reported in the literature.

Jitter

Perhaps the most common method for reporting jitter is in terms of jitter factor (see formula provided earlier). Jitter factor (reported in terms of percent jitter) attempts to account for the influence of vocal F_0 on cycle-to-cycle frequency variability (Baken, 1987; Orlikoff, 1990). A number of sources indicate that jitter (%) may be expected to be <1% in normal subjects (Dworkin & Meleca, 1997; Gelfer & Fendel, 1995; Glaze, Bless, & Susser, 1990; Horii, 1979, 1980, 1982a). For absolute jitter (in ms), normative values in the vicinity of 0.04 ms may be expected. Table 4–1 presents a range of examples of jitter values obtained from normal voice subjects.

Shimmer

Shimmer has been commonly reported in either decibels (dB) or percent (%). When shimmer is reported in dB, it represents the mean absolute difference in cycle-to-cycle amplitude. On the other hand, shimmer reported in percent is a mean-relative measure (Horii, 1980), meaning that the mean difference in cycle-to-cycle amplitude is reported in relation to the overall signal amplitude. These methods are analogous in computation to jitter in milliseconds (an absolute computation) versus percent jitter (a relative measure) (Orlikoff, 1990). Absolute shimmer (in dB) has been observed to be substantially less than 1 dB in normals. Horii (1980) observed overall average shimmer of 0.39 dB with a critical value of 0.98 dB in a group of adult men. Heiberger and Horii (1982) found normal shimmer values to be generally <0.7 dB. Dworkin and Meleca (1997) state that normal voice usually has <0.5 dB shimmer. Normative percent shimmer is considered to be 5% or less of the voice signal (Dworkin & Meleca, 1997). This is consistent with ≤4% level considered normal by Glaze et al. (1990) and Gelfer and Fendel (1995). Table 4–2 presents a range of examples of shimmer values obtained from normal voice subjects.

HNR

HNR is commonly reported in decibels (dB) and is based on the ratio of harmonic to inharmonic (i.e., signal to noise) energy in the voice waveform. Yumoto et al. (1982) reported a mean HNR of 11.9 dB (SD = 2.32) for normal male/female voices, although more recent sources expect normal voice

signals to have an HNR >12 dB (Dworkin & Meleca, 1997). However, depending on the software and algorithm used to compute HNR, normal voices may be observed to have HNRs substantially greater than the cutoff suggested by Dworkin and Meleca (1997). Awan and Frenkel (1994) reported a mean HNR of 15.38 dB (SD = 1.08 dB) in a group of normal adult men and women. Awan and Frenkel (1994) expected that 95% of normal subjects would have HNRs >13.6 dB. Walton and Orlikoff (1994) report mean HNR (as derived using the Kay CSL [Kay Elemetrics, Lincoln Park, NJ] program) of 14.77 dB (SD = 3.38) and 16.32 dB (SD = 2.56) in groups of African-American and Caucasian adult men, respectively. Glaze et al. (1990) indicate that normative SNR (signal-to-noise ratio as derived using the CSpeech program [Paul Milenkovic, Madison, WI]) is in the vicinity of 20 dB. Table 4–3 presents a range of examples of HNR values obtained from normal voice subjects.

Although the voice clinician should be familiar with the aforementioned general normative "cutoffs," it should be remembered that factors such as age, gender, and race may result in considerable variability in what is expected for the "normal" voice.

Age

The effects of functional changes in the larynx and general sensorimotor deficits with increased age may produce changes in voice quality (Kahane, 1990; Liss et al., 1990). Hoarseness may be a characteristic of both aged male and female voices (Honjo & Isshiki, 1980; Ptacek & Sander, 1966). Mueller (1998) presents data indicating that the older voice is often perceived as having quality deviations (*hoarse, crackly*) and is generally perceived with a negative connotation. Ryan and Burke (1974) indicated that both laryngeal tension and air loss perceptions were strong predictors of perceived age. In a study of 227 elderly subjects between the ages of 60 and 96 years, Mueller (1978 cited in Mueller, 1997) reported perceived hoarseness in 30% of the elderly women and 64% of the elderly men. It appears that there may be increased decrements in voice quality (particularly marked by hoarse quality) with advanced age. However, voice quality deviation is not a *necessary* characteristic feature of aging. Heterogeneity of the aging process as it affects voice function is to be expected (Awan & Mueller, 1992).

The possibility of decrement in vocal quality with advanced age is also reflected in measures of perturbation. Linville and Fisher (1985) observed higher mean jitter values in a group of 70- to 80-year-old women compared with young and middle-aged adult women. Linville (1988) reported that elderly women produce significantly higher jitter levels than young women, particularly for the vowels /ɑ/ (2.21% vs. 0.55%) and /u/ (1.21% vs. 0.84%), and observed that aging

Table 4–1 Jitter Values from Sustained Vowel Productions

Author	Gender	No. of Subjects	Age (yr.)	Mean & SD	Range
Horii (1980)	M	31	18–38 ($\bar{x}$ = 26.6)	0.61% (0.20)	N/A
Murry & Doherty (1980)	M	5	55–71 ($\bar{x}$ = 63.8)	0.99% (N/A)	0.76–1.49
Ramig & Ringel (1983)[a]	$M_{Y,G}$	8	26–35 ($\bar{x}$ = 29.5)	0.42% (0.09)	N/A
	$M_{Y,P}$	8	25–38 ($\bar{x}$ = 32.3)	0.50% (0.09)	N/A
	$M_{M,G}$	8	46–56 ($\bar{x}$ = 53.0)	0.50% (0.10)	N/A
	$M_{M,P}$	8	42–59 ($\bar{x}$ = 52.6)	0.70% (0.32)	N/A
	$M_{O,G}$	8	62–75 ($\bar{x}$ = 67.5)	0.60% (0.15)	N/A
	$M_{O,P}$	8	64–74 ($\bar{x}$ = 69.1)	0.65% (0.14)	N/A
Horii (1985)[b]	M	12	24–40	0.085 ms (0.032)	0.035–0.151
				0.87% (0.32)	0.46–1.61
Ludlow et al. (1987)[c]	M	38	$\bar{x}$ = 42.1 (17.5)	0.047 ms (0.028)	0.011–0.163
	F	61	$\bar{x}$ = 40.8 (17.9)	0.033 ms (0.013)	0.011–0.074
Linville (1988)[d]	F	22	18–22 ($\bar{x}$ = 20.32)	0.55% (0.36)	0.15–2.30
Linville et al. (1989)	F	20	67–86 ($\bar{x}$ = 76.0)	2.07% (1.56)	0.48–6.10
Deem et al. (1989)	M	5	26–45	0.56% (0.02)	N/A
	F	7	26–48	0.47% (0.05)	N/A
Orlikoff (1990)[e]	M_Y	6	26–33 ($\bar{x}$ = 30.0)	0.042 ms (0.006)	0.034–0.051
				0.46% (0.067)	0.41–0.59
	M_E	6	68–80 ($\bar{x}$ = 73.3)	0.053 ms (0.015)	0.038–0.081
				0.625% (0.102)	0.468–0.74
Karnell (1991)	M	9		0.62% (N/A)	N/A
	F	9		1.128% (N/A)	N/A
Zwirner et al. (1991)	M&F	12	37–76 ($\bar{x}$ = 58.0)	0.04 ms (0.02)	0.012–0.07
Kent et al. (1992)	F	19	65–80 ($\bar{x}$ = 71.8)	0.073 ms (0.049)	N/A
Walton & Orlikoff (1994)[f]	M_W	50	$\bar{x}$ = 30.0	0.28% (0.12)	0.17–0.89
	M_B	50	$\bar{x}$ = 29.0	0.40% (0.36)	0.14–2.33
Dwire & McCauley (1995)	M	24	18–25	0.38% (0.17)	N/A
	F	25	18–25	0.89% (0.62)	N/A
Gelfer (1995)[g]	F	29	20–39 ($\bar{x}$ = 27:1)	0.333% (0.105)	N/A
Gelfer & Fendel (1995)[h]	F	30	21–36 ($\bar{x}$ = 25.5)	0.34% (0.11)	N/A
				0.016 ms (0.006)	N/A
Martin et al. (1995)	M&F	8	23–65	1.18% (N/A)	N/A
Scherer et al. (1995)	M&F	24	22–81	0.52% (0.23)	N/A
Stemple et al. (1995)[i]	F	10	22–45 ($\bar{x}$ = 25.3)	0.38% (0.18)	N/A
Wolfe et al. (1995)	M&F	20	23–65	1.86% (1.89)	0.33–7.52

continues

Table 4–1 continued

Author	Gender	No. of Subjects	Age (yr.)	Mean & SD	Range
Awan & Ziminsky-Ammon (1996)	F	10	18–30 ($\overline{x}$ = 23.80)	0.36% (0.17)	N/A
	F	10	40–49 ($\overline{x}$ = 43.40)	0.47% (0.30)	N/A
	F	10	50–59 ($\overline{x}$ = 54.80)	0.82% (0.77)	N/A
	F	10	60–69 ($\overline{x}$ = 65.20)	0.51% (0.40)	N/A
	F	10	70–79 ($\overline{x}$ = 72.30)	0.46% (0.33)	N/A
Boltezar et al. (1997)	M&F	8	$\overline{x}$ = 14.50 (1.77)	0.81% (0.59)	N/A
Omori et al. (1997)	M	50	Adult	N/A	0.15–0.53%
	F	50	Adult	N/A	0.07–0.69%
Author	M	20	18–30	0.43% (0.09)	0.27–0.62
				0.25% RAP (0.06)	0.16–0.36
				0.04 ms (0.01)	0.01–0.06
	F	20	18–30	0.50% (0.15)	0.31–0.82
				0.31% RAP (0.10)	0.16–0.51
				0.02 ms (0.01)	0.02–0.04
	M&F	10	5–6	0.61% (0.21)	0.39–1.08
				0.38% RAP (0.12)	0.26–0.65
				0.02 ms (0.01)	0.01–0.05

M = male; F = female; $\overline{x}$ = mean; RAP = relative average perturbation; N/A = not available.

[a] Young ($_Y$), middle age ($_M$), and old age ($_O$) subjects in good ($_G$) and poor ($_P$) condition. Data from vowel /ɑ/ sustained for comfortable duration.

[b] Data reported from modal register phonations.

[c] Jitter converted to ms from microseconds (μsec).

[d] Data from the vowel /ɑ/ only.

[e] Data from healthy young men (M_Y) and healthy elderly men (M_E).

[f] Data from white (M_W) and black (M_B) subjects. Jitter values are based on RAP.

[g] Data from vowel /ɑ/ produced at 70 dB (12-in. mouth-to-microphone distance).

[h] Data from directly digitized voice samples only.

[i] Data from pretest only (prelaryngeal fatigue).

appears to increase intraspeaker variability on measures of jitter. Linville et al. (1989) reported a mean jitter of 2.07% (SD = 1.56%) for a group of elderly women and observed that increased jitter was related to overall vocal frequency instability. Wilcox and Horii (1980) found increased mean perturbation in both male and female elderly subjects.

Variability in perturbation measures from elderly subjects may be strongly related to physical condition. Ramig and Ringel (1983) and Ringel and Chodzko-Zajko (1987) observed lower amounts of vocal jitter and shimmer in healthy versus poor physical condition subjects. Similar findings were observed by Orlikoff (1990), who investigated acoustic characteristics in male voices as a function of age and cardiovascular health. Results indicated that elderly men (mean age >70 years) produced significantly higher shimmer (both in dB and %) than young men (mean age = 30 years). A strong trend was observed for elderly men to have higher jitter (in both ms and %) than younger men, although this

trend was significant only for atherosclerotic elderly men. Measures of jitter (%) were also observed to be significantly lowered in healthy versus atherosclerotic elderly men.

Gender

Gender may affect the perceived voice quality in normal-voiced subjects. In men, the production of an extremely low-pitch voice may be perceived as rough, harsh, or hoarse (Coleman, 1969; Davis, 1981; Wendahl, 1963). In the female voice, perceived breathiness may be an important gender marker (Andrews & Schmidt, 1997; Klatt & Klatt, 1990). In terms of measures of perturbation, several studies have observed lower amounts of jitter in female voices compared with male voices (Milenkovic, 1987; Nittrouer, McGowan, Milenkovic, & Beehler, 1990; Sussman & Sapienza, 1994). The lower jitter in female voices has been attributed to factors such as higher vocal F_0, and differences in vocal fold

Table 4–2 Shimmer Values from Sustained Vowel Productions

Author	Gender	No. of Subjects	Age (yr.)	Mean & SD	Range
Horii (1980)	M	31	18–38 ($\bar{x}$ = 26.6)	0.47 dB (0.34)	N/A
Ramig & Ringel (1983)[a]	$M_{Y,G}$	8	26–35 ($\bar{x}$ = 29.5)	0.27 dB (0.13)	N/A
	$M_{Y,P}$	8	25–38 ($\bar{x}$ = 32.3)	0.27 dB (0.18)	N/A
	$M_{M,G}$	8	46–56 ($\bar{x}$ = 53.0)	0.35 dB (0.16)	N/A
	$M_{M,P}$	8	42–59 ($\bar{x}$ = 52.6)	0.43 dB (0.29)	N/A
	$M_{O,G}$	8	62–75 ($\bar{x}$ = 67.5)	0.36 dB (0.09)	N/A
	$M_{O,P}$	8	64–74 ($\bar{x}$ = 69.1)	0.43 dB (0.25)	N/A
Horii (1985)[b]	M	12	24–40	0.48 dB (0.25)	0.17–1.29
Ludlow et al. (1987)	M	38	$\bar{x}$ = 42.1 (17.5)	5.1% (2.9)	1.4–14.3
	F	61	$\bar{x}$ = 40.8 (17.9)	5.3% (3.9)	1.5–24.1
Deem et al. (1989)	M	5	26–45	0.56 dB (0.02)	
	F	7	26–48	0.47 dB (0.05)	
Orlikoff (1990)[c]	M_Y	6	26–33 ($\bar{x}$ = 30.0)	0.257 dB (0.088)	0.154–0.36
				2.93% (1.0)	1.76–4.11
	M_E	6	68–80 ($\bar{x}$ = 73.3)	0.39 dB (0.113)	0.269–0.562
				4.42% (1.24)	3.12–6.27
Zwirner et al. (1991)	M&F	12	37–76 ($\bar{x}$ = 58.0)	4.1% (3.3)	1.1–12.8
Kent et al. (1992)	F	19	65–80 ($\bar{x}$ = 71.8)	2.6% (1.04)	N/A
Walton & Orlikoff (1994)[d]	M_W	50	M = 30	0.27 dB (0.11)	0.09–0.70
	M_B	50	M = 29	0.33 dB (0.15)	0.11–0.66
Gelfer (1995)[e]	F	29	20–39 ($\bar{x}$ = 27:1)	2.53% (0.86)	N/A
Gelfer & Fendel (1995)[f]	F	30	21–36 ($\bar{x}$ = 25.5)	1.29% (0.34)	N/A
Martin et al. (1995)	M&F	8	23–65	0.24 dB (N/A)	N/A
Scherer et al. (1995)	M&F	18	22–81	1.88% (0.83)	N/A
Wolfe et al. (1995)	M&F	20	23–65	0.29 dB (0.22)	0.12–1.12
Awan & Ziminsky-Ammon (1996)	F	10	18–30 ($\bar{x}$ = 23.80)	4.47% (1.95)	N/A
	F	10	40–49 ($\bar{x}$ = 43.40)	4.60% (1.81)	N/A
	F	10	50–59 ($\bar{x}$ = 54.80)	7.45% (4.66)	N/A
	F	10	60–69 ($\bar{x}$ = 65.20)	6.61% (5.22)	N/A
	F	10	70–79 ($\bar{x}$ = 72.30)	6.57% (3.36)	N/A
Boltezar et al. (1997)	M&F	8	$\bar{x}$ = 14.50 (1.77)	2.52% (1.40)	N/A
Omori et al. (1997)	M	50	Adult	N/A	0.45–4.53%
	F	50	Adult	N/A	0.69–4.52%

continues

Table 4–2 continued

Author	Gender	No. of Subjects	Age (yr.)	Mean & SD	Range
Author	M	20	18–30	0.17 dB (0.05)	0.09–0.27
				0.11 dB RAP (0.02)	0.07–0.15
				1.02% RAP (0.29)	0.54–1.62
	F	20	18–30	0.16 dB (0.06)	0.10–0.33
				0.10 dB RAP (0.03)	0.06–0.20
				1.05% RAP (0.39)	0.61–2.04
	M&F	10	5–6	0.25 dB (0.06)	0.15–0.36
				0.16 dB RAP (0.04)	0.09–0.22
				1.60% RAP (0.37)	0.97–2.35

M = male; F = female; $\bar{x}$ = mean; RAP = relative average perturbation; N/A = not available
[a] Young (Y), middle age (M), and old age (O) subjects in good (G) and poor (P) condition. Data from vowel /ɑ/ sustained for comfortable duration.
[b] Data reported from modal register phonations.
[c] Data from healthy young men (M_Y) and healthy elderly men (M_E).
[d] Data from white (M_W) and black (M_B) subjects.
[e] Data from vowel /ɑ/ produced at 70 dB (12-in. mouth-to-microphone distance).
[f] Data from directly digitized voice samples only.

Table 4–3 Harmonics-to-Noise Ratio (HNR in dB) from Sustained Vowel Productions

Author	Gender	No. of Subjects	Age (yr.)	Mean & SD	Range
Yumoto et al. (1982)	M&F	42	19–60	11.9 (2.32)	7.0–17.0
Zwirner et al. (1991)	M&F	12	37–76 ($\bar{x}$ = 58.0)	20.2 (4.1)	12.6–27.9
Kent et al. (1992)	F	19	65–80 ($\bar{x}$ = 71.8)	21.4 (2.02)	N/A
Awan & Frenkel (1994)	M	10	$\bar{x}$ = 24.2	15.63 (1.26)	N/A
	F	10	$\bar{x}$ = 24.7	15.12 (0.85)	N/A
Walton & Orlikoff (1994)[a]	M_W	50	$\bar{x}$ = 30.0	16.32 (2.56)	10.49–21.45
	M_B	50	$\bar{x}$ = 29.0	14.77 (3.38)	6.68–20.96
Gelfer (1995)[b]	F	29	20–39 ($\bar{x}$ = 27:1)	22.1 (2.9)	N/A
Gelfer & Fendel (1995)[c]	F	30	21–36 ($\bar{x}$ = 25.5)	27.5 (2.3)	N/A
Scherer et al. (1995)	M&F	18	22–81	20.26 (2.81)	N/A
Awan & Ziminsky-Ammon (1996)	F	10	18–30 ($\bar{x}$ = 23.80)	16.90 (3.59)	N/A
	F	10	40–49 ($\bar{x}$ = 43.40)	17.80 (2.73)	N/A
	F	10	50–59 ($\bar{x}$ = 54.80)	15.00 (4.62)	N/A
	F	10	60–69 ($\bar{x}$ = 65.20)	16.42 (3.94)	N/A
	F	10	70–79 ($\bar{x}$ = 72.30)	16.37 (3.89)	N/A
Author	M	20	18–30	16.25 (2.50)	11.36–21.52
	F	20	18–30	17.89 (2.00)	13.54–21.50
	M&F	10	5–6	13.26 (1.63)	11.09–16.28

M = male; F = female; $\bar{x}$ = mean; N/A = not available
[a] Data from white (M_W) and black (M_B) subjects.
[b] Data from vowel /ɑ/ produced at 70 dB (12-in. mouth-to-microphone distance).
[c] Data from directly digitized voice samples only.

length and vibratory characteristics between women and men (Sussman & Sapienza, 1994; Titze, 1989).

Race

Differences in vocal quality may be used to discriminate between different racial groups. Walton and Orlikoff (1994) observed significantly greater jitter and shimmer and lower HNRs in 50 African-American men compared with 50 adult Caucasian men. In addition, listeners were most successful in distinguishing between Caucasian and African-American speakers when substantial differences existed between voice pairs in terms of vocal perturbation and additive noise.

WHAT TO EXPECT: ABNORMAL VOICE

Of course, voice quality deviations are often the hallmark of abnormal voice production. A number of abnormal voice types and conditions have been observed that are commonly associated with the perceived voice quality deviations we have discussed earlier in this chapter. As has been described in this chapter, quantification of perceptual voice quality deviations may be achieved by the use of the various measures of perturbation analysis described (jitter, shimmer, and HNR). It should be realized that the numerical results of jitter, shimmer, and HNR analyses might be accounted for by many different physiological conditions (Gerratt & Kreiman in Orlikoff et al., 1999). Various types of laryngeal behavior and pathological conditions may affect the aforementioned measures in similar ways. This fact exemplifies the notion that objective acoustic analyses must be a part of a comprehensive voice evaluation that includes detailed case history information, perceptual assessment, and physiological measures.

RELATIONSHIP BETWEEN PERCEPTUAL AND ACOUSTIC MEASURES IN QUALITY ASSESSMENT

Several studies have examined the relationships and prediction between perceptual assessment of voice (quality type and severity) and acoustic measures, with varying results reported. Selected studies are reviewed below.

- Wolfe and Steinfatt (1987) examined the ability of various acoustic measures to predict severity of voice disorder in 51 subjects with diverse laryngeal pathological conditions. The best predictor of severity was classification of vocal noise level from sound spectrograms. Because Yumoto and colleagues (1982, 1983, 1984, 1987) had developed HNR as an objective method of quantifying spectrographic noise, the results of this study would appear to support the use of HNR in the prediction of dysphonic severity. Jitter was observed to be a significant secondary factor in the prediction of breathy and strained voice types. However, by itself, a relatively weak correlation of only 0.51 was observed between vocal roughness and jitter obtained from sustained vowels /ɑ/ and /i/.

- Eskanazi et al. (1990) examined the relationship between various voice qualities and acoustic measures in 23 pathological voice patients (8 men, 15 women). Results indicated that HNR was one of the best predictors of vocal quality. Rough voices, vocal fry, and overall quality were characterized in part by decreased HNR. Breathy and hoarse voices were characterized in part by increased jitter. Difficulty was observed in the prediction of breathy voice type, with breathy voices "closer to normal voices" (p. 304) than other voice types.

- Martin, Fitch, and Wolfe (1995) used various acoustic measures to classify voice samples from 60 subjects (9 men and 51 women; mean age = 45 years) diagnosed with unilateral vocal fold paralysis, vocal nodules, or functional dysphonia. Analysis of sustained vowel /ɑ/ productions using the CSL program indicated that dysphonic severity of rough voices was predicted most successfully by HNR, whereas breathy voices were predicted most successfully by combined features of reduced jitter, increased shimmer, and reduced HNR. No combination of acoustic features was successful in the prediction of hoarseness.

- Wolfe et al. (1995) observed significant but weak correlations between measures of shimmer and HNR and severity of dysphonia ($r = 0.54$ and $r = -0.32$, respectively). No significant correlations were observed between jitter and severity.

- Wolfe et al. (1997) examined various time-domain measures (i.e., measures obtained from the time × amplitude oscillogram) and their ability to predict perceptual severity of dysphonia. There were 51 subjects (20 men and 31 women; mean age = 48 years). Results from sustained vowel /ɑ/ and /i/ analyses indicated that NHR (similar in nature to HNR) was the most successful measure of dysphonic prediction across voice types (breathy, hoarse, and rough). Measures of frequency perturbation (e.g., jitter and HNR) were most useful in discriminating vocal roughness, whereas measures of amplitude perturbation (e.g., shimmer) correlated more strongly with breathy/hoarse voices. Overall, the authors concluded that measures that assessed both harmonic and inharmonic components of the voice signal (as found in HNR) may predict perceptual severity better than those that focus solely on inharmonic components.

- Wolfe and Martin (1997) explored the ability to classify dysphonic patients by means of various acoustic measures in 51 dysphonic subjects. Results indicated that hoarse voices differed from breathy and strained voices in having increased jitter and shimmer. Strained voices had decreased SNR but also decreased jitter as compared with breathy voices. Strained voices (i.e., reflective of increased vocal effort) were observed to be relatively normal in terms of perturbation measures, whereas hoarse voices were substantially abnormal in all parameters. Breathy voices were observed to fall between the strained and hoarse types in terms of perturbation measures.

In addition to examining relationships between perturbation measures and degree of perceived dysphonia, a number of studies shown below have examined the ability of isolated perturbation measures to discriminate between normal and disordered groups.

- Zyski, Bull, McDonald, and Johns (1984) assessed the ability of various measures of pitch and amplitude perturbation to differentiate 20 normal subjects from 52 subjects with medically diagnosed laryngeal pathological conditions (various cases including patients with mass lesions, unilateral paralysis, and spastic dysphonia). Results showed that perturbation methods could achieve some degree of discrimination between normal and pathological groups, with pitch perturbation (jitter) more effective than amplitude perturbation (shimmer). However, considerable overlap between the two groups was observed, with between 21% and 77% of pathological cases producing perturbation levels within the "normal" range. These authors concluded that perceptual measures may be able to discriminate some cases of abnormal phonation not identifiable by acoustic measures alone.
- Ludlow et al. (1987) reported on the capability of jitter and shimmer to accurately categorize normal (38 men and 61 women) versus pathological voice cases (17 men and 17 women) of various types. Results indicated that "jitter and shimmer were sensitive to morphological changes associated with carcinoma and partial laryngectomy, but were less sensitive to less marked morphological changes such as nodules, polyps, and edema" (p. 500). Overall correct assignment to normal versus pathologic groups was 78.5%, although percent correct classification for pathological cases on the basis of jitter ranged from only 29% to 47% and from 41% to 53% on the basis of shimmer. The overall conclusion of these authors was that jitter and shimmer were not adequate as indices for the detection of laryngeal pathology.

Perturbation Measures and Various Abnormal Voice Types

Hypoadductive/Hypofunctional Cases

Some inability or inadequacy in effectively approximating the vocal folds during phonation characterizes many voice disorders. One of the results of this disruption to phonation is the excessive leakage of air by way of the glottis perceived as breathiness (see earlier definition). The perceived quality of breathiness may be observed in a variety of disorders of psychogenic, functional, or organic origin. Several authors (Boone & McFarlane, 1988; Case, 1996; Murry, 1982; Prater & Swift, 1984; Stemple et al., 1995) provide examples of disorders that often have breathy voice quality as one of their primary voice characteristics:

- Irregularities of the vocal fold margins
- Additive lesions (e.g., nodules, polyps)
- Vocal fold paralysis or paresis
- Asymmetrical/asynchronous vocal fold vibration
- Vocal fold weakness secondary to fatigue
- Bowing of the vocal folds
- Edematous vocal folds

It may be expected that the degree of incomplete vocal fold closure will be related to the degree of perceived breathiness (Andrews, 1995; Sodersten & Lindestad, 1990). However, the degree of breathiness is also significantly affected by the loudness of voice production (increased breathiness with decreased loudness of phonation [Sodersten & Lindestad, 1990]), and glottal configuration and conditions of the side walls (Bless & Hicks, 1996) (i.e., conditions that may result in increased turbulence in transglottal airflow).

Hyperadductive/Hyperfunctional Cases

In cases in which the patient uses excessive effort and muscular tension during voice production, overadduction of the vocal folds may result. The perceived voice quality in these cases is often one of harshness/roughness (see previous definitions). As with breathiness, the harsh voice may be observed in a variety of voice disorders of varying origins (Andrews, 1995; Askenfelt & Hammarberg, 1986; Bless & Hicks, 1996; Prater & Swift, 1984):

- Personality attributes and conflicts
- Pharyngeal and/or glottal constriction secondary to vocal abuse/misuse
- Structural alterations
- Neurological deficits and configurations (spasticity, focal dystonia/spasmodic dysphonia)
- Irregular vocal fold vibration

- Surface moisture on the vocal folds
- Poor breath support

As previously discussed, the hoarse voice quality is associated with a combination of breathy and harsh quality. Hoarseness may result because of (1) hyperadductive compensation for an initial/primary hypoadductive condition, (2) hypoadduction as a result of fatigue and trauma caused by primary hyperadduction, or (3) hypoadduction from hyperadduction, in which excessive tension in the posterior cricoarytenoid muscle during phonation results in a significant posterior glottal chink (Morrison & Rammage, 1993). Therefore, voice disorders associated with hoarseness are similar to those previously mentioned for breathiness and/or harshness. Prater and Swift (1984) and Andrews (1995) list a number of other disorders/conditions associated with hoarse voice quality:

- Neurological disease
- Structural alterations
- Laryngeal edema (secondary to abuse/misuse)
- Upper respiratory tract infections
- Excessive or thick vocal tract secretions (*wet hoarseness*)

Mass Lesions and Distributed Tissue Change

The addition of mass (e.g., by means of a pathological lesion or from edema) may have key effects on phonation: (1) the lesion may cause aperiodicity in vocal fold vibration associated with perceived roughness and elevated perturbation; and/or (2) the presence of lesion or tissue change may affect the ability to adequately approximate the vocal folds during phonation, resulting in excessive airflow, perceived breathiness, and increased perturbation.

- Murry and Doherty (1980) examined measures of perturbation in discriminating five normal male subjects from five male speakers diagnosed with laryngeal cancer (primary site of lesion was the true vocal folds in all cancer cases). Ten subjects (five men with cancer and five male controls) provided continuous speech and sustained vowel samples. Results indicated that measures of frequency perturbation (mean jitter [%]: 0.99% vs. 3.79% for normals vs. pathological subjects) were the strongest factors in the accurate classification of normal and pathological subjects. The authors speculated that the presence of a laryngeal mass lesion would detrimentally affect vocal fold vibratory pattern.
- Kane and Wellen (1985) examined pitch and amplitude perturbation in 10 children (6 males and 4 females; mean age = 8 years, 8 months) diagnosed with vocal

nodules. Both pitch and amplitude perturbation measures correlated significantly with a 7-point severity scale ($r = 0.68$ and $r = 0.82$, respectively). The authors concluded that jitter and shimmer measures may be more sensitive to small changes in vocal quality than perceptual judgments.

- Hirano (1989) reported on the predictive ability of various measures of voice analysis with 1,563 adult voice patients. Measures of pitch perturbation and amplitude perturbation were observed to vary considerably with disease group. Significant, although weak, positive correlations were observed between perturbation measures and polyp size.
- Milenkovic, Bless, and Rammage (1991) reported on the acoustic characteristics of 38 patients with vocal nodules (ages 18 to 40 years) and 10 age-matched controls. These authors had speculated that "elevated jitter and shimmer may result from unstable patterns of vocal fold oscillations produced by abnormalities in vocal fold structure" (pp. 266–267). The results of this study partially confirmed this speculation by showing a tendency for higher jitter and lower SNR in patients with nodules compared with normal subjects, although the findings showed the means to be within one standard deviation of each other for each measure. The acoustic waveform for many of the patients with nodules was characterized by double-pulsing (a possible sign of diplophonia and roughness). A key reason why Milenkovic et al. (1991) did not observe a greater difference between the nodules and the control groups is that the patients with double-pulsing characteristics were removed from analysis, leaving patients with relatively normal acoustic characteristics for comparison purposes. In addition, irregular vowel onsets were also observed for many patients with nodules.
- Pruszewicz, Obrebowski, Swidzinski, Demenko, Wika, and Wojciechowska (1991) examined the ability of acoustic measures to differentiate organic from functionally dysphonic patients. The organic group was made up of 15 subjects with organic changes confined to the glottis (cases included epithelial changes, polyps, and papilloma). Patients in the functional group (15 subjects) all had normal appearing laryngeal structures and were diagnosed with hyperfunctional dysphonias. Results from acoustic analyses indicated that the speech signal of the organic patients demonstrated a more disturbed harmonic structure than the functional subjects, with the result being substantially higher measured jitter (mean jitter: 8% vs. 4%, respectively). The authors speculated that acoustic disturbances in the organic patients were possibly related to asymmetric growth of vocal fold mass, whereas alterations in the degree

of tension and coordination affected the voices of the functionally disordered patients. Overall, these authors believed that the use of certain acoustic methods could distinguish those voice disorders in which mass lesion was the underlying pathophysiology.

Effects of Smoking

Although several studies have investigated the effects of smoking on vocal fundamental frequency, relatively few have included measures related to the periodicity of the phonatory signal. Awan and Coy (1992) compared the voice characteristics of 15 female smokers and 15 female non-smokers, with mean ages of 24.7 years and 24.4 years, respectively. Although no significant difference was revealed between the two groups for measures of jitter and shimmer, measures of HNR for the smoking group were significantly higher than those of the nonsmoking group, even though subjects in both groups were perceived to have normal vocal quality.

Neurological Disorders

Several sources (as shown below) have summarized the possible effects on vocal quality for a number of neurological states (Colton & Casper, 1996; Darley et al., 1975; Dworkin, 1991):

- Upper motor neuron disorders: Key phonatory characteristics are rough/harsh quality (possibly strained-strangled); possibly breathiness secondary to hypertonia and possible hyperadduction (effects of fatigue and/or significant posterior glottal chink).
- Extrapyramidal disorders (hypokinetic dysarthrias): Rigidity in the laryngeal musculature may result in roughness/harshness and some strain/struggle. Vocal fold bowing may result in breathy quality.
- Hyperkinetic disorders: Uncontrolled contractions may result in harsh/strained-strangled quality, although sudden changes between harshness and breathiness/aphonia are also possible. Severe tremors may result in voice arrest (as in spasmodic dysphonia).
- Ataxia: Harshness, hoarseness, and tremor have been described.
- Lower motor neuron disruptions: Common characteristics are breathiness and hoarseness, inhalatory stridor, and diplophonia (resulting in a rough quality).

Several examples of studies that have reported on vocal quality disruption in neurological disorders can be found below.

- Ramig, Scherer, Klasner, Titze, and Horii (1990) reported acoustic measures obtained from a single 69-year-old patient with amyotrophic lateral sclerosis (ALS). The patient was free of phonatory dysfunction at the start of the study. Acoustic measures (including jitter, shimmer, and HNR) were conducted five times throughout a 6-month period. Increased phonatory instability was reflected in a comparison of initial versus final trial measures, which showed substantial increases in jitter and shimmer and reductions in HNR. Perturbation increases were attributed to factors such as reduction in short-term laryngeal adductory/abductory control, mucus in the glottal flow path, changes in vocal fold tension, and/or breathiness. Decreased HNR was attributed to combined respiratory, laryngeal, and mucous contributions to phonatory instability. The various acoustic findings were believed to support the hypothesis that the progression of ALS affects the vocal mechanism and that vocal mechanism changes are reflected in certain specific acoustic measures. Acoustic measures were believed to provide a method by which early signs of neuromuscular degeneration may be identified and monitored through disease progression.
- Zwirner et al. (1991) examined the phonatory characteristics of three dysarthric groups (Parkinson's disease, Huntington's disease, and cerebellar ataxia). Results showed that all three dysarthric groups had significantly higher jitter than the controls. For measures of shimmer, the Huntington's and ataxic patients showed significantly higher levels than the controls. No difference was observed between the various groups for SNR. In addition to these differences, the neuropathological subjects showed a higher degree of group variability than the control group. Although the aforementioned significant differences between dysarthric and normal subjects were observed, the authors believed that the degree of overlap between normal versus disordered values was relatively high, such that the normal group could not be effectively separated from the dysarthric subgroups. In addition, measures of perturbation and noise were not uniquely attributable to any of the three dysarthric subgroups. Zwirner et al. (1991) concluded that "acoustic measures alone do not add substantially to the differential diagnosis of neuropathologies" (p. 298).
- Kent et al. (1992) described various phonetic and acoustic characteristics in a group of 10 ALS patients. Results showed that, as compared with a group of normal controls, ALS patients exhibited significantly higher jitter and shimmer and lower SNR. As Ramig et al. (1990), Kent et al. (1992) believed that their results indicated that "acoustic analysis...may provide a means by which

early oral-facial and laryngeal signs of disease can be detected" (p. 731).

- Dromey et al. (1995) examined speech and phonatory function in a single Parkinson's disease patient before and after therapy by use of the Lee Silverman Voice Treatment approach (in this approach, the patient is encouraged to increase vocal intensity by increasing phonatory effort, vocal fold adduction, and respiratory support). Results indicated that phonatory stability (as reflected by measures of jitter, shimmer, and HNR) improved with use of increased sound pressure level. These authors speculated that "increased vocal intensity and adduction contributed to more stable vocal fold oscillation" (p. 761).

- Hirano et al. (1995) reported perturbation measures for 240 patients with unilateral vocal fold paralysis before and after transcutaneous intrafold silicone injection (TCIFSI). Pretreatment pitch and amplitude perturbation levels were abnormally high compared with normal expectations in more than 80% of the subjects examined. The authors speculated that asymmetry of the vocal folds resulted in irregular vibration and, thus, increased pitch and amplitude perturbation. After TCIFSI, perturbation measures were substantially decreased, indicating improved periodicity of vocal fold vibration and reductions in turbulent noise.

Muscle Tension Dysphonias (MTDs)/Hyperfunctional Voice

The presence of excessive tension in the extralaryngeal musculature may be reflected in abnormal vocal quality. Hyperfunction and laryngeal rigidity may be combined with conditions such as vocal fatigue and myasthenia larynges (functional vocal fold bowing) to result in variable voice quality deviations (breathiness, roughness, and hoarseness). Increases in jitter and shimmer and decreases in HNR may reflect these quality deviations.

- Roy and Leeper (1993) conducted perceptual and acoustic measures of voice function with 17 functionally dysphonic patients before and after therapy. Treatment focused on a single therapy session including manual laryngeal musculoskeletal tension reduction. Mean jitter (0.312 ms) and mean shimmer (22.35%) were observed to be substantially higher than normal expectations before therapy; mean SNR (12.19 dB) was substantially lower than expected. After treatment, substantial improvements in all measures were observed, although only changes in shimmer and SNR were observed to be statistically significant.

- Gelfer, Andrews, and Schmidt (1991) investigated the effects of prolonged reading on acoustic measures of the voice in trained and untrained singers. Subjects were 50 trained female singers (ages 23 to 48 years) versus 24 young adult female controls who had received no vocal instruction. Prolonged reading resulted in significant decreases in SNR measured from sustained vowel production in the untrained subjects, as well as a trend for deteriorations in jitter. However, results indicated that jitter and shimmer values in sustained vowels actually decreased somewhat before versus after task comparison for the trained singers. The results of this study suggested that the effects of vocal/singing training generalize to speaking situations and that prolonged loud reading may have significant effects on the vocal function of individuals who have not received any type of prior vocal training.

- Stemple et al. (1995) examined acoustic, aerodynamic, and videostroboscopic characteristics associated with laryngeal fatigue as a result of prolonged voice use. Subjects were 10 adult women (mean age = 25.3 years). Analyses were made before and after 2 hours of reading at a SPL of 75 to 80 dB. Results indicated minor changes in jitter, although mean jitter was <1% in both premeasurements and postmeasurements.

- Eustace, Stemple, and Lee (1996) conducted a retrospective study in which acoustic and other data were analyzed from patients who had complained of vocal fatigue. Eighty-eight subjects were reviewed; all had no evident laryngeal pathology. Analysis of measures of jitter showed that the mean perturbation for all but two of the patients had been <1%, even though most of the subjects presented with some type of glottal chink (anterior, anterior and posterior, spindle).

Hearing Impairment/Deafness

Control of the phonatory mechanism occurs (to some degree) by way of the auditory mechanism. The presence of severe hearing loss during the developmental acquisition of speech and voice control may affect the ability to produce normal vocal quality.

- Monsen (1979) reported on the acoustic qualities of phonation in 24 hearing-impaired children versus a group of normal controls. Quality deviations of breathiness and diplophonia were observed in the phonations of a number of the hearing-impaired subjects. Excessive air escape by way of the glottis and temporary irregularities in glottal vibration were speculated as the underlying causes of these quality deviations.

- Thomas-Kersting and Casteel (1989) investigated the relationships between spectral noise and perceived vocal effort in 18 hearing-impaired children. Results from sustained vowel analysis (both acoustic and perceptual) showed that spectral noise levels tended to increase with increases in vocal effort. The average hearing-impaired child was perceived as demonstrating excessive vocal effort during phonation, with the voice being perceptually characterized as "tense," "strained," or "metallic." The authors of this study speculated that harsh voice quality and effortful voice were due to "inappropriate tension and strain in the respiratory, phonatory, and articulatory processes" (p. 134) of hearing-impaired individuals.

VOICE QUALITY: TUTORIAL

In this section, the reader will listen to voice characteristics and review the analyses of several voice samples that will illustrate (1) both normal voice quality and a number of the commonly observed voice quality deviations, and (2) methods of quantitatively analyzing acoustic characteristics that relate to perceived voice quality. In addition, this tutorial section begins with an analysis of several synthesized voice samples that are used to illustrate some of the basic concepts related to the analysis of vocal quality. All the voice samples discussed in this section can be found in the C:\VDP directory.

The examples that will be presented in this tutorial have been analyzed using the EZVoicePlus voice analysis software (VoiceTek Enterprises, Nescopeck, PA). However, the principles to be discussed will be applicable to most any voice analysis program the clinician may choose to use.

Synthesized Vowel /ɑ/ (Negligible Noise Components)

In the Windows Explorer program, double-click on the C:\VDP folder to find the file to be discussed. In this step, we will be analyzing the file Q1.WAV. If you click on the file name using the L. mouse button, you will hear a small sample of a synthesized vowel /ɑ/. Figure 4–6 shows a close-up view of approximately seven cycles of the synthesized vowel. Note that the waveform is extremely periodic

(i.e., the pattern of vibration repeats itself in a consistent manner). Because this is a computer-generated, synthesized voice waveform, there is very little noise in it. Also note that in an example of a voice waveform, we see a complex wave. A complex wave is made up of more than one frequency; in the case of the voice, these frequencies are the fundamental frequency (F_0) and its harmonics (integer multiples of the F_0). A relatively large peak, followed by several smaller peaks and valleys, often initiates each cycle of a normal, human voice acoustic signal. As was described previously, the more complex the waveform (i.e., the more frequencies present in the acoustic signal) the more complex will be the pattern of vibration (i.e., more peaks and valleys will be observed per cycle).

In an attempt to quantify the fact that there is very little noise in this synthesized voice signal, we will compute measures of jitter, shimmer, and HNR. As we have previously learned, these are acoustic measures of the perturbation (i.e., disturbance or noise) in the voice waveform. Computation of the F_0 contour, associated F_0 statistics, and measures of perturbation and noise are shown in Figure 4–7.

The various measures of acoustic quality that have been calculated tell us that this is a highly periodic signal with very little noise in it. The jitter value (0%) tells us that the signal does not vary at all in terms of cycle-to-cycle frequency. As stated previously, this is a computer-generated signal with very little noise mixed into it; in fact, even extremely good quality human voices are not perfectly periodic and, therefore, will be observed to have small amounts of jitter present. The HNR value tells us that the harmonic (i.e., periodic) component of this waveform is 32 dB greater than any noise component. Again, this is a higher value than would be expected in a human voice signal. The shimmer value tells us that there is a very small amount of cycle-to-cycle perturbation in amplitude; however, the shimmer value is still slightly lower than often observed in good-quality human voices. In addition to the measures of noise, we can also see that (1) the F_0 trace/contour is perfectly flat, and (2) the F_0 standard deviation is zero, telling us that there is no

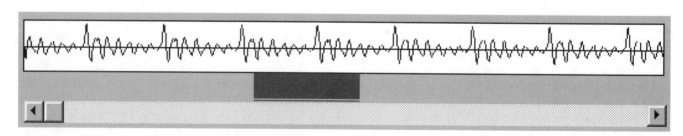

Figure 4–6 Close-up View of Several Cycles of a Synthesized Vowel /ɑ/

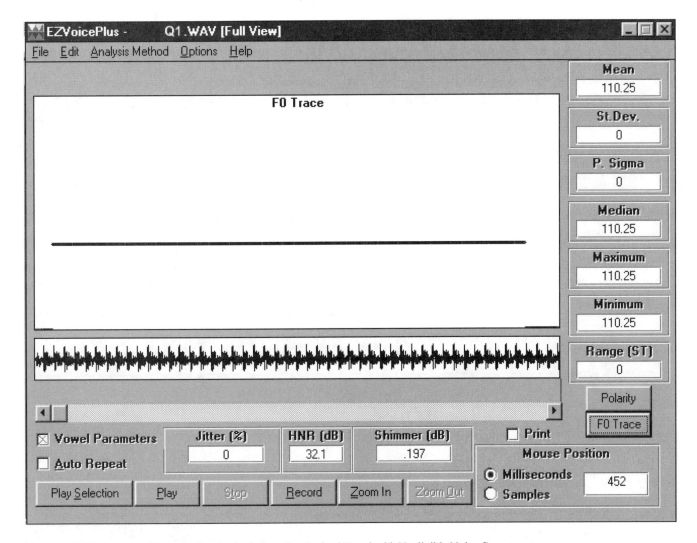

Figure 4–7 Frequency and Perturbation Analysis for a Synthesized Vowel with Negligible Noise Components

variability in the frequency of the signal. These observations also confirm that the synthesized voice signal being analyzed is extremely periodic.

Synthesized Vowel /ɑ/ (Substantial Noise Components)

As an example of the possible effects of noise on the voice signal and measures of voice quality, we will now analyze a sound file in which a considerable amount of noise has been mixed. In the signal we will analyze, the highly periodic synthesized voice signal we previously analyzed has been mixed with white noise (a type of "hissing" noise) to a level of approximately 3 dB HNR (i.e., in this example, the periodic component of the sound wave is only slightly greater in amplitude than the noise component).

In this step, we will be analyzing the file Q2.WAV. If you click on the file name using the L. mouse button, you will hear a synthesized vowel /ɑ/ sample that appears to have a prominent "breathy" quality because of the increased amplitude of the noise component. In Figure 4–8 we see a close-up view of approximately six cycles of the synthesized vowel. Note that, although a repeatable pattern of vibration can be discerned, this time the waveform shows substantial differences in profile (i.e., the shape of the waveform) from cycle to cycle. Also note that the complexity of the waveform has increased tremendously because the addition of considerable noise to the periodic synthesized voice signal has added frequencies inbetween the F_0 and harmonics.

To quantify the fact that there is considerable noise in this synthesized voice signal, the clinician could again compute

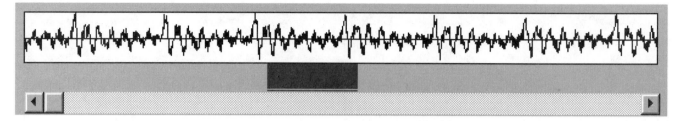

Figure 4–8 Close-up View of Several Cycles of a Synthesized Vowel /ɑ/ Mixed with White Noise to a Harmonics-to-Noise Ratio of 3 dB

measures of jitter, shimmer, and HNR. Computation of the F_0 contour, associated F_0 statistics, and measures of perturbation and noise are shown in Figure 4–9.

This time the analysis confirms that the synthesized voice signal is highly perturbed. Jitter (1.229%) is considerably higher than we would expect in a normal voice signal (often in the 0.4% to 0.6% range), indicating that there is increased variability in cycle-to-cycle frequency. The HNR value (3.223 dB; considerably lower than the 15- to 20-dB HNR often observed in the normal voice) confirms that

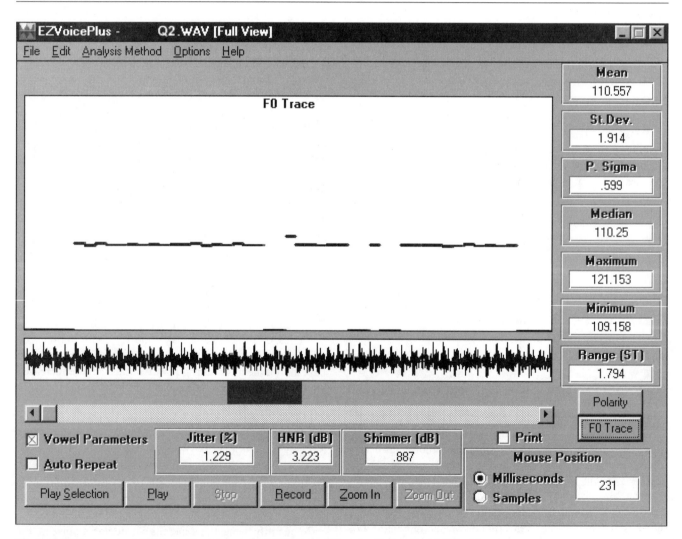

Figure 4–9 Frequency and Perturbation Analysis for a Synthesized Vowel with Substantial Noise Components

the noise level is competing with the periodic sound wave. The shimmer value (0.887 dB) tells us that the additive noise has also affected the consistency of the cycle-to-cycle amplitudes. In addition to the measures of noise, it can also be seen that the F_0 trace/contour is variable; the blank sections ("dropouts") in the F_0 trace/contour indicate that certain cycles were so indistinct that the program could not calculate an estimate of F_0 for that portion of the waveform (i.e., the cycle boundaries [peaks] were not clear). The F_0 standard deviation (1.194 Hz) is quite high for a sustained vowel (often observed to be 1% or less in normal voice production), also indicative of increased variability in the frequency of the waveform. All in all, these observations confirm that the synthesized voice signal being analyzed is quite aperiodic and verify the perceptual impression of abnormal voice.

Sustained Vowel /ɑ/ (Normal Adult Male)

The previous examples have used synthesized vowel samples to introduce the reader to the use of the quantitative measures used in the analysis of vocal quality. Let us now examine some samples of normal voice starting with an adult male example.

✎ Click on the file Q3.WAV using the L. mouse button; you will hear a sample of a normal adult male sustaining the vowel /ɑ/. You should not hear any substantial degree of breathiness, roughness, or hoarseness in this voice.

Computation of the F_0 contour, associated F_0 statistics, and measures of perturbation and noise are shown in Figure 4–10.

The human voice is *quasiperiodic* (i.e., it closely approximates periodicity, but there are very slight variations cycle to cycle, even in normal voices). The analysis of this normal male voice sample shows these characteristics. The perturbation measures (jitter = 0.317%; shimmer = 0.131 dB) indicate very small amounts of cycle-to-cycle frequency and amplitude variability that are well within normal expected levels. These small amounts of perturbations are not enough to significantly disturb the HNR (19.141 dB, well within expected levels), indicating that the periodic component of this signal is significantly greater in amplitude than any noise component. Although the F_0 contour has some slight variation in it, the F_0 standard deviation is considerably less than 1% of the mean F_0.

Sustained Vowel /ɑ/ (Normal Adult Female)

✎ Click on the file Q4.WAV using the L. mouse button; you will hear a sample of a normal adult female sustaining the vowel /ɑ/. Computation of the F_0 contour, associated F_0 statistics, and measures of perturbation and noise are shown in Figure 4–11.

This example of a typical young adult female voice again shows all the characteristics of periodic phonation with very little perturbation or noise. You should not have heard any substantial degree of breathiness, roughness, or hoarseness in this voice. Compared with the previously analyzed male voice, the adult female voice may be perceived as having less "rumble" and perhaps a somewhat steadier pitch.

Disordered Samples

A variety of different disordered conditions (functional vs. organic disorders, hypofunction vs. hyperfunction) may have similar perceptual and acoustic characteristics (Behrman & Orlikoff, 1997; Gerratt & Kreiman in Orlikoff et al., 1999). In addition, there is tremendous heterogeneity of voice characteristics even within a single diagnostic category (e.g., functional dysphonia). With this in mind, it would appear to be somewhat amiss to present voice samples as being representative of a particular disorder (e.g., "Here is a voice sample for unilateral vocal fold paralysis," "Here is a voice sample for muscle tension dysphonia," etc.). The final accepted diagnostic hypothesis must be derived from a synthesis of information from a variety of sources (case history, medical background information, perceptual/acoustic/ physiological signs and symptoms). Therefore, the voice samples we will look at in this next section will focus more on the perceptual qualities of the voice and the possible effects on acoustic analyses rather than on examples supposedly attributable to specific disorders.

Samples Characteristic of Hypoadduction: Mild Breathiness (Sustained Vowel Production)

✎ In this step, we will be analyzing the file Q5.WAV. If you click on the file name using the L. mouse button, you will hear a sample of an adult female who had been diagnosed with a functional dysphonia (excessive musculoskeletal tension) sustaining the vowel /ɑ/. This patient's voice had been characterized as having a mild degree of breathiness. Figure 4–12 shows a small portion of the acoustic signal; we see that the cycle boundaries are quite clear in the mild breathy voice, although small deviations cycle to cycle can be observed. Several authors have noted that the breathy voice appears to be more similar acoustically to normal voices.

Computation of the F_0 contour, associated F_0 statistics, and measures of perturbation and noise are shown in Figure 4–13.

This particular example very nicely shows how acoustic measures of perturbation and noise can be effective in documenting voice disorders, particularly when they are mild in nature. Perceptually, the breathy quality in this voice is quite subtle; many clinicians (particularly inexperienced ones) would miss detection of this quality deviation. However,

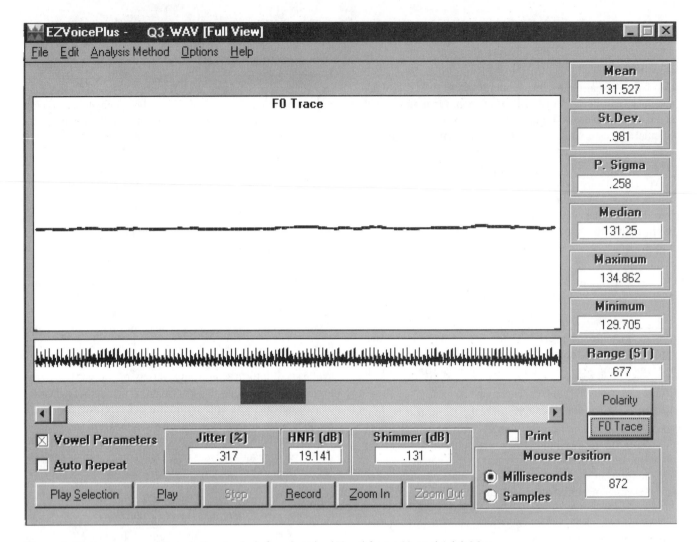

Figure 4–10 Frequency and Perturbation Analysis for a Sustained Vowel from a Normal Adult Man

the acoustic analysis of the vowel shows that there is actually a high degree of jitter (1.754%). On the other hand, the shimmer (0.338 dB) is only slightly elevated compared with normal expectations, and the HNR (13.607 dB) is only slightly depressed. The F_0 standard deviation (3.59 Hz) is substantially greater than 1% or less of the mean F_0, confirming that the average variability of vocal frequency is increased.

In mild or "borderline" cases of voice disorder, it has been my clinical experience that, of several acoustic measures computed, only one or two may be clearly abnormal, whereas others may be at low-normal to normal levels. This example exemplifies the importance of redundancy in our diagnostic protocol, in which abnormalities missed by one method of analysis may be detected by an alternative method. The acoustic analysis for this mild breathy sustained

vowel sample clearly shows the clinician that there is some type of abnormality in the voice signal and, at the very least, may cause the clinician to reexamine the perceptual attributes of the patient's voice.

Sample Characteristic of Hypoadduction: Moderate Breathiness (Sustained Vowel Production)

✎ Click on the file Q6.WAV using the L. mouse button; you will hear a sustained vowel /ɑ/ sample from an adult female who had been diagnosed with chronic laryngitis. This patient's voice had been characterized as having a moderate degree of hoarseness (stronger breathy component). The quality was deemed to be highly noticeable during her phonation and occasionally caused phonation breaks to occur. In Figure 4–14, the voice waveform shows that there is substantially more cycle-to-cycle deviation in profile than

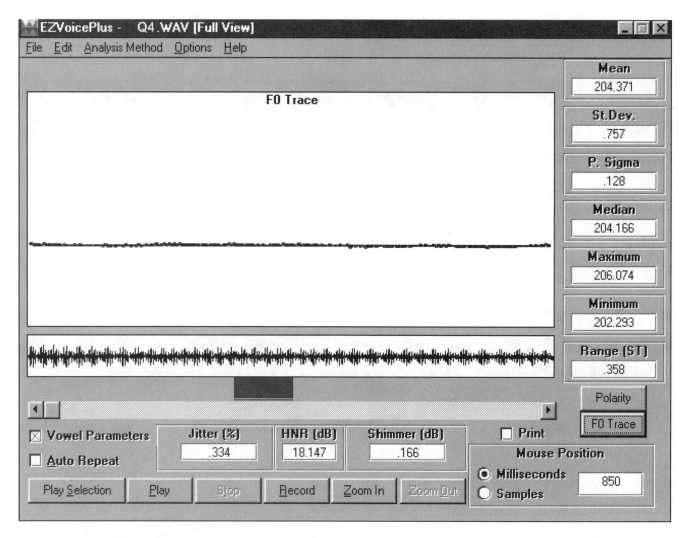

Figure 4–11 Frequency and Perturbation Analysis for a Sustained Vowel from a Normal Adult Woman

was observed in the previous example of mild breathiness. Each cycle has a "jagged" appearance that is due to the addition of substantial amounts of turbulent noise (secondary to increased transglottal airflow) to the periodic voice signal.

Computation of the F_0 contour, associated F_0 statistics, and measures of perturbation and noise are shown in Figure 4–15.

This moderately hoarse-breathy voice has substantially greater jitter than expected (3.003%), as well as a much lower HNR than expected (9.039 dB). Shimmer (0.249 dB) has remained within normal limits, perhaps because the increased flow of air through this patient's glottis has remained relatively constant. Again, this patient's F_0 standard deviation is elevated (greater than 1% of the mean F_0); this high degree of average variability is clearly reflected in a F_0 trace/contour that has a "splintered" appearance.

Sample Characteristic of Combined Hypoadduction and Hyperfunction: Moderate Hoarseness (Continuous Speech Segment)

Vocal quality should be judged not just from sustained vowels but from continuous speech as well. To illustrate this point, we will next examine a continuous speech segment from a patient who presented with a moderate degree of hoarseness.

✎ In this step, we will be analyzing the file Q7.WAV. If you click on the file name using the L. mouse button, you will hear a continuous speech segment (second sentence of "The Rainbow Passage") for the same adult female analyzed in the previous example. This patient's voice had been characterized as having a moderate degree of hoarseness (stronger

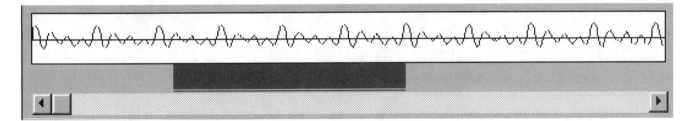

Figure 4–12 Close-up of the Acoustic Waveform for a Mild Breathy Voice Sample

breathy component) as a result of chronic laryngitis. The quality was deemed to be highly noticeable during her phonation and occasionally caused phonation breaks to occur. You will hear phonation cease prematurely during production of the last word of the sentence ("colors"). The patient's voice also has an effortful quality to it. It is the combination of hypoadduction and hyperfunction (perhaps compensatory in nature) that results in the perceived hoarse quality.

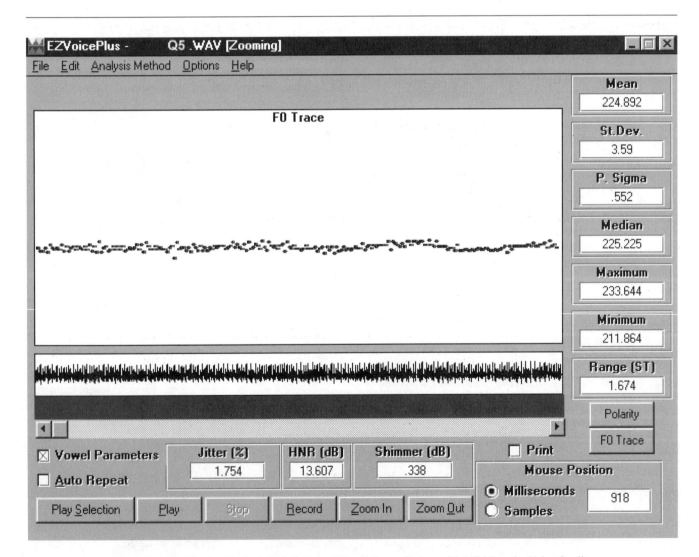

Figure 4–13 Frequency and Perturbation Analysis for a Sustained Vowel from a Patient with Mild Breathy Voice Quality

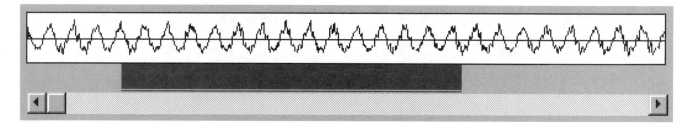

Figure 4–14 Close-up of the Acoustic Waveform for a Moderate Breathy Voice Sample

Although fundamental frequency analysis has been addressed in greater depth elsewhere is this book, we will examine the F_0 contour so that the absence of F_0 information during the phonation break segment can be observed.

Computation of the F_0 contour and associated F_0 statistics are shown in Figure 4–16. Measures of perturbation and noise will not be conducted in this sample because factors such as natural voiced/voiceless distinctions and the pres-

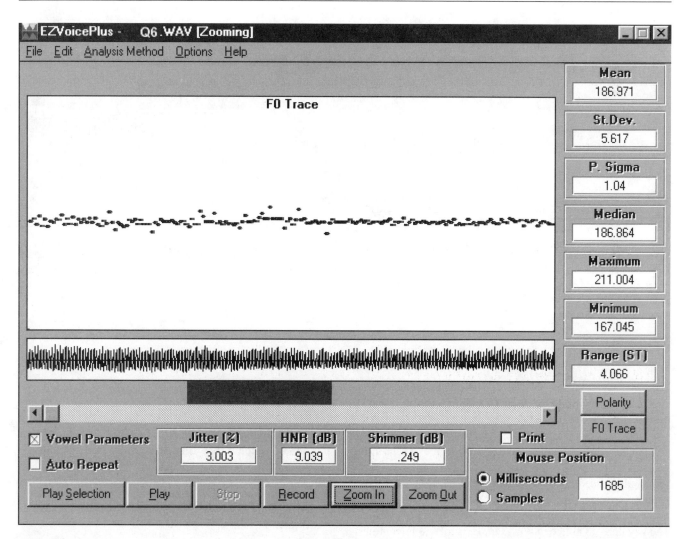

Figure 4–15 Frequency and Perturbation Analysis for a Sustained Vowel from a Patient with a Moderate Degree of Hoarse Voice Quality (Strong Breathy Component)

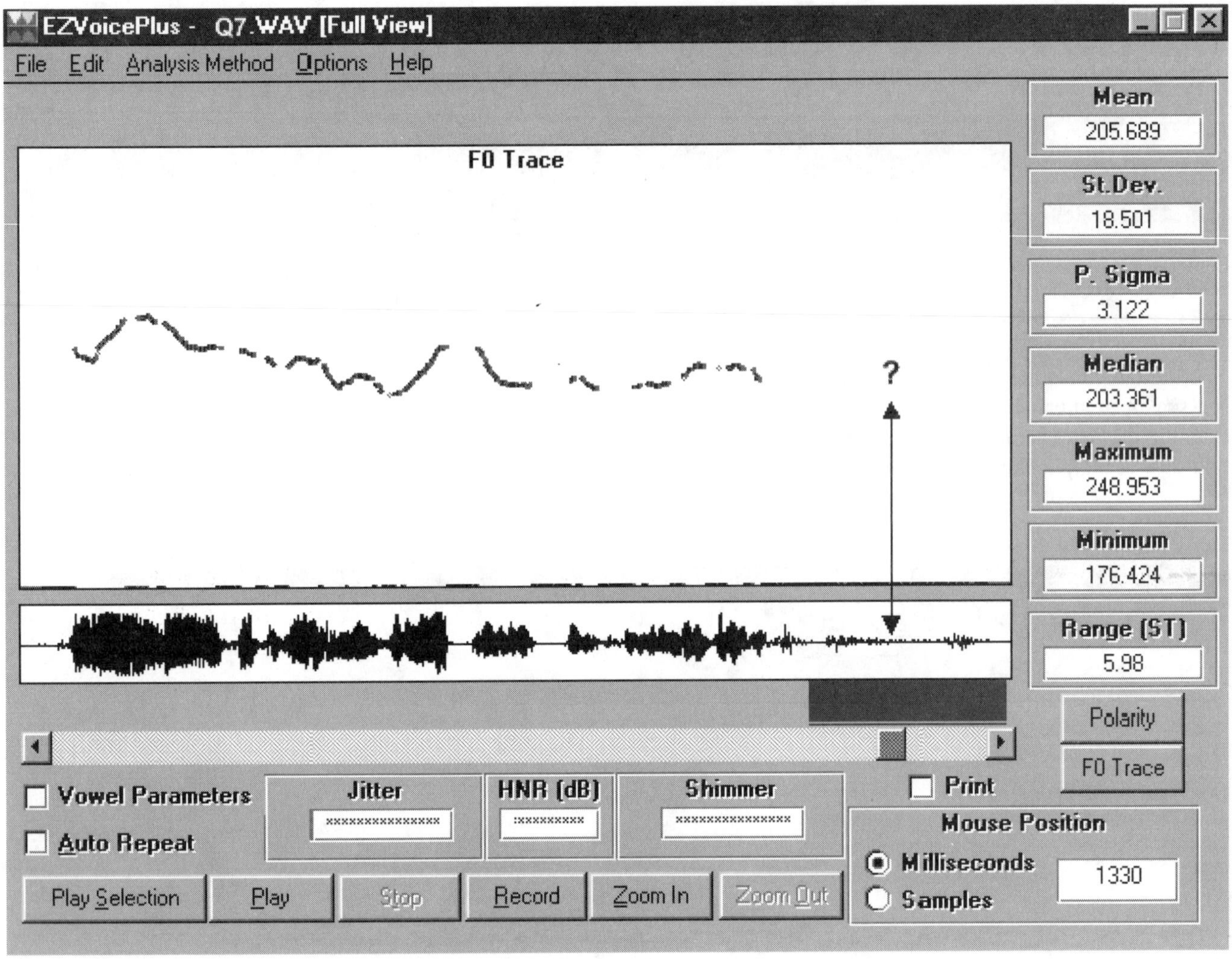

Figure 4–16 Frequency Contour and Associated Statistics for a Continuous Speech Sample Analysis from a Patient with a Moderate Degree of Hoarse Voice Quality (Strong Breathy Component). The arrow indicates a portion of the sentence in which a phonation break (intermittent aphonia) occurred. The computer program has not calculated a F_0 contour for the aphonic portion because no periodic pattern in the voice waveform could be identified.

ence of frequency and amplitude variations during intonation patterns could invalidate measures of jitter, shimmer, and HNR.

Note that the F_0 contour shows a great degree of variation in it compared with what we have observed in sustained vowel analysis. This is to be expected because there are natural variations in frequency and amplitude (i.e., intonation patterns) that accompany continuous speech production. The key thing to notice in this example is that no F_0 contour was computed for the final word of the sentence ("colors") because the patient has a phonation break on this word,

resulting in aphonic production. The patient was characterized as moderate in terms of severity because of (1) breathy-hoarse quality that was highly noticeable and (2) occasional periods of aphonia that affected her ability to effectively communicate.

Sample Characteristic of Hyperadduction: Mild-to-Moderate Roughness (Sustained Vowel Production)

✎ Click on the file Q8.WAV using the L. mouse button; you will hear a sample of an adult male who had been diagnosed with a unilateral vocal polyp sustaining the vowel /ɑ/. This patient's voice had been characterized as having a mild-to-moderate degree of roughness; although his quality deviation was quite noticeable, it was intermittent in nature. Listen closely to the end portion of his sustained vowel; you will hear an improved quality emerge in his voice as he nears the end of the phonation. In particular, the patient has a diplophonic (i.e., double pitch) quality to his voice that contributes to the rough quality and also gives the perception of a lower pitch.

Computation of the F_0 contour, associated F_0 statistics, and measures of perturbation and noise are shown in Figure 4–17.

We see that both jitter (2.58%) and shimmer (0.422 dB) are elevated in this patient's voice, reflecting the underlying cycle-to-cycle frequency and amplitude perturbation. The overall HNR (12.465 dB) is somewhat low compared with normal expectations (15 to 20 dB). In addition, the F_0 standard deviation is substantially higher than the 1% or less of the mean F_0 often seen in normal sustained vowel productions. All these measures reflect the perception of a disordered voice. However, there are two acoustic characteristics of this rough voice that were not observed in the previous breathy examples. First of all, two very distinct frequencies are present in the F_0 trace/contour versus the consistent "splintered" look of the breathy voice F_0 contours. This

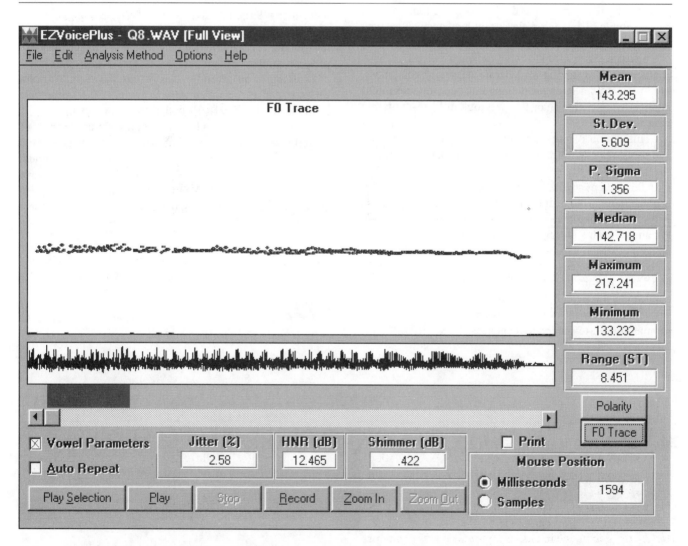

Figure 4–17 Frequency and Perturbation Analysis for a Sustained Vowel from a Patient with a Mild-to-Moderate Degree of Rough Voice Quality. Note that the F_0 contour stabilizes near the end of the phonation, corresponding with improvement in voice quality.

shows us the diplophonic component of the voice, often a key characteristic of rough quality. The second characteristic is observed in Figure 4–18, in which we see a close-up view of several individual cycles of the voice signal corresponding with a section of a diplophonic section of the F_0 contour.

In Figure 4–18, we see that the individual cycles of vibration are highly variable in terms of profile. In addition, the cycle-to-cycle amplitude varies such that large versus small amplitude peaks alternate throughout sections of the waveform. This may be evidence of a subharmonic, in which the periodicity of the voice waveform actually occurs every second or third cycle rather in a cycle-to-cycle manner.

Sample Characteristic of Hyperadduction: Moderate Roughness (Sustained Vowel Production)

In this step, we will be analyzing the file Q9.WAV. If you click on the file name using the L. mouse button, you will hear a sample of an adult male sustaining the vowel /ɑ/ who had been diagnosed with L. vocal fold weakness as a result of neck trauma and MTD. This patient's voice had been characterized as having a moderate degree of roughness. This patient as a stronger diplophonic (i.e., double pitch) quality to his voice than the previous mild-to-moderate patient.

Computation of the F_0 contour, associated F_0 statistics, and measures of perturbation and noise are shown in Figure 4–19.

In this patient's voice sample, the diplophonic component is much more prominent than in the previous patient's voice, with the two frequencies of vibration (approximately 156 Hz and 170 Hz) clearly shown as two distinct F_0 traces/contours. All the measures of perturbation are considerably higher than expected (jitter = 6.181%; shimmer = 0.568 dB), and HNR is considerably lower than expected (9.06 dB), confirming the perceptual judgment that this voice sample shows an increased severity of disruption than the previous sample of mild-to-moderate roughness.

Sample Characteristic of Hyperadduction: Severe Roughness (Sustained Vowel Production)

Click on the file Q10.WAV using the L. mouse button; you will hear a sample of an adult female patient who had been diagnosed with functional dysphonia. Her voice quality was judged to be severe, because the quality deviation was highly noticeable, disruptive of communication, and judged to be extremely effortful.

Computation of the F_0 contour, associated F_0 statistics, and measures of perturbation and noise are shown in Figure 4–20.

In this sample, the periodicity of the voice signal has become so disrupted that the computer program has had a great deal of difficulty identifying any cyclic behavior. This has resulted in a F_0 trace/contour that is highly variable. Measures of perturbation and noise reflect the perception of a severe voice disorder, with all measures highly abnormal (jitter = 9.653%; HNR = –0.625 dB; shimmer = 3.318 dB). The negative HNR indicates that the amplitude of the inharmonic (i.e., aperiodic) component is greater than any periodic component that may be present.

Zooming in on several cycles of this waveform shows a series of pulses occurring approximately 20 ms intervals apart (see Figure 4–21). However, there is no definitive pattern of vibration; each pulse looks quite different in terms of overall profile. In addition, each pulse is actually composed of a series of peaks, many of which are similar in amplitude. The characteristics of this severely rough voice waveform have made it difficult for the computer program to identify any consistent periodic component. Any estimates that have been made are extremely variable in nature.

It has been said that traditional measures of perturbation and noise (such as jitter, shimmer, and HNR) may not be valid with severely dysphonic voices (Bielamowicz et al., 1996; Rabinov et al., 1995). However, this example illustrates that, *if a computer algorithm has been demonstrated to be effective at identifying cyclic behavior in most voice signals analyzed (normal and near-normal samples), its*

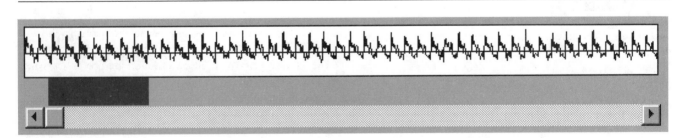

Figure 4–18 A Close-up View of Several Cycles of the Diplophonic Portion of This Patient's Vowel Sample. Note how the cycle-to-cycle amplitude alternates throughout this waveform (perhaps indicative of a subharmonic).

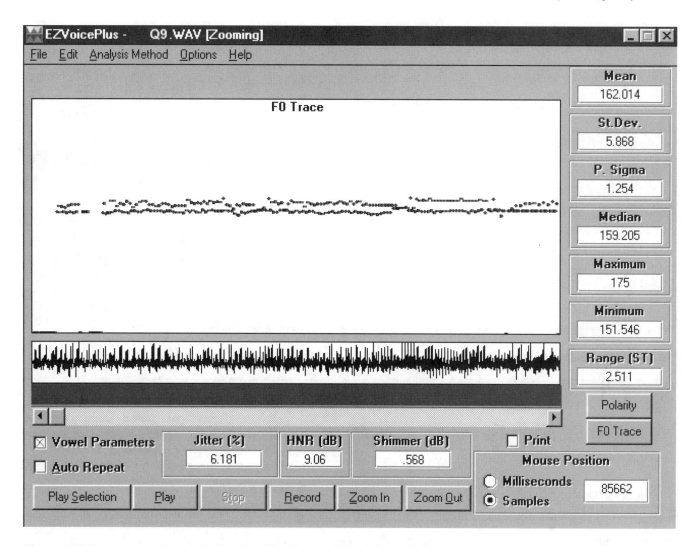

Figure 4–19 Frequency and Perturbation Analysis for a Sustained Vowel from a Patient with a Moderate Degree of Rough Voice Quality. Note the consistent "double pitch" (diplophonia) evident in the F_0 contour.

apparent ineffectiveness at dealing with severely disrupted signals is informative in itself. The fact that a computer program appears to be having trouble identifying periodicity in a voice waveform should alert the clinician (and probably confirm his or her judgment) that there is some type of severe deviation from the norm in the voice signal under analysis.

Sample Characteristic of Extreme Hyperfunction: Instability and Effort (Sustained Vowel Production)

In this chapter on voice quality deviations, it was indicated that quality could be disturbed in ways other than breathiness, harshness/roughness, or hoarseness. In the final example for this tutorial, we shall examine a voice sample that demonstrates vocal instability and strain/effort.

Click on the file Q11.WAV using the L. mouse button; you will hear a sample of an adult female patient who had been diagnosed with spasmodic dysphonia (adductor type). Her voice quality was judged to be severe (obtrusive voice quality deviation, highly effortful, phonation absent at times because of extreme hyperadduction), with instability present. In this particular voice sample, you can hear that the initiation of the phonation has much better quality (although still deviant) than the mid-to-end of the production. By the end of this sample, you will hear a strained-strangled quality in the patient's voice.

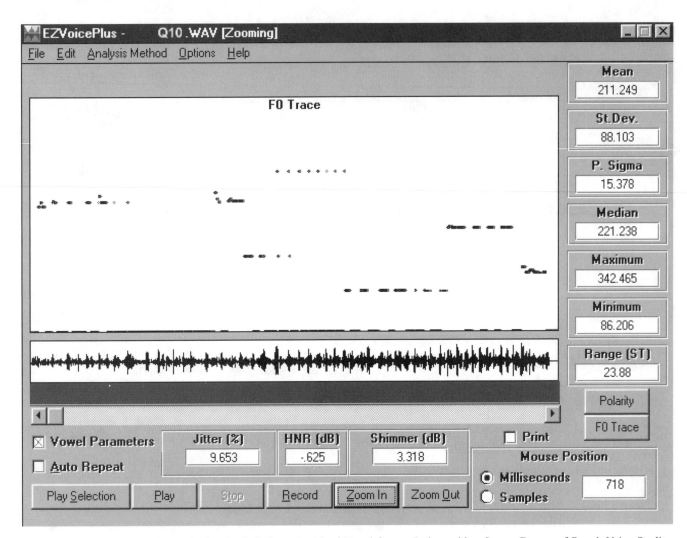

Figure 4–20 Frequency and Perturbation Analysis for a Sustained Vowel from a Patient with a Severe Degree of Rough Voice Quality. The extreme variability in the F_0 contour (highly abnormal jitter, shimmer, and HNR measurements) reflects the extreme aperiodicity in this voice sample.

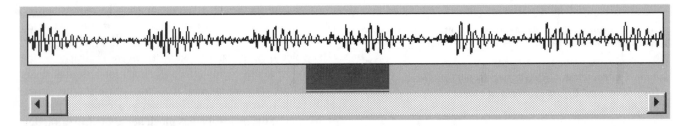

Figure 4–21 A Close-up View of Several Cycles of the Vowel Sample from a Severely Rough Voice. The waveform shows no definitive repeating pattern of vibration.

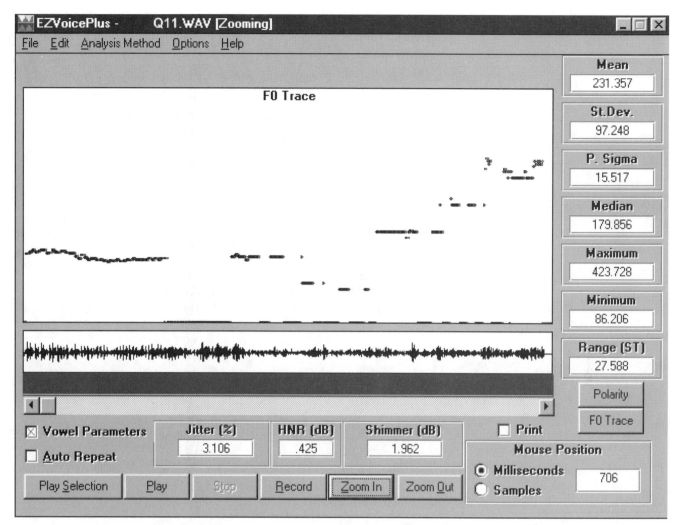

Figure 4–22 Frequency and Perturbation Analysis for a Sustained Vowel from a Patient with Adductor Spasmodic Dysphonia. Instability of phonation is evident, with a relatively stable F_0 contour (reflecting relatively periodic vibration) observed at the beginning of the phonation transforming into a highly disrupted contour (reflecting aperiodic voicing during the "strained-strangled" portion of the vowel) near the end of the production.

Computation of the F_0 contour, associated F_0 statistics, and measures of perturbation and noise are shown in Figure 4–22.

The relatively smooth F_0 trace/contour confirms improved periodicity of phonation at the start of the sample. However, the strained-strangled portion of the sample shows the same extreme variability in vibratory behavior as was observed in the previous severely rough patient. As expected, measures of perturbation and noise are all substantially different from normal expectations (confirming the perception of a severe disorder). However, the key characteristics to note in this sample are (1) the instability of phonation (i.e., highly variable) and (2) the extreme amount of perceived strain/effort in the patient's voice.

CHAPTER 5

Evaluation of Duration: Respiratory/Phonatory Control

DEFINITION

During continuous speech production or sustained vowel production (e.g., in singing), coordinated function of the respiratory and phonatory mechanisms is essential. To extend the duration of phonatory activity, the following key activities must be successfully carried out:

- An increase (slight to substantial) in inspiratory air.
- Production of the outgoing (expiratory) airstream using checking action (activity in which inspiratory muscle forces are used to counteract or "check" passive expiratory forces [Zemlin, 1988]).
- For voiced productions, the vocal folds must adduct and approximate at the midline of the glottis. This action serves to (1) generate and control subglottal pressure required to put the vocal folds into vibration and (2) also aids in control and conservation of the outgoing airstream.

If the ability to generate and control the outgoing airstream is disrupted, the following noticeable effects on speech production may be observed:

- An inability to maintain appropriate duration of respiratory/phonatory function, resulting in inappropriate phrase length and inappropriate breath groups
- Effortful speech/voice function as a result of excessive muscular force to compensate for poor respiratory/phonatory control and function
- Eventual fatigue

In this chapter, we will focus on perceptual and quantitative methods that assess the durational aspects of the speech/voice signal. The ability to coordinate respiratory and laryngeal mechanisms to sustain voicing and control utterance duration is an essential aspect of normal voice/speech function.

PERCEPTUAL ASSESSMENT OF THE DURATIONAL ASPECTS OF SPEECH/VOICE

In the normal voice, the speaker must be able to produce sufficient airflow to effect efficient phonation within an utterance. The termination of a sentence or phrase should coincide with the termination of exhalation (Prater & Swift, 1984). When respiratory support is inadequate or uncontrolled by adequate laryngeal valving, the patient may not be able to sustain speech/voice function adequately, with the following possible results:

- The patient needs to breathe (inspire) more frequently, resulting in fewer words or syllables per breath groups (inappropriately short utterances) and/or inappropriate breath groups (i.e., pauses for inspiration occur at illogical places in the utterance).
- In the absence of adequate respiratory support, the patient attempts to build subglottal pressure and sustain voicing by increased musculoskeletal tension and hyperfunctional voice.
- The patient who attempts to continue speaking on residual air often leaves the listener with the impression of a tense, effortful voice production.

HOW TO DO IT: PERCEPTUAL ASSESSMENT OF THE DURATIONAL ASPECTS OF SPEECH/ VOICE

The durational aspects of speech/voicing may be observed from a standard reading, as well as from conversational speech. In particular, the clinician should rate utterance length. The durational characteristics of the utterance may be scaled on a categorical/equal-appearing interval (EAI) scale such as:

-3	-2	-1	0	+1	+2	+3

| Severe | Moderate | Mild | Normal Duration | Mild | Moderate | Severe |

| Short Utterances with Frequent Respiratory Replenishment per Utterance | | | | Speech beyond the Point of Expected Respiratory Replenishment |

Although the scale incorporates 7 points, note that the central point of the scale is zero (i.e., no substantial difference from normal expectations), with ratings of utterance duration beyond the point of expected respiratory replenishment (positive numbers) and ratings of inappropriately short breath groups (negative numbers) rated on either side of the normal expectation point. Definitions for mild, moderate, and severe are the same as those presented in the Introduction (Chapter 1). In addition to noting the length of utterance in relation to expected point of inspiration, the clinician should also note perceptions of tension/effort (particularly on the "+" side of the scale) and signs of laryngeal hypofunction (particularly on the "−" side of the scale [e.g., breathy voice]). Inhalatory stridor (excessive noise during inspiration [Prater & Swift, 1984]) is a particularly important observation, because it is associated with narrowing/stenosis of the airway (Colton & Casper, 1996).

A key observation that must be made during the patient's conversational speech and/or reading sample is the type of respiratory pattern the patient uses. Deviations from normal (i.e., appropriate coincidence of utterance length, expiratory airflow, and efficient phonation) in either direction on our perceptual scale may be due to an underlying inefficient respiratory pattern or a lack of coordination between inspiratory and expiratory movements. Three basic types of respiratory pattern have been described.

Clavicular Breathing

This type of breathing pattern mainly uses the secondary/accessory muscles of respiration (upper thoracic and neck muscles such as the scalenes and the sternocleidomastoid [Zemlin, 1988]) to elevate the shoulders and upper chest during inspiration. This type of breathing pattern results in a weak, shallow inspiration and, therefore, poor respiratory support for speech and voice. In addition, because many of

these muscles course in the vicinity of the larynx, overuse of these muscles may effect an increase in laryngeal tension (Prater & Swift, 1984). According to Haynes et al. (1992), many hyperfunctional voice cases use this inefficient form of breathing.

Thoracic Breathing

This type of breathing has been described as being "somewhere between clavicular and diaphragmatic-abdominal breathing" (Boone & McFarlane, 1988, p. 100) and is characterized by expansion of the midthoracic region (Colton & Casper, 1996; Prater & Swift, 1984). In thoracic breathing "expansion of the chest, not the shoulders, in a slight heaving motion is more observable…" (Haynes et al., 1992, p. 297). This is a commonly used breathing pattern that should be adequate to support most speaking situations. It may not be sufficient to support the demands of the actor or singer (Prater & Swift, 1984).

Diaphragmatic-Abdominal Breathing

In this breathing pattern, thoracic enlargement is achieved by expansion of the lower thoracic and abdominal cavities during inspiration. Little noticeable upper chest movement will be noticed in this pattern (Boone & McFarlane, 1988). Diaphragmatic-abdominal breathing allows for the greatest exchange of air during the respiratory cycle, while being a mechanically efficient form of breathing (Prater & Swift, 1984). However, voice patients should not necessarily be required to learn this breathing pattern; it is particularly useful for those who make heavy demands on the respiratory system for singing, acting, etc. (Boone & McFarlane, 1988; Prater & Swift, 1984).

Reading a Standard Passage on One Breath

In addition to noting the type of respiratory pattern, it is also important for the clinician to observe the coordination between expiration and the onset of phonation. The control of expiratory airflow and generation of adequate subglottal pressure for phonation depend to a large degree on the coordination between laryngeal valving and expiration. If adequate laryngeal valving does not take place, air loss can occur, and the patient may respond to this by altering the durational aspects of speech and voice. Prater and Swift (1984) state that poor respiratory/phonatory coordination may occur as a result of (1) neurological disorders and (2) poorly learned speaking patterns. The patient's ability to control and coordinate expiratory and phonatory functions may be observed by having him or her read as much of a standard passage as possible in one breath at a normal/acceptable reading rate (normal adult speaking rate is approximately 150 to 200 words per minute or approximately 3 to 5 syllables per second [Dworkin, 1991]). This task provides the clinician an indication of adequacy of both respiratory support and control of the expiratory airflow in a continuous speech task. Prater and Swift (1984) suggest that the number of words and the length of time (in seconds) be recorded. Because reading rate would clearly affect results, it is suggested that reading rate be governed by a metronome beat and/or by example of the clinician. In addition to number of words and sample time, Prater and Swift (1984) state that (1) the respiratory pattern should be noted and (2) the degree of phonatory control (hypofunctional, hyperfunctional, etc.) should also be noted during the task.

5 FOR 5 TESTING

Hixon, Hawley, and Wilson (1982) described the construction of a simple device by which an estimate of the patient's ability to generate respiratory driving force could be obtained. This method is included in this section because the method emphasizes the clinician's judgment regarding the patient's capability to maintain a steady respiratory force during the task.

HOW TO DO IT: 5 FOR 5 TESTING

The materials below are required to construct Hixon et al.'s (1982) respiratory pressure indication device.

- A transparent drinking glass.
- A strip of adhesive tape (that can be written on) approximately as long as the glass is tall. This strip of tape should be marked in 1-cm increments.
- A drinking straw (with a flexible/bendable tip or accordion-style elbow).
- A large paper clip.

Figure 5–1 shows an example of what the pressure-indicating device should look like after construction.

To construct the device and carry out 5 for 5 testing, use the steps below.

1. Attach the tape to the side of the drinking glass in a vertical orientation so that the first 1-cm increment on the tape is approximately 1 cm down from the rim of the glass. Mark this increment as "0" (zero) and each increment proceeding toward the bottom of the glass in ascending numerical order (1, 2, 3…).
2. Fill the glass with water up to the "0" mark.
3. Slip the barrel of the straw through one loop of the paper clip.
4. Place the straw into the water. Slide the paper clip over the edge of the glass so that the straw

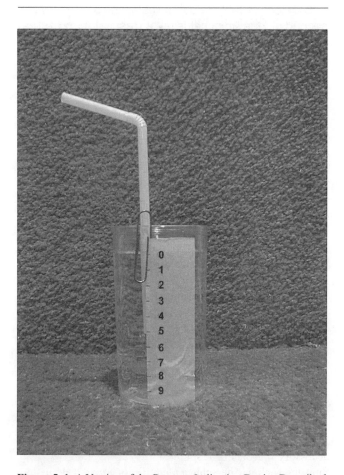

Figure 5–1 A Version of the Pressure Indicating Device Described by Hixon, Hawley, and Wilson (1982). The adhesive tape on the side of the glass is marked in 1-cm increments. Water is filled to the 0-cm mark. The submerged end of the bendable straw is placed at the 5-cm mark.

can be suspended at various depths within the water.

5. Lower the end of the straw so that the end is 5 cm deep in the water.
6. Give your patient the following instructions: "I want you to blow gently and steadily through the straw so that you can produce a steady stream of bubbles in the water. Keep blowing until I tell you to stop."
7. Time your patient carrying out the blowing task for at least 5 seconds.

When the end of the straw is 5 cm below the surface of the water, a pressure of at least 5 cm H_2O must be generated by the patient to create a bubble in the liquid. The capability to generate and sustain 5 cm H_2O for 5 seconds (i.e., "5 for 5") is believed to reflect sufficient pressure-generation capability and control for most speech situations (Hixon et al., 1982). Dworkin and Meleca (1997) state that sustaining 5 cm H_2O for 5 seconds is the "minimal level of (respiratory pressure) needed to support vocal fold vibration" (p. 45). It should be noted that because 5 cm H_2O is a minimal pressure for phonation, even patients with relatively severe voice disorders may be able to achieve this pressure. It may be expected that patients with respiratory dysfunctions may have difficulty with pressure generation for this task (e.g., severe asthma, emphysema, tuberculosis, lung cancer, and neuromuscular disability affecting the respiratory system). In addition, the *control* of a steady respiratory driving force over time may be more likely to be compromised than the actual pressure that can be produced at any point in time. Therefore, during the 5 for 5 task, the clinician should monitor the following:

- The patient's ability to generate the required pressure
- The patient's ability to maintain the required driving force for at least 5 seconds
- The patient's ability to control a steady driving pressure for the required duration (i.e., no sudden drops or rises in pressure generation that may indicate a lack of control over respiratory forces)

QUANTITATIVE EVALUATION OF THE COMPONENTS OF DURATIONAL CONTROL

We have seen that the interaction of expiratory airflow and laryngeal valving allows the speaker to control speech and voice for the variable durations required to complete an intended utterance. In this section, we will discuss several simple objective methods that allow us to quantify several aspects of respiratory/phonatory control. All the tests mentioned in this section of the chapter are referred to as *maximum performance tests* (or are derived from maximum performance tests, as in the case of the S/Z ratio and the Phonation Quotient). The term *maximum performance test* refers to the fact that these tests attempt to assess some of the limits of speech mechanism capability. Although speech performance is generally well within the overall limits of capability, it can be clinically important to assess the extent of the speech resources of a patient. As Kent et al. (1987) point out, "A reduced reserve can impair a talker's flexibility and can also mean that speaking for such an individual is a taxing process" (p. 382).

VITAL CAPACITY

Vital capacity (VC; also known as forced vital capacity [FVC]) is defined as the maximum amount of air that can be exhaled after maximum inhalation. Vital capacity is commonly measured with a spirometer and is generally reported in milliliters (ml) or liters (L). VC is measured as a basic indicator of respiratory ability and indicates that amount of air available for phonation (Andrews, 1995). Although only a portion of VC is used for most speaking situations (Hixon, Goldman, & Mead, 1973), it is important to assess the maximum capabilities of the speech system to determine the system's ability to function under stress (e.g., maximum exhalation, maximum phonation). It is these "stressful" situations and tasks that often (1) reveal underlying deficits possibly responsible for a presenting voice disorder and (2) enable the clinician to discriminate between normal versus disordered speech/voice function. In the case of VC, we also have a simple procedure by which we may be able to rule out any significant respiratory disorder that may be affecting voice (Bless and Hicks [1996] state that one of the main purposes of measuring laryngeal aerodynamics is to differentiate between respiratory and laryngeal problems). Colton and Casper (1996) state that the control of the respiratory capacity during speech may be of more importance than measures of respiratory volumes. However, it would seem that knowledge of the basic capacity of a system is a prerequisite to (1) the assessment of control and (2) the determination of whether it is a factor underlying the patient's voice disorder.

HOW TO DO IT: MEASUREMENT OF VITAL CAPACITY

As previously stated, the most common method for obtaining a measure of VC is to use a spirometer. A number of hand-held spirometers (both digital and analog) are available for relatively low cost (see Figure

5–2). Rau and Beckett (1984) investigated the validity of using portable, hand-held spirometers in the assessment of VC. Data collected from 19 young adult speakers indicated that VC results from hand-held spirometry correlated very strongly (*r*'s from 0.94 to 0.97) with results from wet spirometry. In addition, test-retest reliability was also very strong for hand-held spirometers. Rau and Beckett (1984) concluded that hand-held spirometry could be used to provide valid aerodynamic assessment of vocal function.

Instructions for the measurement of VC are found below.

1. Turn the spirometer on (assuming you are using some type of digital spirometer) and insert a new disposable tube (most spirometers use disposable cardboard mouthpiece tubes for sanitary purposes).
2. Provide the following instructions to the patient: "I want you to take a deep breath and blow out as long and as hard as possible into the spirometer tube." In most cases, the patient should place the tube between the lips and form a tight seal around the tube. The clinician should pay close attention to respiratory movements during this task. Hixon and Hoit (1998) state that extensive outward movement of the rib cage wall and abdominal wall should characterize maximum inspiration (such as that observed during the VC task). The movement of the abdominal wall is moderately fast, smooth, and symmetrical.
3. It is useful to verbally encourage the patient into exhaling as maximally as possible. The patient should probably feel a "tightness" in the chest (particularly near the end of this task) as he or she exhales as long and as hard as possible.
4. Record the patient's VC (in ml or L). Repeat this procedure two more times for a total of three trials minimum. Use the maximum value from the three trials as the patient's VC.

Figure 5–3 provides an example of a clinician eliciting vital capacity from a patient.

Appropriate VC must be interpreted in light of the patient's age, gender, and height. In the event that a spirometer is not available, predictive equations have been developed by Baldwin, Courand, and Richards

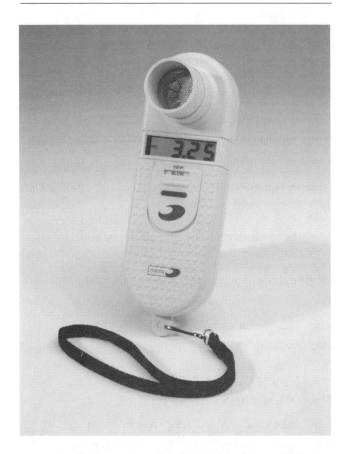

Figure 5–2 Hand-held Digital Spirometer. Courtesy of Micro Medical, Ltd., Kent, England.

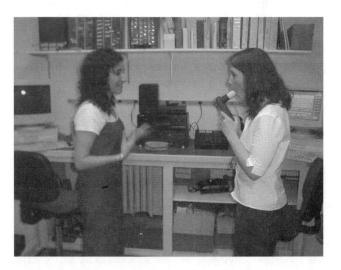

Figure 5–3 Clinician Eliciting Maximum Exhalation during Vital Capacity (VC) Testing. The patient is generally asked to stand for this task.

(1948, in Kent et al., 1987) by which VC may be estimated:

$$VC \text{ (Males)} = (27.63 - 0.112 \times Age) \times Height$$

$$VC \text{ (Females)} = (27.78 - 0.101 \times Age) \times Height$$

An alternative formula by Dockery, Ware, Ferris, Glicksberg, Spiro, and Speizer (1985) is:

$$FVC = HT^2 (1.75 - 0.287 \text{ } Sex - 0.000135 \text{ } Age - 0.0001008 \text{ } Age^2)$$

where FVC is in liters; HT is in meters; age is in years; and sex = 0 for men and 1 for women. These VC prediction formulas should be used with caution because considerable difference may exist between estimated and actual VC (Kent et al., 1987).

WHAT TO EXPECT: NORMAL VOICE

Gender

During early childhood, males and females may be expected to be quite similar in terms of VC. However, as children approach and then complete puberty, increased VC is generally observed in males versus females. Trullinger and Emanuel (1989) observed overall mean vital capacity to be significantly greater in 8- to 10-year-old males versus females (2.16 L vs. 1.88 L). Of course, body size/type must always be taken into account when judging the normalcy of VC. In addition, factors such as extensive athletic experience (e.g., swimmers), formal singing training, or extensive musical experience with woodwinds or brass instruments may also result in increases in normal VC.

In general, adult men are expected to have a VC in the range of 4 to 5 L, whereas adult women may be expected to have VCs in the 3 to 4 L range (Case, 1996; Prater & Swift, 1984). Data from several studies that support this conclusion are presented in Table 5–1. Enright, Vaz Fragoso, and Sly (1996) indicate that normal VC should be greater than 80% of the predicted value. Predicted values may be computed by use of the aforementioned formulas of Baldwin et al. (1948) or Dockery et al. (1985). Kent et al. (1987) caution that there is a tremendous amount of variation in normative values for VC, as well as for other pulmonary measures, making clinical interpretations problematic.

Aging

Advancement of the aging process may be observed to have a substantial effect on VC. In a study of young (<40 years old) versus elderly men (>65 years old), Ptacek et al. (1966) observed the geriatric men to have significantly lower VCs than the younger subjects (mean VC: 3.1 L vs.

4.8 L). Ptacek et al. (1966) attributed the decrease in VC to a decrease in the power of the respiratory muscles and loss of elasticity in lung tissue. Similar findings were observed for women in a study by Awan and Ziminsky-Ammon (1996), who reported a significant reduction in VC in postmenopausal women, with 18- to 30- and 40- to 49-year-old groups observed to produce significantly greater VCs than 50- to 59-, 60- to 69-, and 70- to 79-year-old groups. In addition, a strong inverse correlation between age and VC ($r = -0.81$; $p < .001$) was also reported (see Figure 5–4). In Figure 5–5, the mean VC of the young adult group (18 to 30 years of age) minus 2 standard deviations was used as a value to judge VC change for the older subjects (i.e., Z-scores were calculated for each subject using the mean and standard deviation of the young adult female group as the control group). Results show increasing percentages of each aging group with subjects producing mean VCs substantially lower than the mean VC of the young adult group.

Table 5–1 presents a range of examples of VC elicited from normal voice subjects.

WHAT TO EXPECT: ABNORMAL VOICE

Most patients with voice disorders will show adequate respiratory capacity as reflected in measures of VC. We are conducting VC testing primarily to *rule out* any significant reduction in respiratory capacity. However, reduced vital capacity may be observed in patients with the following characteristics (Aronson, 1990a; Dworkin, 1991):

1. Patients with pulmonary diseases that increase airway resistance (e.g., severe asthma, emphysema, tuberculosis).
2. Patients with diseases that reduce the elasticity and compliance of the lungs and chest wall (e.g, asbestosis, pneumonia, lung cancer).
3. Patients who may be using inefficient breathing patterns (shallow breathing or clavicular breathing).
4. Patients with neuromuscular disorders may also present with reduced respiratory capacity. All major groups of dysarthria (spastic, ataxic, hyperkinetic, hypokinetic, and flaccid) may have shallow inhalations. In addition, poor respiratory postures, incoordinated inspiratory-expiratory patterns, and rigidity of the respiratory musculature may also result in reduced capacity.

MAXIMUM PHONATION TIME

The maximum phonation time (MPT) (also known as the maximum phonation duration [MPD]) adds phonation to a task similar in nature to the aforementioned procedures used to elicit VC. Prater and Swift (1984) state that the MPT may

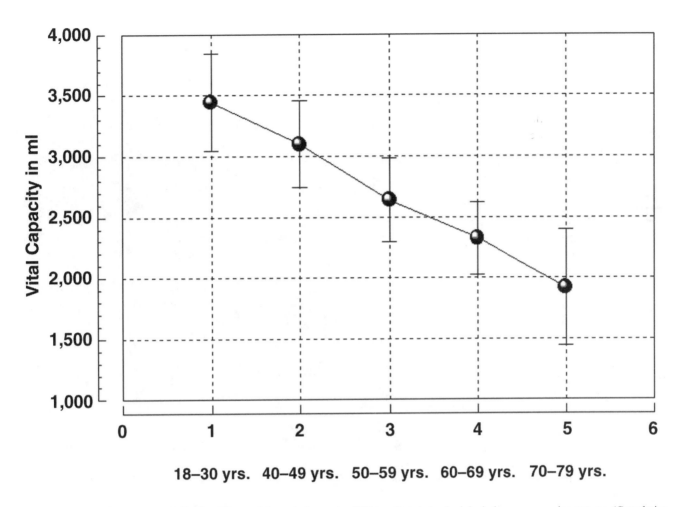

18–30 yrs.   40–49 yrs.   50–59 yrs.   60–69 yrs.   70–79 yrs.

Figure 5–4 Mean Vital Capacity of Aging Women. Mean vital capacity (VC in ml) and standard deviations across aging groups. (Correlation between aging and vital capacity: $r = -0.81$, $p < .001$.)

be used "as a measure of the efficiency of glottal closure and efficiency of the respiratory system" (p. 39). As with VC, the MPT is a maximum performance test meant to assess the limits of respiratory/phonatory function. As such, it may reveal weaknesses not apparent at lower levels of functioning (Colton & Casper, 1996). Tanaka, Hirano, and Terasawa (1991) have indicated that the MPT directly relates to the inconvenience of voice disorders and is one of the most sensitive tasks to phonatory dysfunction.

Methodological Considerations

A number of studies as shown below have examined effects of factors such as number of trials, task instructions, and coaching of the subjects.

- Shanks and Mast (1977) investigated methodological variables influencing MPT in 30 male and 30 female subjects between the ages of 20 and 25 years. Patients were asked to sustain the vowel /ɑ/ for as long as possible at a comfortable pitch and loudness. Ten trials were elicited from each subject. Results showed that the duration of MPTs was not significantly different across trials. However, increased variability in MPT was observed with more trials. In addition, MPTs did not increase significantly after three trials. Shanks and Mast (1977) suggest the use of four trials of MPT with the first trial ignored.
- Neiman and Edeson (1981) examined the effects of modeling on MPT productions in 20 male and 20 female subjects. Subjects were asked to produce 15

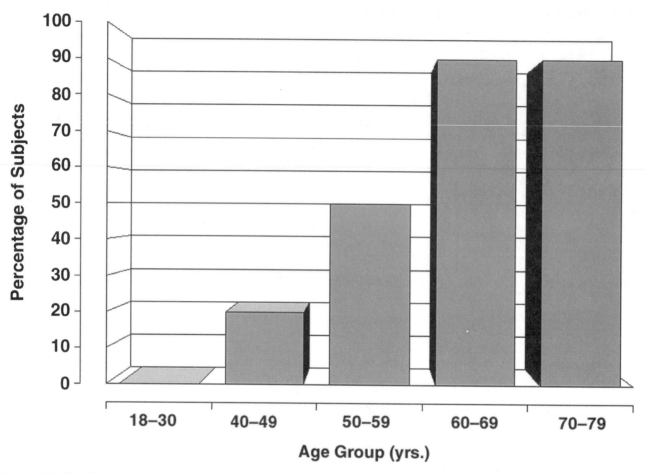

Figure 5–5 Vital Capacity. Percentage of subjects per aging female group with mean pitch sigma ≤2 standard deviations below the mean vital capacity (VC) of the young adult female group. (Percentage of subjects with Z-scores ≤ –2.0 re: young adult comparisons [18–30 yr.])

trials of MPT using the vowel /ɑ/ with a 10 s rest between trials. Subjects were cued to prolong the sustained vowel production for a longer duration with each subsequent trial. In addition, a subgroup of the subjects was also provided with a clinician demonstration (modeling). Results indicated that the modeled subjects achieved MPT at a significantly earlier trial than the unmodeled subjects. Fifty percent of the modeled group achieved MPT by the third trial versus only 10% in the unmodeled group. In addition, the modeled group reached 90% of MPT by the third trial and showed decreased variability compared with the unmodeled group. The authors concluded that (1) all subjects should receive verbal and visual modeling before eliciting MPT; (2) at least three trials should be elicited; and (3) instructions should be standardized across subjects.

- Lewis, Casteel, and McMahon (1982) examined the effect of 20 trials on MPT in 40 prepubescent children. Results showed that only 1 of the 40 subjects produced their maximum MPT in three trials; 50% of their subjects needed 14 trials to achieve MPT. On the basis of their findings, Lewis et al. (1982) believed that three trials would be inadequate in the elicitation of MPT.
- In a study of the effects of multiple trials on MPT, Stone (1983) observed increases in MPT up to the 15th trial in 21 adult subjects. The author concluded that early trials of the MPT task may not actually elicit the maximum performance of the subject and that the MPT task may be susceptible to a strong practice effect.
- Finnegan (1984) studied the effects of multiple trials on MPT in 286 male and female children (age 3.6 to 17.11 years.). In this study, the maximally sustained vowel

Table 5–1 Vital Capacity (in Liters) from Normal Voice Subjects

Author	Gender	No. of Subjects	Age (yr.)	Mean & SD	Range
Ptacek et al. (1966)	M	31	18–39 ($\bar{x} = 27.6$)	4.80 (0.60)	3.40–6.00
	M	27	68–89 ($\bar{x} = 76.9$)	3.10 (0.70)	2.00–4.80
	F	31	18–38 ($\bar{x} = 23.5$)	3.50 (0.60)	2.40–4.60
	F	35	66–93 ($\bar{x} = 76.9$)	1.90 (0.40)	1.10–2.90
Yanagihara et al. (1966)	M	11	30–43 ($\bar{x} = 36.0$)	4.73 (0.65)	3.86–5.76
	F	11	21–41 ($\bar{x} = 28.0$)	3.63 (0.38)	3.10–4.30
Ramig & Ringel (1983)[a]	$M_{Y,G}$	8	26–35 ($\bar{x} = 29.5$)	5.16	4.52–6.47
	$M_{Y,P}$	8	25–38 ($\bar{x} = 32.3$)	5.04	3.77–6.25
	$M_{M,G}$	8	46–56 ($\bar{x} = 53.0$)	5.02	4.16–7.30
	$M_{M,P}$	8	42–59 ($\bar{x} = 52.6$)	4.26	3.23–6.00
	$M_{O,G}$	8	62–75 ($\bar{x} = 67.5$)	3.97	2.68–5.05
	$M_{O,P}$	8	64–74 ($\bar{x} = 69.1$)	3.41	2.03–4.26
Rau & Beckett (1984)	M	10	19–28 ($\bar{x} = 21.10$)	4.18 (0.87)	3.10–6.15
	F	9	21–29 ($\bar{x} = 24.33$)	3.02 (0.32)	2.42–3.37
Reich & McHenry (1987)[b]	F	5	16.50–18.50 ($\bar{x} = 17.8$)	3.42 (0.30)	3.04–3.73
Trullinger & Emanuel (1989)	M	5	8.1–8.11	1.82 (0.38)	1.22–2.38
	F	5	8.1–8.11	1.79 (0.23)	1.56–2.16
	M	5	9.0–9.10	2.22 (0.57)	1.50–2.93
	F	5	9.0–9.10	1.88 (0.12)	1.68–2.04
	M	5	10.1–10.9	2.42 (0.57)	1.55–2.73
	F	5	10.1–10.9	1.96 (0.24)	1.72–2.42
Sperry & Klich (1992)[c]	F_Y	9	20–28 ($\bar{x} = 23.6$)	3.36 (0.62)	N/A
	F_O	9	62–70 ($\bar{x} = 65.5$)	2.46 (0.58)	N/A
Awan & Ziminsky-Ammon (1996)	F	10	18–30 ($\bar{x} = 23.80$)	3.45 (0.40)	2.95–4.00
	F	10	40–49 ($\bar{x} = 43.40$)	3.10 (0.42)	2.50–3.75
	F	10	50–59 ($\bar{x} = 54.80$)	2.64 (0.35)	2.25–3.20
	F	10	60–69 ($\bar{x} = 65.20$)	2.33 (0.30)	1.70–2.65
	F	10	70–79 ($\bar{x} = 72.30$)	1.92 (0.48)	1.10–2.80
Author	M	37	18–30 ($\bar{x} = 23.94$)	4.63 (0.51)	3.65–6.05
	M	14	31–77 ($\bar{x} = 52.05$)	3.89 (0.83)	1.64–5.00
	F	6	8–13 ($\bar{x} = 10.28$)	2.01 (0.60)	1.45–3.11
	F	166	18–30 ($\bar{x} = 22.87$)	3.39 (0.52)	1.57–5.15
	F	10	36–41 ($\bar{x} = 38.49$)	3.23 (0.40)	2.69–3.95
	F	16	46–80 ($\bar{x} = 54.25$)	2.61 (0.62)	1.58–3.60

M = male; F = female; $\bar{x}$ = mean; N/A = not available.

[a] Young (Y), middle age (M), and old age (O) subjects in good (G) and poor (P) condition.

[b] Subjects with minimal history of dysphonic episodes only.

[c] Young (Y) vs. older (O) subjects.

/ɑ/ was elicited over 14 trials. Results showed that most of the children did not achieve their maximum MPT until the ninth trial. Finnegan (1984) concluded that the extensive use of repeated trials to obtain maximum MPT may not be clinically feasible.

• Reich, Mason, and Polen (1986) examined the effects of task instructions and coaching on MPT in 28 third grade females. Each subject was asked to produce three maximal effort prolongations of the vowel /ɑ/ in each of two experimental conditions (coached [i.e., given verbal encouragement] vs. noncoached). The vowel /ɑ/ was used because it represents a low-impedance pathway to the laryngeal sound source and because it had been traditionally used in MPT studies. Results showed that coaching applied during the MPT task resulted in significantly longer maximum and mean MPTs. However, coaching did not reduce within-subject variability in MPT production across trials. The authors speculated that the application of comprehensive instructions and verbal encouragement/coaching may have increased task motivation and/or task comprehension in their subjects. Reich et al. (1986) state that adequate pretrial practice combined with three MPT trials is sufficient to evoke optimal MPT performance.

HOW TO DO IT: MEASUREMENT OF MPT

On the basis of the findings of the aforementioned studies, the suggestions are given below for the elicitation of MPT.

1. Provide the following instructions to the patient: "I want you to take a deep breath and sustain/hold out the vowel "ah" (/ɑ/) as long as possible." The clinician should model the MPT task for the patient. The MPT is timed using a stopwatch.
2. The sustained vowel is generally produced at a comfortable pitch and loudness level (Colton & Casper, 1996) with some degree of pitch/loudness variability to be expected, particularly near the end of the task.
3. As in the case of VC, it is useful to verbally encourage the patient into sustaining the MPT as long as possible.
4. Three trials will be elicited with the maximum sustained vowel duration from the three trials used as the patient's MPT.

Assuming acceptable elicitation of the task, when MPTs are lower than expected for a patient's age and gender (see "What To Expect"), three clinical possibilities must be considered:

1. The patient may present with poor/insufficient respiratory functioning. VC testing and perceptual determination of respiratory support for speech may provide some indications as to this possibility.
2. The patient is unable to sustain the expiratory flow of air (and, therefore, phonation) because of inefficient laryngeal valving.
3. Some combination of factors 1 and 2 may be present.

Although most attention is paid to short MPTs, it is also possible that MPTs will be substantially greater than expected. This may be the case in patients with hyperadduction of the vocal folds during phonation (Colton & Casper, 1996). Darley et al. (1975) present several striking examples of patients with spastic dysphonia in which vowel productions are sustained to inordinate lengths as a result of substantially reduced airflow during phonation.

It has been stated that MPT productions may also be used for other types of analysis. Certainly, perceptual assessment of the sustained vowel production is appropriate, with quality variations (e.g., breathiness, harshness/roughness) and pitch variation (e.g., vocal tremor) being noted. Although it has been suggested (Kent et al., 1987) that MPT productions could be used for quantitative evaluation of vocal quality (e.g., jitter, shimmer, and HNR), I would not recommend it. The MPT is not controlled for vocal pitch or loudness levels (i.e., the short duration sustained vowels used in perturbation analysis are elicited with as steady a pitch and loudness level as possible). The pitch and loudness (and for that matter, quality) variations that would be expected in MPT productions (particularly toward the end of the task) would inevitably be analyzed as increased perturbation/noise components by standard algorithms and, thus, may give the clinician invalid results.

By itself, MPT assessment cannot delineate between insufficient respiratory functioning and insufficient laryngeal valving. However, in conjunction with other tests (VC or the S/Z ratio) and perceptual judgment of voice quality (e.g., breathiness), the clinician should be able to accurately identify the specific area(s) of dysfunction.

WHAT TO EXPECT: NORMAL VOICE

Gender

Expectations for gender effects on MPT are similar to those described for VC. Significant differences in MPT are expected between genders, although this difference does not appear to become significant until the approach of puberty (Colton & Casper, 1996). As an example, Harden and Looney (1984) observed no gender effect on MPT in kindergarten age (mean age = 6.2 years) males and females (mean MPT: 10.4 s vs. 10.6 s). However, after the onset of puberty, males are generally observed to have longer MPTs than females. Trullinger and Emanuel (1989) observed longer mean MPTs in 8- to 10-year-old males versus similar-aged females, regardless of vowel type (mean MPT range: 10.6 to 11.25 s vs. 9.03 to 10.0 s). A significant gender effect was also reported by Finnegan (1984), who observed a mean MPT of 18.23 s versus 15.79 s in male versus female children between the ages of 3:6 and 17:11 years. In general, prepubescent males and females are both expected to be able to produce MPTs of at least 10 s in duration (Andrews, 1995; Haynes et al., 1992; Kent et al., 1987).

Adult men have been consistently observed to have significantly greater MPTs than adult women. Kent et al. (1987) indicate that minimal expectations for MPT are approximately 15 s for women versus 20 s for men. However, studies dealing with adult MPT show a great deal of variability in normative MPT for both genders, making judgment regarding normalcy of MPT problematic. Several studies have observed mean MPT to approach 30 s for men versus 25 s for women (Hirano, Koike, & von Leden, 1968; Rau & Beckett, 1984; Yanagihara, Koike, & von Leden, 1966). Perhaps a more effective means of judging the normalcy of MPT is to derive a ratio of the actual to predicted MPT. Beckett (1971) reports that predicted MPT may be calculated by means of the following formulas:

$$Predicted\ MPT\ (Males) = \frac{VC(ml)}{100} \times 0.67$$

$$Predicted\ MPT\ (Females) = \frac{VC(ml)}{100} \times 0.59$$

Beckett (1971) indicates that the patient's actual MPT divided by the patient's predicted MPT should be greater than 0.70, whereas a ratio less than 0.70 is an indicator of abnormality.

Aging

A general increase in MPT is expected from childhood to adulthood (Case, 1996; Kent, 1994), although "definite monotonic increases" (Finnegan, 1984, p. 312) in MPT may not be apparent across all age levels. MPT is generally stable until the approach of older age. Ptacek et al. (1966) observed significantly lower MPTs in geriatric versus young adult males (mean MPT: 18.1 s vs. 24.6 s). Ptacek et al. (1966) surmised that decrements in respiratory function combined with degenerative laryngeal changes to produce the decreased MPTs observed in the elderly subjects observed in their study. Kreul (1972) and Mueller (1982) have also reported reductions in MPT for elderly men, and similar decrements in MPT were observed for groups of aging women by Mueller (1982) and Awan and Ziminsky-Ammon (1996). In the Awan and Ziminsky-Ammon (1996) study, a group of 70- to 79-year-old women was observed to produce significantly lower MPTs than 18- to 30-, 40- to 49-, and 50- to 59-year-old comparison groups (no difference observed between 60- to 69- and 70- to 79-year-old subjects; see Figure 5–6). A significant (although weak) correlation ($r = -0.42$, $p < .05$) was observed between age and MPT. In Figure 5–7, Z-scores were calculated for each subject using the mean maximum phonation time and standard deviation

of the young adult female group as the control group. Results show increasing percentages of the 50- to 59-, 60- to 69-, and 70- to 79-year-old group producing mean MPTs substantially lower than the mean MPT of the young adult group.

Table 5–2 presents a range of examples of MPT elicited from normal voice subjects.

WHAT TO EXPECT: ABNORMAL VOICE

The MPT has been observed to be inversely related to mean flow rate (Beckett, 1971; Yanagihara et al., 1966). Therefore, conditions that affect glottal airflow will also affect MPT. However, it must be remembered that MPT is not solely a function of laryngeal valving but is also affected by respiratory function. It is the responsibility of the clinician to accurately determine in which area (respiratory vs. phonatory) the patient's dysfunction lies by interpreting MPT in relation to perceptual judgments of the voice quality and other tests (e.g., VC, S/Z ratio).

Mass Lesions and Distributed Tissue Change

Low MPTs are expected for those patients in whom masses/lesions on the margin(s) of the vocal folds cause persistent chinks (i.e., openings) in the glottis during phonation (Dworkin & Meleca, 1997). Hypoadduction of the folds is associated with breathy voice quality, rapid expenditure of air, and subsequent decreased duration of a sustained vowel (Andrews, 1995; Prater & Swift, 1984). Olsen, Perez, Burk, and Platt (1969, in Harden and Looney, 1984) reported reduced MPTs in groups of children with vocal nodules versus normal individuals. On the basis of a review of 1,536 patients, Hirano (1991) observed MPTs to be reduced in patients with a mass lesion (nodule, polyp, Reinke's edema, cyst, and glottic carcinomas), although many were able to produce MPTs within normal expectations. In addition, a significant (although weak) inverse relationship between MPT and size of the glottic gap in 122 patients with polyps was also observed.

Neurological Disorders

Those neurological disorders resulting in hypoadduction and hypofunctional voice may be expected to have increased MFRs and, therefore, decreased MPTs. This has been reported for cases of vocal fold paralysis (Beckett, 1971; Dworkin & Meleca, 1997; Prater & Swift, 1984). Hirano (1991) observed MPTs to be reduced in a majority of 46 cases with vocal fold paralysis. A significant inverse relationship between MPT and size of the glottic gap in patients with paralysis was also observed. In addition, neurological disorders that result in insufficient respiratory function and/or incoordination of inspiratory/expiratory

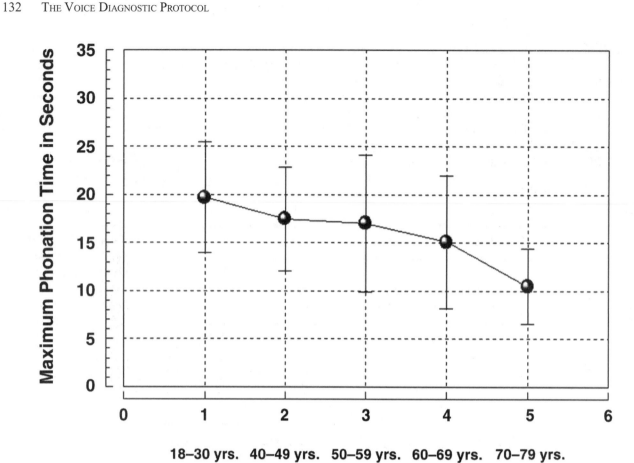

Figure 5–6 Mean Maximum Phonation Time of Aging Women. Mean maximum phonation time (MPT in seconds) and standard deviations across aging groups. (Correlation between aging and MPT: $r = -0.42, p < .05$.)

function would also be expected to have decreased MPTs (Prater & Swift, 1984).

Disorders characterized by hyperadduction/hyperfunction may show greatly increased glottal resistance and, therefore, may be expected to have decreased MFRs and increased MPTs (Beckett, 1971). However, Wit, Maassen, Gabreels, and Thoonen (1993) observed significantly reduced MPTs in a study of children with spastic dysarthria caused by cerebral palsy. It may be that the increased effort required to prolong phonation in the presence of increased glottal resistance results in fatigue and, therefore, decrements in MPT in some patients.

Functional Voice Disorders

Functional voice disorders may present with either hyperfunctional or hypofunctional characteristics. Hyperfunctional voice may be expected to show hyperadduction of the folds during phonation, as well as lateral and/or anteroposterior squeezing of the larynx. The result may be a decrease in

mean flow rate and an increase in MPT. However, hyperfunction may also result in hypoadduction of the vocal folds in instances in which contraction of the posterior cricoarytenoid muscles during phonation results in a significant posterior glottal chink. In this case, increased transglottal airflow may result in a decreased MPT. Functional voice disorders may also have a hypofunctional component in which inadequate vocal fold adduction occurs during phonation. Again, the result may be a decreased MPT.

THE S/Z RATIO

As previously stated, the MPT may be affected by respiratory and/or phonatory disruptions. Boone (1977) introduced the S/Z ratio as a means of expanding the information derived from MPT and as a method by which respiratory inefficiencies could be distinguished from those of a laryngeal nature. The interpretation of the S/Z ratio is based on the assumption that a person with normal/adequate laryngeal

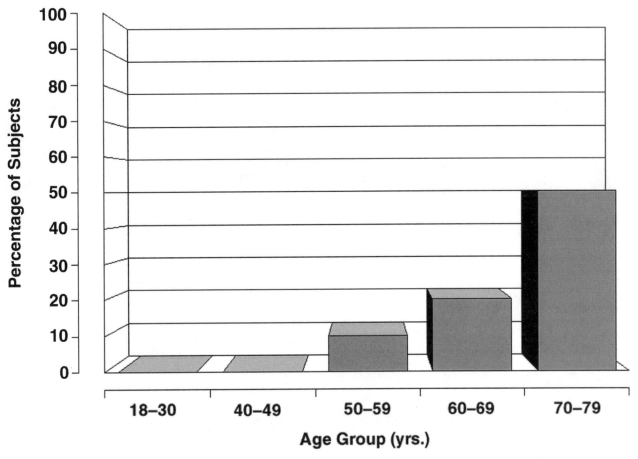

Figure 5–7 Maximum Phonation Time. Percentage of subjects per aging female group with mean maximum phonation times ≤ 2 standard deviations below the mean MPT of the young adult female group. (Percentage of subjects with Z-scores ≤ –2.0 re: young adult comparisons [18–30 yr.]).

valving will be able to sustain a voiced phoneme (/z/) for approximately the same duration as an unvoiced production (/s/). As an explanation of the S/Z ratio, consider the following:

- /s/: This phoneme is produced by means of a respiratory component (expiratory airflow) and an articulatory component (lingua-alveolar constriction resulting in turbulent friction noise). The airflow is unmodulated (i.e., the expiratory airflow is *not* periodically interrupted by vocal fold vibration). Therefore,

$$\text{Duration}_{/s/} = \text{Duration}_{\text{expiratory airflow}}$$

- /z/: This phoneme is produced by means of a respiratory component (expiratory airflow), a laryngeal component (vocal fold vibration), and the aforementioned articulatory component. In /z/ production, the airflow

is modulated (i.e., vocal fold vibration does periodically interrupt the expiratory airflow). *If the phonatory mechanism is functioning effectively, there is no waste of the expiratory air (i.e., no air escapes between the vocal folds without first effecting vocal fold vibration) and all of the expiratory airflow is transformed into vocal fold vibration (i.e., phonation)*; therefore

$$\text{Duration}_{/z/} = \text{Duration}_{\text{phonation}}$$

Because in the normal voice,

$$\text{Duration}_{\text{expiratory airflow}} = \text{Duration}_{\text{phonation}}$$

then

$$\text{Duration}_{/s/} = \text{Duration}_{/z/}$$

and

$$\text{Duration}_{/s/} \div \text{Duration}_{/z/} \approx 1.0$$

Table 5–2 Maximum Phonation Time (MPT in seconds) from Normal Voice Subjects

Author	Gender	No. of Subjects	Age (yr.)	Mean & SD	Range
Ptacek & Sander (1963)[a]	M	40	17–41 ($\bar{x}$ = 24.6)	25.7 (7.86)	14.30–48.00
	F	40	18–40 ($\bar{x}$ = 21.9)	17.9 (6.37)	8.40–39.70
Ptacek et al. (1966)	M	29	18–39 ($\bar{x}$ = 27.6)	24.60 (6.70)	12.50–36.00
	M	20	68–89 ($\bar{x}$ = 76.9)	18.10 (66.00)	10.00–37.20
	F	29	18–38 ($\bar{x}$ = 23.5)	20.90 (5.70)	11.80–32.00
	F	24	66–93 ($\bar{x}$ = 76.9)	14.20 (5.60)	7.00–24.80
Yanagihara et al. (1966)	M	11	30–43 ($\bar{x}$ = 36.0)	30.20 (9.70)	20.40–50.70
	F	11	21–41 ($\bar{x}$ = 28.0)	22.50 (6.10)	16.4–32.7
Hirano et al. (1968)[b]	M	25	N/A	34.6 (−11.4 & +12.1)	N/A
	F	25	N/A	25.7 (−6.5 & +7.5)	N/A
Shanks & Mast (1977)	M	30	20–25	23.37 (9.32)	N/A
	F	30	20–25	18.39 (5.71)	N/A
Neiman & Edeson (1981)[c]	M_a	10	$\bar{x}$ = 23.9	29.05 (5.50)	N/A
	M_b	10	$\bar{x}$ = 21.9	22.20 (11.63)	N/A
	F_a	10	$\bar{x}$ = 20.8	19.65 (4.74)	N/A
	F_b	10	$\bar{x}$ = 23.7	16.65 (4.82)	N/A
Lewis et al. (1982)	M	10	7.5–8.5	13.80	8.00–24.50
	M	10	9.5–10.5	20.00	13.50–34.40
	F	10	7.5–8.5	14.0	8.20–17.10
	F	10	9.5–10.5	12.4	8.20–14.60
Mueller (1982)	M	10	85–92	13.0	7.0–12.0
	F	29	85–96	10.0	6.0–18.0
Finnegan (1984)	M	5	3.6–3.11	7.9 (1.81)	4.38–11.46
	F	5	3.6–3.11	6.3 (1.76)	2.84–9.72
	M	10	4.0–4.11	10.0 (3.05)	4.15–16.09
	F	10	4.0–4.11	8.7 (1.84)	5.26–12.46
	M	10	5.0–5.11	10.1 (3.05)	4.15–16.09
	F	10	5.0–5.11	10.5 (2.57)	5.44–15.50
	M	9	6.0–6.11	13.9 (2.98)	8.06–19.74
	F	9	6.0–6.11	13.8 (3.65)	6.66–20.96
	M	9	7.0–7.11	14.6 (2.82)	9.11–20.15
	F	10	7.0–7.11	13.7 (2.45)	8.88–18.48
	M	10	8.0–8.11	16.8 (6.07)	4.94–28.72
	F	10	8.0–8.11	17.1 (4.62)	7.07–21.87
	M	10	9.0–9.11	16.8 (6.07)	4.94–28.72
	F	10	9.0–9.11	14.5 (3.78)	7.07–21.87
	M	10	10.0–10.11	22.2 (4.74)	12.91–31.49
	F	10	10.0–10.11	15.9 (5.99)	4.14–27.62
	M	10	11.0–11.11	19.8 (3.79)	12.43–27.27
	F	10	11.0–11.11	14.8 (2.06)	10.73–18.79
	M	9	12.0–12.11	20.2 (5.72)	9.02–31.44
	F	10	12.0–12.11	15.2 (3.87)	7.58–22.74
	M	10	13.0–13.11	22.3 (8.19)	6.29–38.29
	F	10	13.0–13.11	19.2 (4.58)	10.27–28.21
	M	10	14.0–14.11	22.3 (6.89)	8.84–35.84
	F	10	14.0–14.11	18.8 (5.15)	8.76–28.94
	M	10	15.0–15.11	20.7 (5.32)	10.32–31.16
	F	10	15.0–15.11	19.5 (4.66)	10.40–29.93
	M	10	16.0–16.11	21.0 (4.40)	12.43–29.66
	F	10	16.0–16.11	21.8 (4.47)	13.09–30.61
	M	10	17.0–17.11	28.7 (7.08)	14.83–42.57
	F	10	17.0–17.11	22.0 (6.30)	9.65–34.33

continues

Table 5–2 continued

Author	Gender	No. of Subjects	Age (yr.)	Mean & SD	Range
Harden & Looney (1984)[d]	M	44	$\bar{x} = 6{:}1$	10.4 (5.1)	3.80–16.80
	F	58	$\bar{x}$ 6:2	10.6 (6.3)	6.20–30.60
Rau & Beckett (1984)	M	10	19–28 ($\bar{x} = 21.10$)	31.60 (7.94)	20.00–47.50
	F	9	21–29 ($\bar{x} = 24.33$)	24.60 (5.45)	19.00–37.50
Linville et al. (1989)	F	20	67–86 ($\bar{x} = 76.0$)	16.8 (5.3)	7.5–30.6
Trullinger & Emanuel (1989)[e]	M	5	8.1–8.11	10.57 (2.93)	N/A
	F	5	8.1–8.11	10.96 (3.60)	N/A
	M	5	9.0–9.10	11.98 (5.21)	N/A
	F	5	9.0–9.10	8.33 (0.85)	N/A
	M	5	10.1–10.9	8.30 (1.81)	N/A
	F	5	10.1–10.9	10.47 (3.58)	N/A
Kent et al. (1992)	F	19	65–80 ($\bar{x} = 71.8$)	11.8 (N/A)	N/A
Stemple et al. (1995)[f]	F	10	22–45 ($\bar{x} = 25.3$)	26.0 (8.0)	N/A
Awan & Ziminsky-Ammon (1996)	F	10	18–30 ($\bar{x} = 23.80$)	19.70 (5.79)	14.10–34.22
	F	10	40–49 ($\bar{x} = 43.40$)	17.48 (5.41)	10.89–28.03
	F	10	50–59 ($\bar{x} = 54.80$)	17.02 (7.10)	7.60–31.10
	F	10	60–69 ($\bar{x} = 65.20$)	15.09 (6.87)	4.66–29.48
	F	10	70–79 ($\bar{x} = 72.30$)	10.49 (3.95)	7.50–18.91
Author	M	52	18–30 ($\bar{x} = 24.13$)	25.45 (7.30)	14.38–46.00
	M	14	41–58 ($\bar{x} = 52.75$)	24.56 (7.95)	15.00–39.00
	F	7	8–13 ($\bar{x} = 10.38$)	14.40 (3.99)	9.00–21.00
	F	205	18–30 ($\bar{x} = 22.83$)	22.31 (5.50)	9.25–44.00
	F	17	32–42 ($\bar{x} = 37.69$)	21.33 (6.29)	15.00–34.00
	F	19	46–80 ($\bar{x} = 57.01$)	20.57 (8.51)	7.00–48.43

M = male; F = female; $\bar{x}$ = mean; N/A = not available.
[a] The maximum mean MPT selected from three trials is reported.
[b] SD differs between negative and positive sides caused by calculation based on a square root transformation.
[c] Modeled (M_a & F_a) vs. unmodeled (M_b & F_b) groups.
[d] Mean and SD for the vowel /ɑ/.
[e] Mean and SD for the vowel /ɑ/.
[f] Data from pretest only (prelaryngeal fatigue).

When laryngeal valving is incomplete (i.e., hypoadduction), some portion of the expiratory airflow escapes without being translated into vocal fold vibration. Because less expiratory airflow is being translated into vocal fold vibration (as a result of escaping air), the duration of /z/ will be less than expected in an efficient larynx and, in particular, less than observed in /s/ production. Therefore,

$$\text{Duration}_{/s/} > \text{Duration}_{/z/}$$

and

$$\text{Duration}_{/s/} \div \text{Duration}_{/z/} > 1.0$$

These examples indicate the following:

- The expected S/Z ratio in the case of a normal, efficient phonatory mechanism is approximately 1.0.
- Difficulty adducting the vocal folds results in a shorter duration /z/ than /s/, and, therefore, the S/Z ratio is >1.0.

In addition to aiding in the identification of laryngeal valving difficulties, the S/Z ratio can also be used to identify possible deficits in respiratory support. In the event that respiratory support is weak and laryngeal valving is adequate, the

S/Z ratio is expected to be normal (i.e., approximately 1.0), but the individual durations of each phoneme will be much shorter than expected.

Methodological Considerations

Several studies as shown below have examined methodological issues relevant to the elicitation of maximum /s/ and /z/ durations and subsequent computation of the S/Z ratio.

- Tait, Michel, and Carpenter (1980) examined /s/ and /z/ durations and S/Z ratio in 53 children (ages 5 to 9 years). The subjects were separated into groups in which productions were elicited with only verbal instructions versus those in which a feedback device (a device containing a series of lights that were illuminated as long as the subject produced a predetermined intensity of production) was used during elicitation. Although no statistical difference was observed between elicitation conditions, it was observed that phoneme durations tended to be longer using only verbal instructions versus the use of a feedback device. Therefore, these authors indicate that too much control or complexity in an elicitation task may actually cause maximum phoneme durations to decrease on subsequent trials.
- Fendler and Shearer (1988) examined test-retest reliability of the S/Z ratio in 78 school-aged children. S/Z ratios were computed on two separate occasions by two different clinicians. In computing the S/Z ratio, three trials were elicited for maximum sustained /s/ and /z/, and the longest individual /s/ and /z/ productions were used to compute the ratio. Results indicated no difference in test-retest S/Z ratios (mean S/Z ratio: 1.12 vs. 1.16) and no significant effect of clinician.
- Larson, Mueller, and Summers (1991) studied elicitation variables for the S/Z ratio in 88 subjects (mean age: 24.46 years). Each subject was asked to produce three sustained /s/ and three sustained /z/ productions in four conditions: /s,s,s/ /z,z,z/; /z,z,z/ /s,s,s/; /s,z/ /s,z/ /s,z/; and /z,s/ /z,s/ /z,s/. Results showed no significant difference in overall /s/ vs. /z/ durations and no significant difference between productions from the four conditions. In addition, no significant differences were observed in method of calculating the ratio (i.e., use of the longest vs. shortest vs. mid vs. average durations from the three trials). Finally, no significant difference was observed between S/Z ratios computed from a single trial versus those obtained from multiple elicitations.
- Mueller, Larson, and Summers (1991) examined the variability of the S/Z ratio in 54 male and female children (mean age: 65.96 months) and 22 young adults (mean age: 24.46 years). Three productions of /s/ and /z/ were elicited in the order /s,z/ /s,z/ /s,z/. Consider-

able variability was observed between trials in both age groups. Although the children produced mean S/Z ratios within normal expectations (≤ 1.0) on each trial, the adult subjects showed increasing durations for sustained /z/ from trial 1 to trial 3, resulting in a normalization of the S/Z ratio only by the third trial. This possible practice effect in maximum /s/ versus /z/ durations should be accounted for by either (1) eliciting multiple trials or (2) using the single longest /s/ and /z/ productions from the three trials in computing the S/Z ratio.

HOW TO DO IT: ELICITATION OF MAXIMUM /S/ AND /Z/ DURATIONS AND COMPUTATION OF THE S/Z RATIO

On the basis of the findings of the aforementioned studies, the suggestions below are given regarding the elicitation of maximally sustained /s/ and /z/ productions and computation of the S/Z ratio.

1. Provide the following instructions to the patient: "I want you to take a deep breath and hold out the sound /s/ ("Sssss...") as long as possible." The clinician should provide a model for the patient. Time and record the duration using a stopwatch. As with previous tasks (VC and MPT), it is useful to verbally encourage the patient into sustaining the productions for as long as possible.
2. "Now I want you to take a deep breath and sustain the sound /z/ ("Zzzzz...") as long as possible." Time and record the duration.
3. Elicit three trials of maximally sustained /s/ and /z/ in the following order: /s,z/ /s,z/ /s,z/.
4. Calculate the S/Z ratio using the single longest /s/ and single longest /z/ durations from the three trials.

Only S/Z ratios ≥ 1.0 are of clinical significance. Ratios substantially <1.0 do not make clinical sense, because, according to the underlying assumptions of this task, the duration of /s/ should always be equal to or greater than /z/. However, actual norms often provide S/Z ratios slightly less than 1.0, because an efficient phonatory mechanism results in voiced durations slightly longer than voiceless durations (Case, 1996). If the ratio is substantially <1.0, it probably indicates that the patient did not carry out the task maximally for the /s/ production.

Although the S/Z ratio would appear to supplant the use of MPT, I suggest incorporation of both tasks into the voice diagnostic protocol, because (1) these tasks provide beneficial redundancy in our assessment of the durational aspects of the voice, and (2) MPT provides an extended opportunity to focus on phonatory variability and "smoothness of continuous vibration" (Andrews, 1995, p. 56) not present in the S/Z ratio.

WHAT TO EXPECT: NORMAL VOICE

As previously described, the ideal S/Z ratio is expected be approximately 1.0. However, for clinical decision making, S/Z ratios greater than 1.2 in children or 1.4 in adults may indicate a deficit in adducting the vocal folds (Boone, 1980; Eckel & Boone, 1981; Haynes et al., 1992; Prater & Swift, 1984).

Aging and Gender

The S/Z ratio appears to be relatively unaffected by gender or aging in normal subjects. However, the individual durations of the /s/ and /z/ phonemes may be affected in similar ways as previously discussed for MPT. Possible effects on individual /s/ and /z/ durations are as shown below.

- Individual /s/ and /z/ durations may increase with age during childhood. Tait et al. (1980) examined S/Z ratios in groups of 5-, 7-, and 9-year-old children. Results showed a tendency for /s/ and /z/ durations to increase with age. Tait et al. (1980) state that these increases in /s/ and /z/ durations are consistent with height and lung capacity increases with age. Regardless of the possible increases in individual /s/ and /z/ durations, overall S/Z ratio appears quite stable in young children (Fendler & Shearer, 1988; Tait et al., 1980).
- Individual /s/ and /z/ durations may decrease with advanced age. Mueller (1993) compared S/Z ratios in young (40 men and women: mean age = 23.9 years) and older (44 men and women: mean age = 76.9 years). The young subjects were observed to produce significantly greater duration /s/ and /z/'s than their elderly counterparts. Mueller (1993) attributed this difference to age-related decreases in pulmonary function and laryngeal efficiency. However, S/Z ratios by both groups were considered within normal limits (mean S/Z ratios = 1.07 vs. 0.89 for young vs. elderly adults, respectively).
- Gender may interact with age to affect the duration of /s/ and /z/ productions. Studies by Fendler and Shearer (1988) and Hufnagle and Hufnagle (1988) observed no effect of gender in young children on individual /s/ and /z/ durations, whereas Tait et al. (1980) observed a strong tendency for males to have longer duration /s/ and /z/ productions than females

in a group of 9-year-old children. Mueller (1993) showed males to have longer /s/ productions than females, regardless of age (i.e., young vs. elderly subjects). However, all these studies have shown that overall S/Z ratio appears to be unaffected by gender.

Table 5–3 presents a range of examples of maximum /s/ and /z/ durations and S/Z ratios from normal voice subjects.

WHAT TO EXPECT: ABNORMAL VOICE

Mass Lesions and Distributed Tissue Change

The studies below have examined the effectiveness of the S/Z ratio in the identification of patients presenting with vocal nodules:
- Eckel and Boone (1981) examined the S/Z ratio in 28 patients with laryngeal pathological conditions (nodules/polyps); 36 functional dysphonia patients (no vocal fold pathology); and 86 normal controls. Results showed no significant difference in /s/ durations between the three groups; however, a significant difference in maximally sustained /z/ production was observed between the nodules group and the normal controls. In addition, the nodules group was observed to have a significantly higher mean S/Z ratio (1.65) than the functional dysphonia group or the normal controls (1.03 and 0.99, respectively). In addition, 95% of the nodules group had S/Z ratios >1.40. The authors concluded that the S/Z ratio appears to be an excellent indicator of poor laryngeal function as a result of glottal margin lesions. (*Author's Note:* It was this statement (i.e., indicator of glottal margin lesions) that has resulted in controversy regarding the S/Z ratio. It is perhaps more accurate to say that an increased S/Z ratio may be an indicator of an inability to valve the glottis rather than attach this ratio to any specific disorder type).
- Rastatter and Hyman (1982) examined the S/Z ratio in 8 male and 8 female children previously diagnosed with bilateral vocal fold nodules. The subjects had been enrolled in voice therapy for 1 month before testing. Results showed mean S/Z ratios of 0.81 in males versus 0.93 in females (well within normal expectations), although the overall durations for each phoneme were much lower than expected (generally in the 4- to 6-s range), indicating more difficulty with respiratory control than laryngeal valving. In addition, /z/ durations were highly variable across trials as compared with /s/. The overall results indicated that the S/Z ratio was not a sensitive measure of vocal nodules in children. Rastatter and Hyman (1982) conclude that variability in /z/ productions and reduced overall durations of both

Table 5–3 Maximum /s/ and /z/ Durations (in seconds) and S/Z Ratios from Normal Voice Subjects

Author	Gender	No. of Subjects	Age (yr.)	/s/	/z/	S/Z Ratio Mean & SD	Range
Tait et al. (1980)[a]	M	6	5	7.9 (1.4)	8.6 (2.1)	0.92 (N/A)	0.82–1.08
	F	9	5	8.3 (4.0)	10.0 (3.3)	0.83 (N/A)	0.50–1.14
	M	6	7	9.3 (1.7)	13.2 (3.6)	0.70 (N/A)	0.52–0.97
	F	8	7	10.2 (2.6)	13.1 (4.0)	0.78 (N/A)	0.51–1.10
	M	15	9	16.7 (8.5)	18.1 (6.8)	0.92 (N/A)	0.66–1.50
	F	8	9	14.4 (3.1)	15.8 (5.2)	0.91 (N/A)	0.75–1.26
Eckel & Boone (1981)	M & F	86	8–88 ($\bar{x}$ = 27.7)	17.73 (7.65)	18.60 (6.97)	0.99 (0.36)	0.41–2.67
Fendler & Shearer (1988)[b]	M	N/A	1st grade	N/A	N/A	1.42 (0.52)	0.51–2.66
	F	N/A	1st grade	N/A	N/A	1.31 (0.38)	0.48–2.02
	M	N/A	2nd grade	N/A	N/A	1.13 (0.33)	0.53–2.13
	F	N/A	2nd grade	N/A	N/A	1.19 (0.31)	0.52–2.34
Larson et al. (1991)[c]	M & F	22	19–41 ($\bar{x}$ = 24.46)	25.45 (8.35)	22.65 (8.25)	1.18 (0.31)	N/A
Mueller et al. (1991)[d]	M & F	54	5–6 ($\bar{x}$ = 5.50)	4.70 (2.48)	5.72 (3.37)	0.89 (0.33)	N/A
	M & F	22	19–41 ($\bar{x}$ = 24.46)	26.24 (9.78)	24.37 (9.46)	1.13 (0.32)	N/A
Sorenson & Parker (1992)	M & F	11	5.1–9.11	12.33 (N/A)	12.74 (N/A)	0.97 (N/A)	0.84–1.27
Mueller (1993)	M	20	20–30 ($\bar{x}$ = 23.9)	25.13 (9.64)	23.22 (7.23)	1.10 (0.33)	0.56–1.81
	M	22	65–87 ($\bar{x}$ = 76.9)	12.75 (7.21)	15.93 (8.40)	0.85 (0.33)	0.46–1.78
	F	20	20–30 ($\bar{x}$ = 23.85)	22.98 (5.45)	23.05 (6.32)	1.05 (0.30)	0.66–1.50
	F	22	65–92 ($\bar{x}$ = 78.0)	9.62 (3.37)	11.32 (4.24)	0.89 (0.23)	0.56–1.44
Author	M	53	18–30 ($\bar{x}$ = 23.89)	25.86 (7.69)	27.53 (8.75)	0.95 (0.15)	0.58–1.41
	M	14	41–58 ($\bar{x}$ = 52.75)	28.07 (9.68)	26.66 (7.70)	1.05 (0.16)	0.86–1.54
	F	7	8–13 ($\bar{x}$ = 10.38)	11.46 (2.86)	11.26 (3.34)	0.99 (0.14)	0.82–1.25
	F	206	18–30 ($\bar{x}$ = 22.83)	23.94 (7.30)	24.75 (6.68)	0.98 (0.13)	0.44–1.50
	F	17	32–42 ($\bar{x}$ = 37.69)	28.17 (8.88)	29.12 (7.78)	0.93 (0.12)	0.74–1.16
	F	20	46–80 ($\bar{x}$ = 55.06)	20.79 (6.8)	20.57 (5.15)	1.01 (0.22)	0.79–1.86

M = male; F = female; $\bar{x}$ = mean; N/A = not available.
[a] Maximal durations obtained using verbal instructions only (Condition I).
[b] Total n = 78; actual ages of the subjects are not provided in the study.
[c] Results from the /s,z/ /s,z/ /s,z/ elicitation procedure only.
[d] Results from trial 3 of /s,z/ elicitation.

/s/ and /z/ phonemes may be indicative of vocal fold pathological condition.

- Hufnagle and Hufnagle (1988) observed the S/Z ratio in 123 dysphonic children (69 with nodules; 54 with no vocal fold pathosis). Results showed mean S/Z ratios to be close to 1.0 in both groups (functional males and females: 0.87 and 0.97, respectively; nodules males and females: 0.84 and 1.03, respectively). The authors concluded that the S/Z ratio could not discriminate the presence of mass lesions in children. Their findings were attributed to the presence of early stage, small, nonfibrous nodules that may not have affected the degree of vocal fold approximation (although all subjects were judged as dysphonic, the specific identification of breathy voice quality is not reported for these subjects). Shorter than expected durations were observed for both /s/ and /z/ phonemes, suggesting that these subjects may have had reduced phonation volumes.

- Sorenson and Parker (1992) examined S/Z ratios in children with and without vocal pathological conditions. Eleven children (mean age: 7.9) with verified nodules/polyps (7 with bilateral lesions and 4 with unilateral lesions) were matched with 11 children without pathological conditions. Results showed the pathological group to have significantly lower maximally sustained /z/ productions and significantly higher overall S/Z ratios (mean S/Z ratio: 1.24 vs. 0.97). However, only seven of the children with vocal pathological conditions had S/Z ratios >1.1 and four normals also had S/Z ratios >1.1. Sorenson and Parker (1992) calculated a critical S/Z ratio value of 1.06 as the discriminant value between the pathological versus nonpathological groups. Overall, these authors concluded that the S/Z ratio was significantly increased in children with vocal pathological conditions.

- In an investigation of the basic assumptions underlying the S/Z ratio, Trudeau and Forrest (1997) studied the contributions of phonatory volumes and transglottal airflow to the S/Z ratio. Subjects were 32 adults (7 men and 25 women) with mass lesions on the vibrating edge of one or both folds. Results indicated the following:

1. The duration of /s/ exceeded /z/ to produce an overall mean S/Z ratio of 1.09 (mean S/Z ratio = 1.15 for women vs. 0.99 for men). The authors claimed that the S/Z ratio failed to identify abnormal performance in subjects with vocal fold pathological conditions.

2. Similar phonation volumes were observed for both /s/ and /z/ (an assumption basic to the S/Z ratio).

3. No significant difference in mean flow rate (MFR) was observed between /s/ and /z/ productions, indicating the rate of transglottal airflow was apparently unaffected by the presence or absence of vocal fold adduction or presence of mass lesions.

4. The MFR difference between /s/ and /z/ correlated strongly (r = 0.84) with the S/Z ratio, indicating that as airflow for /z/ increased over airflow for /s/, the ratio also rose.

Trudeau and Forrest (1997) speculated that many adults with vocal fold lesions appear able to compensate and therefore maintain similar rates of airflow for /s/ and /z/. Therefore, the ratio may not be sensitive to the presence of mass lesions on the vocal fold margins; clinicians are not justified in using the S/Z ratio as an indicator of glottal lesion. The authors do note that overtraining for the task may have affected results. In conclusion, Trudeau and Forrest (1997) state that the S/Z ratio may be used as a measure of glottal competence. They recommend laryngoscopy as a better method for identifying lesions, but also state that electroglottography (EGG) or photoglottography (PGG) could also be used to identify lesions. It is their belief that precision should not take precedence over simplicity in the diagnostic situation. (*Author's Note:* (1) Although the mean S/Z ratios observed in the Trudeau and Forrest (1997) study did not exceed the 1.2 to 1.4 "cutoff" suggested by Eckel and Boone (1981), the 1.11 ratio observed for the female dysphonic patients did exceed the 1.06 suggested cutoff used by Sorenson and Parker (1992); (2) the requirement for laryngological examination and obvious benefits of the procedure do not negate the use of the S/Z ratio as a diagnostic measure that may provide an indication of inefficient laryngeal valving; (3) the comments by Trudeau and Forrest (1997) regarding EGG and PGG are highly questionable because the literature does not appear to show that EGG/PGG waveforms are disease specific, and use of compensation methods on the patient's behalf could also affect EGG and PGG waveforms; (4) the "precision" of the S/Z ratio is difficult to ascertain in this study because the authors presented no data regarding size and location of lesion(s), duration of lesion(s), incidence and type of compensatory activity, or perceptual characteristics of the patients' voices. The low S/Z ratios may have actually been quite accurate if interpreted to mean that the patients in the Trudeau and Forrest (1997) study did not have any significant difficulties with laryngeal valving).

Neurological Disorders

Disorders in which the patient is unable to adequately adduct the vocal folds during phonation (e.g., flaccid dysphonia resulting in unilateral or bilateral vocal fold paresis/

paralysis) may be expected to show elevated S/Z ratios. Neurological conditions in which laryngeal function is either relatively unaffected or in which hyperadduction is the key characteristic (e.g., spasticity) may show S/Z ratios within normal expectations. A study by Wit et al. (1993) observed no significant differences in S/Z ratio between a group of children with spastic dysarthria and a group of normal controls.

THE PHONATION QUOTIENT

The rate at which air is expelled during sustained phonation is another indicator of glottal efficiency (Prater & Swift, 1984) and may be strongly correlated with the degree of laryngeal dysfunction (Dworkin & Meleca, 1997). The measurement of airflow rate during phonation requires the use of a pneumotachograph. Unfortunately, the pneumotachograph and associated instrumentation (e.g., amplifiers, recording equipment) can be quite expensive and/or may not be available in every clinical situation. In addition, the instrumentation setup for this procedure can be extensive and, perhaps, intimidating for clinicians who may have limited exposure to the use of such instrumentation.

Fortunately, the phonation quotient (PQ) is a method by which a "reasonable clinical substitute" (Hirano et al., 1968, p. 199) for airflow rate may be obtained without the use of a pneumotachograph. In addition, the PQ is calculated using the VC and MPT data previously discussed. The PQ is calculated by means of the following formula:

$$PQ\ (ml/s) = \frac{VC\ (ml)}{MPT(s)}$$

The term *phonation quotient* was initially coined by Hirano et al. (1968) to describe the ratio of VC to MPT as an indicator of air consumption (Yanagihara et al., 1966). Hirano et al. (1968) observed that PQ correlated with MFR at $r = 0.86$ in men and $r = 0.75$ in women (both significant at $p < .01$). Studies by Hirano et al. (1968) and Iwata and von Leden (1970) established the PQ as a simple test able to provide valuable clinical information for a variety of laryngeal disorders. Hirano et al. (1968) observed that many pathological conditions resulted in a reduction in MPT, an increase in mean airflow rate, and a subsequent increase in the PQ. These tendencies were particularly true for those cases in which insufficient vocal fold approximation was a key underlying physiological disruption.

It should be emphasized that, although the PQ correlates well with mean flow rate (Hirano et al., 1968), it is generally observed to overestimate actual mean flow rate as obtained by means of a pneumotachograph. This is because the PQ is computed using the VC of the patient rather than the phonation volume (PV; the total air volume used during sustained phonation). Because phonation volume is considerably less than vital capacity (approximately ⅔ to ¾ of VC [Yanagihara et al., 1966]), PQ overestimates actual MFR.

WHAT TO EXPECT: NORMAL VOICE

Gender

Men have been consistently observed to have greater PQ levels than women. This finding is generally attributed to the larger VC of the men compared with women. Normative values for PQ as reported by Hirano et al. (1968) and Rau and Beckett (1984) confirm this gender effect on PQ. Hirano et al. (1968) observed that adult men produced a mean PQ of 145 ml/s, with measures less than 69 ml/s or greater than 307 ml/s considered abnormal. For women, the mean PQ was 137 ml/s, with measures less than 78 ml/s or greater than 241 ml/s considered abnormal.

Aging

Data on PQ as a function of aging are sparse in the literature. Mean flow rate (and, therefore, PQ) has been reported to be lower in children than in adults because children have a smaller VC than adults (Murry, 1982). Although they did not directly compute PQ, Ptacek et al. (1966) did report VC and MPT data for young (<40 years) versus elderly (>65 years) men. A review of the Ptacek et al.'s (1966) data indicates that the young men would have produced a mean PQ of approximately 195.12 ml/s versus 171.27 ml/s for the elderly subjects, with this difference in PQ mainly attributable to a significantly lower VC in the elderly subjects.

Table 5–4 presents a range of examples of phonation quotient (in ml/s) from normal voice subjects.

WHAT TO EXPECT: ABNORMAL VOICE

Changes in PQ (and related MFR) have been particularly associated with disruptions in the ability to valve the airflow through the glottis. Those disorders that result in hypoadduction are expected to result in increased MFR and PQ; those in which hyperadduction is a primary component will be expected to show reduced MFR and PQ.

Mass Lesions and Distributed Tissue Change

Increased airflow rates, and therefore increased PQs, have been associated with the lack of complete vocal fold closure as a result of the presence of vocal fold masses/lesions affecting the margin(s) of the folds (Boone & McFarlane, 1988; Dworkin & Meleca, 1997; Haynes et al., 1992; Murry, 1982). Hirano et al. (1968) studied PQ in 25 men and 25 women with normal voice characteristics versus 73 subjects with diverse voice disorders. These authors observed that

Table 5–4 Phonation Quotient (in ml/s) from Normal Voice Subjects

Author	Gender	No. of Subjects	Age (yr.)	Mean & SD	Range
Yanagihara et al. (1966)[a]	M	11	30–43 ($\bar{x}$ = 36.0)	166.27 (33.71)	103.86–230.30
	F	11	21–41 ($\bar{x}$ = 28.0)	170.21 (36.55)	94.80–210.98
Hirano et al. (1968)[b]	M	25	N/A	145.0 (−44 & +62)	N/A
	F	25	N/A	137.0 (−32 & +42)	N/A
Iwata & von Leden (1970)	M	N/A	N/A	N/A	101–207
	F	N/A	N/A	N/A	105–176
Rau & Beckett (1984)[c]	M	10	19–28 ($\bar{x}$ = 21.10)	135.00 (19.30)	93.00–156.00
	F	9	21–29 ($\bar{x}$ = 24.33)	125.80 (16.40)	87.00–148.00
Awan & Ziminsky-Ammon (1996)	F	10	18–30 ($\bar{x}$ = 23.80)	186.75 (50.75)	115.43–283.69
	F	10	40–49 ($\bar{x}$ = 43.40)	202.52 (52.62)	114.16–272.65
	F	10	50–59 ($\bar{x}$ = 54.80)	182.58 (70.34)	72.35–315.79
	F	10	60–69 ($\bar{x}$ = 65.20)	198.81 (112.51)	85.95–461.37
	F	10	70–79 ($\bar{x}$ = 72.30)	200.18 (63.96)	97.83–303.69
Author	M	36	18–30 ($\bar{x}$ = 24.02)	190.94 (50.01)	95.64–303.89
	M	13	31–58 ($\bar{x}$ = 50.12)	173.71 (46.50)	107.50–248.71
	F	6	8–13 ($\bar{x}$ = 10.28)	146.20 (27.65)	93.53–169.63
	F	166	18–30 ($\bar{x}$ = 22.87)	157.84 (31.71)	95.45–275
	F	10	36–41 ($\bar{x}$ = 38.49)	137.02 (29.82)	102.73–182.56
	F	15	46–80 ($\bar{x}$ = 54.60)	150.57 (35.77)	95.00–225.71

M = male; F = female; $\bar{x}$ = mean; N/A = not available.
[a] Mean and SD are calculated from the raw VC and MPT data provided in the study.
[b] SD differs between negative and positive sides caused by calculation based on a square root transformation.
[c] Results provided from the Collins P-900 respirometer.

organic and functional voice disorders are often associated with increased air consumption during phonation. As confirmation of this, Hirano et al. (1968) observed that both PQ and MFR indicated the same clinical category (normal vs. abnormal) in 86% of the pathological cases examined. Iwata and von Leden (1970) investigated PQ in patients with laryngeal disease, as well as the relationship between PQ and MFR during maximally sustained phonation. Observations with disordered subjects showed slightly increased PQs in cases of laryngeal inflammation, abnormally high PQs in patients with inflammatory benign tumors (nodules, polyps), increased PQs for other benign tumors (papilloma, leukoplakia), and low normal PQs in cases of contact ulcers. In addition, PQ was observed to decrease after radiation therapy in patients with carcinomas of the larynx. Overall, a close relationship was observed between PQ and MFR in most pathological groups, although the authors concluded that PQ was not specific for laryngeal diseases and was a less sensitive indicator than actual MFR.

Neurological Disorders

The ability to valve the glottis during phonation may be affected by various neurological dysfunctions. High airflow rates, and therefore increased PQs, would be expected in those disorders in which hypoadduction would be expected (e.g., flaccid dysphonia) (Haynes et al., 1992; Iwata & von Leden, 1970; Murry, 1982). In contrast, neurological dysfunctions resulting in a highly constricted glottis (e.g., spastic dysphonia, spasmodic dysphonia) would be expected to have low MFRs and, therefore, low PQs (Boone & McFarlane, 1988; Dworkin & Meleca, 1997; Murry, 1982). Boone and McFarlane (1988) stress that measurements of airflow are usually substantiated by perceptual assessment of the voice, with breathy vocal quality related to increased flow, and harsh, constricted voice quality associated with decreased flow.

Functional Voice Disorders

Hyperfunctional voices may be expected to show reduced PQs secondary to hyperadduction of the folds during phonation. Hypoadduction caused by a hypofunctional component or significant posterior glottal chink may be expected to produce increased PQs.

MAXIMUM PERFORMANCE TESTS

This chapter has discussed several procedures that have been referred to as maximum performance tests (VC, MPT, and S/Z ratio) or are derived from maximum performance tests (PQ). These procedures have been seen to potentially provide the clinician with important information regarding the patient's respiratory and/or laryngeal status. However, the clinician must also be aware of methodological issues that may weaken the validity of these procedures. A number of pros and cons for the use of maximum performance tests are presented for consideration:

Pros and Cons

Kent et al. (1987) and Wit et al. (1993) have described a number of beneficial aspects of maximum performance tests that are shown below.

- Maximum performance tests may be useful in determining the relative degree of involvement of the functional systems of speech (for our purposes, the respiratory and phonatory systems).
- Maximum performance tests may be used to either confirm a diagnosis or to exclude an alternative diagnosis.
- Maximum performance tests may be useful indices of change.
- Maximum performance tasks aid in identifying diminished speed, strength, and range, which may have negative effects on the intelligibility and naturalness of disordered speech.

- By separately testing the performance capability of individual components of the speech mechanism, the "locus and general pathophysiologic consequence of a particular impairment" (Wit et al., 1993, p. 452) may be identified.
- With appropriate instruction, maximum performance tasks may be applied by the clinician in a highly standardized and objective manner (i.e., strong intraclinician administration).

Kent et al. (1987) have also summarized several cons of maximum performance tests that the clinician should be aware of during diagnostic testing and while interpreting the results of these procedures as shown below.

- The unfortunate lack of standardized procedures has resulted in considerable normative variability from study to study (i.e., poor interclinician administration).
- The effects (both individual and combined) of factors such as practice, motivation, or task instructions may prevent the patient from actually producing the maximum performance. This factor not only affects possible diagnostic decision making but also may affect the validity of pre- and post-therapy decisions regarding patient improvement.
- Normative data focus primarily on young adult data, with relatively little data on children or elderly subjects available. Because aging appears to have a substantial effect on several of the tests discussed in this chapter (VC and MPT), more extensive data are required for effective clinical use.
- Maximum performance tests do not assess speech in the conventional sense (i.e., although these tests may either correlate with speech behavior or present a form of simplified speech, they do not actually measure respiratory and/or phonatory system function in continuous speech itself).

It is clear that there are limitations in the use of maximum performance tests that the clinician must be aware of. However, a body of literature exists that shows that these tests can provide valuable diagnostic information for a variety of voice disorders. If the clinician takes into account the various methodological considerations discussed herein, these tests can add a valuable dimension to the *VDP*.

CHAPTER 6

Evaluation of Muscle Tension Dysphonia

DEFINITION

Functional voice disorders often present with excessive amounts of laryngeal musculoskeletal tension as either the primary cause of the voice dysfunction or as a maintaining factor of the dysfunction (Roy & Leeper, 1993). These types of functional dysphonias have alternatively been referred to as hyperfunctional in nature or as muscle tension dysphonias (MTDs). Patients with MTDs often provide symptoms such as tightness/tension in the laryngeal region; neck and shoulder tightness; full body tension; headaches; effortful voice and fatigue; and multifaceted pitch, loudness, and quality deviations. Other characteristics consistent with MTD may be head or hand tremors, abnormal breathing patterns, visible tightness in the neck or jaw region, abnormal facial expression and gaze, and inconsistency of voice characteristics (Andrews, 1995; Boone & McFarlane, 1988; Stemple, 1993). Unusual downward or upward excursions of the larynx during speech have also been reported in MTD (Boone & McFarlane, 1988).

It should be noted that a wide variety of voice disorders may present with excessive laryngeal musculoskeletal tension as part of their symptom complex. Stemple (1993) has compiled a number of case studies described as hypofunctional (both functional and organic in nature) that have also described elements of increased laryngeal tension and vocal hyperfunction, which were addressed in their respective therapy plans.

CHARACTERISTICS OF MTD

In MTD, the presenting voice disorder is affected (either primarily or secondarily) by misuse of the voluntary muscles affecting phonation, as well as misuse of associated muscles of the speech mechanism (muscles of the larynx, pharynx, jaw, tongue, neck, and respiratory system) (Morrison & Rammage, 1993). Several causative scenarios may account for the presence of excessive musculoskeletal tension as shown below.

- Psychological and/or personality factors may induce tension. According to Aronson (1990a), factors such as anxiety, anger, irritability, impatience, frustration, and depression may be responsible for hypercontraction. This hypercontraction may arise as a result of a release of subcortical centers under situations of emotional stress. This subcortical emotional release may result in reduced control over respiratory and phonatory mechanisms (Aronson, 1990a). Psychological distress contributes to pressor responses in the nervous system that, in turn, affect hypertonicity of the voluntary musculature (Morrison & Rammage, 1993).

- Technical misuse of the vocal mechanism, particularly in face of extensive and extraordinary vocal demands, may incorporate or lead to the development of excessive musculoskeletal tension and MTD (Morrison & Rammage, 1993; Roy, Ford, & Bless, 1996). Poor technical use of the phonatory mechanism may include such factors as poor coordination between respiratory, phonatory, resonatory, and articulatory gestures; excessive or inadequate laryngeal valving; improper resonance focus; and improper control of pitch and/or loudness dynamics (Morrison & Rammage, 1993).

- Excessive musculoskeletal tension may be a learned adaptation after upper respiratory tract infection or other organic triggers (e.g., gastroesophageal reflux disease, allergic reactions, asthma) (Morrison & Rammage, 1993; Roy et al., 1996).

- Excessive musculoskeletal tension may be a compensatory adaptation for some underlying organic or neurologically based dysfunction (e.g., vocal fold lesions, vocal fold paralysis or paresis) (Roy et al., 1996).

It can be seen that excessive musculoskeletal tension has an insidious nature and may be (1) the cause of a voice disorder, (2) an accompanying factor in a voice disorder, or (3) the outcome of a voice disorder and thus a perpetuating factor in voice dysfunction (Morrison & Rammage, 1993; Roy et al., 1996). Figure 6–1 graphically depicts the inter-relationships between excessive muscle tension, psychological and emotional stress, and voice dysfunction.

Roy and Bless (1998) provide an extensive review of the signs and symptoms of increased laryngeal musculoskeletal tension as shown below.

1. Voice quality deviations are quite variable in terms of both severity and type. Voice characteristics range from those indicative of hyperadduction (tension, pressed voice, rough quality) to those commonly associated with hypoadduction (breathiness). Roy and Bless (1998) state that the patient may be "pitch- and loudness-locked" (p. 152), indicative of restriction in both pitch and loudness/dynamic range. The patient will often report increased effort in voice production.

2. Excessive laryngeal tension may be associated with symptoms such as a dull to severe ache in the anterior neck, laryngeal, and shoulder regions, as well as neck swellings/lumps (sites of nodularity). The presence of MTD is suspected when patients report a feeling of a lump, a ball, or tension in the larynx or pharynx; occasionally, pain may also be reported.

3. Feelings of tension and restriction are not necessarily restricted to the laryngeal region; they may extend to the jaw and tongue, as well as to the thoracic regions.

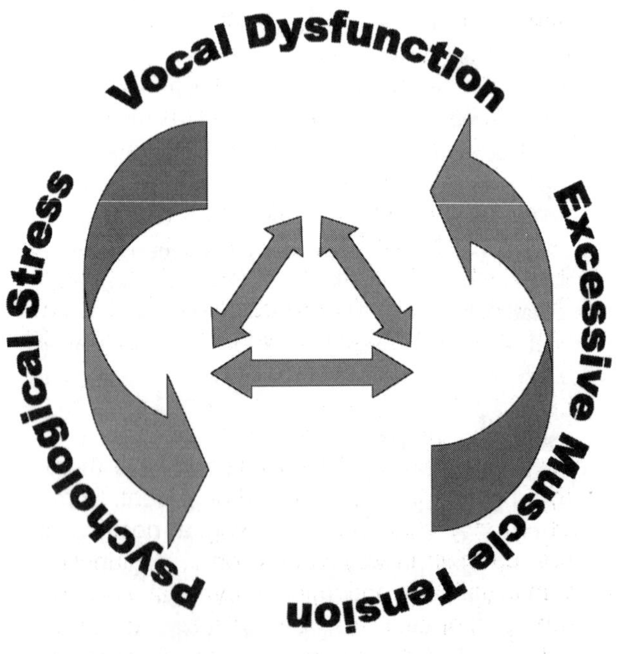

In addition to the characteristics mentioned by Roy and Bless (1998), several other key characteristics consistent with MTD have been reported as shown below.

- It is often observed that these patients have (1) structurally normal larynges or (2) secondary pathological conditions generally associated with vocal hyperfunction and abuse (nodules, polyps, etc.) (Morrison & Rammage, 1993).
- Neurotic tendencies (Aronson, 1990a).
- Elevation of the tongue, which contributes to tension and pain in the submental musculature (Aronson, 1990a).

Morrison and Rammage (1993) prefer the term "muscle misuse voice disorder" (p. 428) to the term "functional dysphonia," because "functional dysphonia" has often been used synonymously with "psychogenic." Morrison and Rammage (1993) described six classes of dysphonia in which muscle misuse was a key factor. These are listed below.

1. Muscular tension dysphonia—the laryngeal isometric: This class of muscle misuse was observed in untrained occupational and professional voice users. These patients showed a generalized increase in muscular tension throughout the laryngeal and suprahyoid regions. Laryngoscopic findings often show the presence of a posterior glottal chink caused by significant contraction of the posterior cricoarytenoid muscle during adduction. The result may be whispery/breathy phonation. However, strong adductive forces may be used to overcome the presence of the posterior glottal chink, thereby adding a rough aspect to the phonation.

2. Lateral contraction and/or hyperadduction: These patients often have a tense-sounding voice and complaints of vocal fatigue and discomfort, particularly near the end of the day. Laryngoscopically, this class of patient often shows laryngeal squeezing in a side-to-side manner and hyperadduction. Morrison and Rammage (1993) hypothesize that this type of patient does not adequately coordinate respiratory and phonatory function. This may result in "surges of uncontrolled respiratory air" (p. 431), which the patient attempts to control by means

Figure 6–1 The Complex Interaction between Vocal Dysfunction, Psychological Stress, and Excessive Muscle Tension

of excessive laryngeal valving. The result is an effortful, harsh voice and rapid fatigue. Decreased vocal pitch may be observed due to laryngeal compression (indicative of possible anterior-posterior squeezing of the larynx in addition to the lateral squeezing).

3. Anterior-posterior contraction of the supraglottal larynx: As previously mentioned, this type of laryngeal posture often results in a lowering of vocal pitch. This type of patient was observed to complain of effortful voice and fatigue but was able to improve voice quality and phonation with less effort at a higher pitch.

4. Conversion aphonia: Morrison and Rammage (1993) state that "the anxiety that leads to conversion aphonia/hysteria has produced such mental pain that a physical symptom such as aphonia is much more bearable to the individual" (p. 432). The voice (if any) produced by this patient was observed to be high pitched, squeaky, or breathy. However, this patient shows the capability for normal adduction of the vocal folds by producing a normal cough or other type of vegetative function (e.g., laughter).

5. Psychogenic dysphonia with bowed vocal folds: Although bowed vocal folds are often associated with presbyphonia (i.e., voice changes associated with advanced aging), this glottal configuration was also observed in cases of psychogenic functional dysphonia. Morrison and Rammage (1993) indicate that this type of patient may have habituated hoarseness initiated by upper respiratory tract infection or other organic trigger.

6. Adolescent transitional aphonia: More commonly referred to as mutational falsetto or puberphonia, this class of muscle misuse was characteristically observed in patients who had experienced pitch or register breaks and accompanying embarrassment during normal adolescent voice change during puberty. As a result of lack of physical control over phonation and subsequent psychological stress, the patient may attempt to inhibit the normal voice change and establish "perpetual falsetto phonation" (Morrison and Rammage, 1993, p. 433). In maintaining the high-pitch, falsetto voice, the patient often has increased laryngeal tension and laryngeal elevation.

Morrison and Rammage (1993) summarize the possible causes of excessive muscular tension and muscle misuse by stating that "if the central basal ganglia control and the laryngeal sensorimotor reflexes are relatively constant, then the main clinically important factors which may account for shifts in muscular tension are (1) technical ability, (2) psychological tension, and (3) reflux" (p. 433). The third factor mentioned (reflux) may be better termed "organic triggers" to also include factors such as upper respiratory tract infections, allergies, etc.

HOW TO DO IT: CLINICAL ASSESSMENT OF EXCESSIVE MUSCULOSKELETAL TENSION

Aronson (1990a) stressed the diagnostic importance of muscle tension assessment by stating that "all patients with voice disorders, regardless of etiology, should be tested for excess musculoskeletal tension, either as a primary or a secondary cause of the dysphonia" (p. 314). Musculoskeletal tension evaluation should enable the clinician to subjectively determine (1) degree of laryngeal elevation, (2) patient response to pressure in the laryngeal region, and (3) the presence of palpable tension in the extrinsic laryngeal musculature and sites of focal nodularity (i.e., areas that are distinctly harder or prominent) (Roy et al., 1997a). The aforementioned characteristics of excessive musculoskeletal tension may be determined through focal palpation of the laryngeal region. This palpation provides the clinician with direct tactile assessment of the possible presence of MTD. Roy and Bless (1998) describe a number of procedures beneficial in the initial assessment of MTD and pertinent diagnostic observations below.

- During laryngeal palpation, the pressure applied should be similar to that "required to cause the thumbnail to blanch when pressed against a firm surface" (Roy & Bless, 1998, p. 152). The clinician cannot be too timid during this procedure. Only firm palpation of the extralaryngeal region will allow the clinician to detect underlying muscle tension and rigidity and elicit discomfort and/or tenderness that is considered abnormal and a key characteristic of MTD. When specific points of excessive tension or nodularity are palpated, the patient may wince, withdraw, or verbalize feelings of discomfort.

- Palpation should include the thyrohyoid space. When the larynx is abnormally elevated (i.e., suspended high in the neck region), the thyrohyoid space will be narrowed or absent. Some cases may show normal laryngeal position at rest but high laryngeal position in conjunction with initiation of phonation. Laryngeal elevation during phonation may be indicative of the involvement of the extrinsic laryngeal musculature during voice production.

- The clinician should attempt to move the larynx side-to-side. The lack of lateral mobility is also indicative of extralaryngeal hypertonicity.
- Morrison (1997) suggests palpation of the cricothyroid space during rest and during pitch glides from low to high pitches and vice versa. An absent space during these conditions may indicate excessive tension in the cricothyroid musculature. If the clinician has trouble detecting the cricothyroid, the clinician may be able to detect movement of the anterior portion of the cricoid cartilage superiorly toward the thyroid during pitch elevation.

Several of the key areas of laryngeal palpation are identified in reference to a model of the hyoid-laryngeal complex in Figure 6–2.

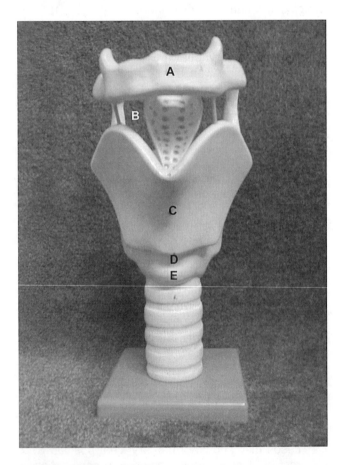

Figure 6–2 Anterior View of a Model of the Hyoid-Laryngeal Complex. Key anatomical sites during evaluation of muscle tension dysphonia (MTD) and laryngeal palpation are (A) the hyoid bone, (B) the thyrohyoid space, (C) the thyroid cartilage, (D) the cricothyroid space, and (E) the cricoid cartilage.

Laryngeal Reposturing

The presence of extralaryngeal hypertonicity often alters the posture of the larynx both at rest and during phonation, with the aforementioned signs and symptoms of MTD produced. It has been described that reposturing/repositioning of the larynx often results in rapid and significant change in vocal functioning. Roy and Bless (1998) describe laryngeal reposturing maneuvers that (1) may aid the clinician in verifying the effects of inappropriate posture on voice and (2) may reveal the extent of voice change possible after reposturing:

1. During phonation, the clinician may physically impede the elevation of the larynx by applying downward pressure over the superior border of the thyroid lamina.
2. During phonation, the larynx may be compressed in an anterior-to-posterior direction by applying pressure over the inferior portion of the hyoid bone or within the thyrohyoid space. This laryngeal compression may reduce excess tension and vocal fold stiffness. This component has similarity to the techniques of anterior-posterior compression (Blaugrund, Taira, & Isshiki, 1991) and digital manipulation (Boone & McFarlane, 1988), in which external pressure exerted on the thyroid cartilage is used to relieve stiffness and tension and elicit pitch change.
3. During phonation, medial compression may be combined with downward pressure in the region of the superior horns of the thyroid cartilage.

It should be noted that these reposturing methods may fail for reasons such as (1) ineffectively applied pressure, (2) wrong position on the laryngeal structures, and (3) patient intolerance to pressure (Blaugrund et al., 1991). However, when done correctly, Roy and Bless (1998) state that "by manually repositioning or stabilizing the larynx during a sustained 'ah,' the clinician can stimulate improved voice and briefly interrupt patterns of muscle misuse" (p. 153). In the event that voice change is observed after reposturing of the larynx, the clinician should bring voice improvement to the immediate attention of the patient. Voice change may be reinforced by the use of biofeedback (e.g., auditory and visual feedback by means of computerized voice assessment) and extending use of the improved voice through a hierarchy of speech tasks (vowels, syllables, words, sentences).

Circumlaryngeal Massage—Diagnostic Therapy Description

In the event that excessive musculoskeletal tension is suspected but reposturing has had limited effect on the patient's voice, the clinician should move on to other approaches that may effect changes in muscular tension. Several voice therapy techniques have been described by which tension in the laryngeal region may be relieved. Approaches such as the chewing approach, the yawn-sigh method, and techniques of progressive relaxation have all been advocated in the relief of excessive tension (Boone & McFarlane, 1988; Prater & Swift, 1984). Aronson (1990a) has described one of the more active/direct forms of therapy advocated for the relief of excessive laryngeal tension. Aronson (1990a) advocates a form of circumlaryngeal massage in which the extrinsic laryngeal musculature is palpated and kneaded in an attempt to relieve excessive muscle tension. In addition to the kneading action, attempts are made to actively lower the position of the larynx within the neck (incorporating an aspect of the previously described laryngeal reposturing).

Although circumlaryngeal massage has been used effectively as a voice therapy technique (Roy & Leeper, 1993; Roy et al., 1996; Roy et al., 1997a; Stemple, 1993), *it is stressed that this method should be also incorporated into the voice diagnostic.* One of the most effective ways in which we can determine whether vocal hyperfunction and excessive musculoskeletal tension are components underlying the patient's voice disorder is to attempt to relieve the tension. If the voice improves after a period of diagnostic therapy that has focused on the relief of laryngeal tension, the clinician may assume that tension must have been present. Aronson (1990a) stated that "the degree of voice improvement following therapy for musculoskeletal tension is proportional to the reduction of the muscle tension" (p. 314).

There are several basic principles regarding the use of circumlaryngeal massage as a diagnostic therapy technique (Aronson, 1990a; Peifang, 1991 in Roy & Bless, 1998):

1. Excessive tension/tightness in the extrinsic laryngeal musculature most probably affects intrinsic muscle function.
2. Reducing musculoskeletal tension releases the inherent capability of the larynx to produce voice.
3. When massaged, muscles relax, become less painful, and less restricted in motion.
4. Lowering laryngeal position permits more normal phonation.
5. Massage of the extralaryngeal region is believed to stretch muscle and connective tissue, improve local circulation, promote muscle relaxation, and relieve pain and discomfort resulting from muscle spasm and/or tension.

As previously stated, perhaps the essential diagnostic sign of the presence of MTD is the extent of voice improvement after tension reduction (Aronson, 1990a). Therefore, it is suggested that the circumlaryngeal massage technique be used as *both* a diagnostic and a therapeutic technique. The procedures used to relieve MTD that I have had success with are based on those described by Aronson (1990a). In the event that MTD is suspected, explain the procedures used in circumlaryngeal massage and the possible benefits of the procedure. Before beginning the massage/manipulation procedure, clearly explain to your patient that (1) you will be touching him or her in the neck area, and (2) there may be some temporary discomfort. It is essential that the therapist display a confident manner to the patient during this procedure; tentative approaches to this treatment will surely result in a lack of certainty in the skills of the therapist and may result in even more tension in the patient. When the therapist is ready to begin, these basic steps should be followed:

1. Identify the region of the horns of the hyoid bone (approximately lateral and slightly inferior to the angle of the mandible; see Figure 6–3).
2. Exert *firm pressure* in the region of the horns of the hyoid bilaterally; begin rotary massage with the fingertips (thumb and index/middle finger; see Figure

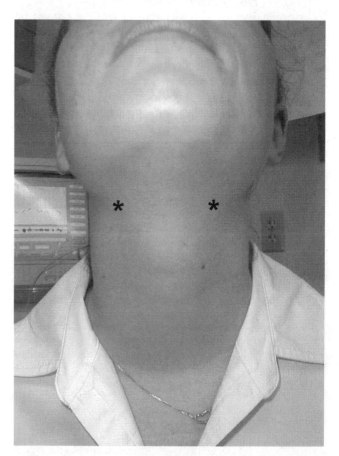

Figure 6–3 The Region of the Horns of the Hyoid Bone Are Indicated (*)

6–4 for an example of hand position). This step is, perhaps, the largest deviation from the procedure as described by Aronson (1990a). I have had the most success using firm, direct pressure rather than the light pressure described by Aronson.

3. Ask the patient about the presence of pain/discomfort; note sites of discomfort or nodularity and focus your massage in these areas.

4. Continue rotary massage with the fingertips for several minutes; while still massaging, start to flatten the thumb and forefingers into the thyrohyoid space.

5. After several minutes of massage, find the margins (posterior borders) of the thyroid cartilage just medial to the sternocleidomastoid; continue rotary massage in this area (see Figure 6–5).

6. Continue massage; now begin to work the larynx downward, as well as laterally. After several minutes of this massage, you should be able to easily move the larynx laterally, as well as feel a widening of the thyrohyoid space.

7. Ask the patient to prolong vowels during these procedures. The clinician should be keenly aware of changes in perceived voice characteristics (quality, pitch, etc.). I also recommend that the patient be instructed on the following facets of voice production before phonation:

- Deep breath support
- A feeling of relaxation and easy onset
- Front focus (i.e., encourage vocal resonance in the anterior oral cavity; vowel production initiated with a nasal phoneme such as /mɑ/ is often useful in encouraging this effect)

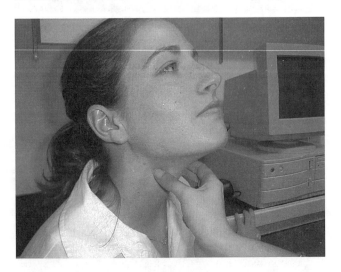

Figure 6–4 Hand and Finger Position for Laryngeal Massage in the Region of the Horns of the Hyoid Bone Bilaterally

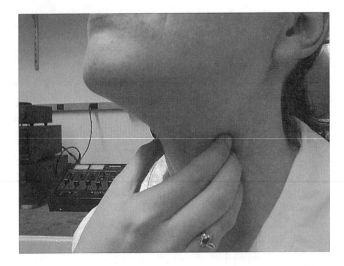

Figure 6–5 Massage Position along the Margins (Posterior Borders) of the thyroid. Rotary massage is applied in this area with the larynx manipulated downward as well as laterally.

Before having the patient produce a phonation after the initial massage, the instructions below are provided to the patient.

"When I ask you, you will sustain the vowel /ɑ/. Take a deep breath; when you are ready to produce voice, know that nothing is going to prevent or block the flow of air as it travels from your lungs and out the mouth. I want you to focus the vibrations you will produce in the front of the mouth, face, and nasal region."

Computerized visual and audio feedback of the patient's voice production by means of voice analysis software provides rapid feedback and "unbiased" confirmation of voice change. Aronson (1990a) notes that "the voice rarely changes from aphonia or dysphonia to normal without first passing through several dysphonic stages" (p. 315). Therefore, the clinician must be prepared to provide immediate feedback regarding voice improvements and to repeat the circumlaryngeal massage procedure several times within a session, with rest periods provided.

The Pros and Cons of Evaluating the Presence of Excessive Musculoskeletal Tension

Several key positive aspects ("pros") of the application of laryngeal musculoskeletal tension evaluation methods are listed below.

- Palpation of the laryngeal region provides the clinician with a method of evaluating the possible presence of increased musculoskeletal tension rather than depending solely on patient symptoms.
- Because these methods are therapeutic, as well as diagnostic in nature, they have the capability to reveal the effects of underlying muscle misuse and/or poor laryngeal posture on the voice.
- The detection of underlying muscle misuse leads to the development of specific treatment goals.
- The revelation of underlying muscle misuse leads to increased clarity in reference to the prognosis for the patient.

Although there are definite benefits to the evaluation of MTD by means of laryngeal palpation, there are also several issues that may contraindicate the use of these methods or limit their potential benefits as shown below.

- Both clinician and patient may be tentative regarding the safety of this technique. However, Aronson (1990a) states that "maneuvering the patient's laryngeal and hyoid anatomy as described is safe as long as it is performed with good judgement" (p. 315). Roy (personal communication, April 2000) states that manual circumlaryngeal techniques would be contraindicated in patients with history of cerebral or cardiovascular episodes due to manipulation/ massage in close proximity to major veins and arteries that course in the vicinity of the laryngeal region. Similar caution should be exercised with elderly patients.
- The clinician should remember that pain in the laryngeal region is not just a symptom of excessive muscle tension but can also be associated with other significant disorders (e.g., contact ulcer, arytenoid fixation). As previously stressed, *appropriate medical referral (ideally before the voice evaluation, but certainly afterward and before initiating any treatment) is essential*.
- Although several studies have described the benefits of circumlaryngeal techniques as both diagnostic and therapeutic methods, it has been questioned whether voice changes that may occur after laryngeal manipulation are due to decreased muscular tension or other factors (e.g., placebo effects, clinician instructions, expectations, experience, and confidence). Roy et al. (1997b) state that the fact that some subjects improve seconds after the initiation of the circumlaryngeal treatment may indicate that factors other than tension reduction are responsible for voice change. In particular, postural adjustment of the larynx may explain the sudden changes in voice

characteristics. Roy (personal communication, April 2000) believes that the perturbation of the larynx (i.e., disruption of inappropriate laryngeal posture and muscle tension) may be responsible for the sudden changes in voice characteristics often observed.

WHAT TO EXPECT

In those cases in which MTD is a significant component of the voice disorder, drastic changes in voice characteristics may be observed within a single therapy session by use of the massage/manipulation technique. Rapid voice improvement may be observed in those cases in which the dysphonia has been of relatively short duration, and the primary cause of the dysphonia is excessive musculoskeletal tension. In other cases, several hours of therapy over multiple sessions may be required (Aronson, 1990a). Substantial improvements in voice quality, as well as pitch, loudness, and duration, may be perceived and may be objectively displayed to the patient by measures such as vocal F_0 and measures of phonatory periodicity (e.g., jitter, shimmer, and harmonics-to-noise ratio).

A number of studies shown below have attempted to document the effects of the circumlaryngeal massage technique on patients with functional dysphonias.

- Stemple (1993) describes a case of direct digital massage in an adult female patient diagnosed as having a functional voice disorder characterized primarily by the presence of strained, raspy phonation. This patient showed improvement to normal voice quality "within 3 weeks of the (initial) evaluation" (p. 102).
- Roy and Leeper (1993) investigated the perceptual and acoustic effects of manual laryngeal musculoskeletal tension reduction in patients with functional dysphonias. The results of the Roy and Leeper (1993) study were derived from a single session, before-after therapy design, with session length for each of 17 patients varying from 1 to 3 hours. As a group, the dysphonic patients showed significant improvement in perceptual ratings of their voice quality, as well as significant reductions in jitter and shimmer and significant increases in SNR. Although the authors do report that 93% of the patients were judged to have maintained voice quality change as determined by phone conversation 1 week after therapy, the authors provide no objective measurement data to substantiate this observation.
- Roy et al. (1996) described the role of manual laryngeal tension reduction in the management of three cases of laryngeal hyperfunction. The authors describe relief of tightness and pain in the laryngeal region and subse-

quent voice improvement in a single case of a patient diagnosed with MTD; the other two cases presented with accompanying spasmodic dysphonia and showed limited and temporary improvements in vocal characteristics.

- Roy et al. (1997a) reported significant improvements in perceived vocal severity and acoustic measures of perturbation and spectral noise (jitter, shimmer, and SNR) in a single voice diagnostic/treatment session with 25 adult female patients diagnosed with functional dysphonia. Improvements were also maintained in two follow-up sessions (follow-up session 1 was approximately 3 months after the initial session; follow-up 2 was 16.5 months ± 11.4 months after the initial session). Although no direct measures of muscular tension were conducted, the authors did believe that there was indirect evidence to support Aronson's view's on MTD: (1) most patients reported a decrease in laryngeal pain immediately after the manual circumlaryngeal procedure; and (2) during the treatment, subjects progressed through stages of decreasing dysphonia until symptoms remitted.

Positive changes in voice characteristics are generally maintained; often when the patient hears and sees that he or she has the capability to produce improved voice, confidence and enthusiasm for continued therapy drastically improve and the ability to control the phonatory mechanism is enhanced. The previously described findings by Roy and Leeper (1993) and Roy et al. (1997a) confirm this observation. Although before and after comparison designs are often effected by historical effects that may contribute to voice change between the two measurement points (Kazdin, 1982; Schiavetti & Metz, 1997), the observation of significant changes in both perceptual and acoustic measures of the dysphonic voice in the single sessions described in the Roy and Leeper (1993) and Roy et al. (1997a) studies would appear to lend validity to the use of the manual laryngeal musculoskeletal tension reduction technique. The authors of these studies stress that caution must be exercised in attributing voice change particularly to reductions in muscle tension because no objective measures of muscle activity were used. In addition, other considerations such as placebo effects, clinician instructions, expectations, experience, and confidence may have contributed to their results (Roy et al., 1997a). Notwithstanding, it may be concluded that Aronson's (1990a) technique deserves serious consideration.

SUMMARY

Laryngeal massage/digital manipulation provides a "hands-on" approach to voice diagnosis and therapy that has the capability of revealing the effects of excessive mus-

culoskeletal tension and producing positive changes in voice characteristics within a relatively short time. Of course, this technique should be applied as part of a comprehensive voice treatment protocol that would include factors such as (1) educational information regarding normal and abnormal voice production, (2) the identification and reduction of vocal abuses and misuses, and (3) encouragement of vocal hydration. However, because MTD may be a primary or secondary factor in a multitude of voice disorders (functional or organic in nature, hyperfunctional, or hypofunctional), speech pathologists dealing with voice-disordered patients would be strongly encouraged to further investigate this method of voice assessment and therapy.

CASE STUDY

The following case study focuses on the diagnostic evaluation of a patient who had many characteristics consistent with a muscle misuse disorder. Because the circumlaryngeal techniques described herein have the capability of producing significant and lasting change in the patient's voice, data relating to the within-diagnostic session voice changes, as well as data pertaining to postdiagnostic follow-up sessions, are provided.

Subject Characteristics

Patient MTD was a 33-year-old woman referred for voice evaluation and treatment by her family physician. The patient was a teacher at a local elementary school who had a history of chronic voice difficulties that had persisted for 5 to 6 years. At the time of the initial evaluation, patient MTD had a moderate degree of hoarseness with a strong breathy component. Intelligibility of the patient's speech was occasionally disrupted because of intermittent periods of aphonia.

Approximately 4½ years previously, the patient had been diagnosed as having bilateral vocal nodules. A more recent ear, nose, and throat (ENT) evaluation had indicated that the patient's vocal nodules had diminished in size and did not present a significant factor in affecting vocal fold vibration. However, the more recent ENT evaluation did indicate the presence of reflux esophagitis and some degree of accompanying vocal fold irritation. In response to the presence of possible reflux difficulties, patient MTD had been prescribed ranitidine (Zantac). In addition, she reported extensive diet changes to avoid foods that may have resulted in reflux difficulties. Unfortunately, patient MTD reported that the medication and diet changes had had no substantial effect on improving her voice quality.

Patient MTD also reported undergoing approximately 1 year of voice therapy with a speech pathologist at a local hospital. Therapy reports from the previous therapist indicated that the focus of remediation was on improving breath support and on the monitoring of vocal abuses. Patient MTD reported that any improvements in her voice as a result of this period of therapy were temporary in nature.

Overall, patient MTD was a very personable and conscientious patient with no hesitations in discussing her medical or personal history as it pertained to her voice disorder. She reported that one of her main concerns was whether she would be able to continue with her profession as an elementary school teacher.

Initial Diagnostic Results

The initial session was separated into a diagnostic session (case history and collection of perceptual, acoustic, and respiratory data, approximately 45 minutes in duration), followed by a period of diagnostic therapy (approximately 45 minutes in duration). As previously stated, patient MTD had moderate hoarseness (strong breathy component). During the initial case history/questioning session, the patient described the presence of muscular tension in the suprahyoid region, as well as effort and strain to produce voice. Patient MTD related this tension to a feeling of "a ball in the throat" during voice production. Generally, voice production became more effortful later in the day. The patient also described occasional headaches, as well as tension in the shoulder region. During discussion with the patient, visible tension in the suprahyoid and sternocleidomastoid regions was noted. The patient denied any history of smoking and also reported adequate daily hydration (4 to 6 8-oz. glasses of water per day).

After the case history period, the voice evaluation focused on collecting objective data that would aid in characterizing the patient's voice disorder. The following acoustic measures were conducted.

Continuous Speech Analysis

The patient was asked to read "The Rainbow Passage" (Fairbanks, 1960) at a comfortable pitch and loudness. The second sentence of the passage was recorded using a PC-compatible computer, SoundBlaster16 (Creative Labs, Milipitas, CA) sound card, and high-quality microphone. The voice productions were sampled at 44,100 Hz with 16 bits of resolution and saved to disk using the EZVoice (Voice-Tek Enterprises, Nescopeck, PA) voice analysis software program.

Measures of F_0 and Perturbation

The patient's mean speaking F_0 was measured at 194.9 Hz (SD = 37.5 Hz). This mean speaking F_0 was considered within normal limits for the patient's age and gender but possibly slightly lower than might be expected in consideration of her height (61 in.).

The patient was asked to sustain three trials of the vowel /ɑ/ at a comfortable pitch and loudness for 2 to 3 seconds. Vowel recordings were made in an identical manner to the continuous speech sample. The middle 1 s of each vowel was selected for further analysis and results averaged: mean F_0 = 174 Hz (SD = 7.17 Hz); jitter = 3.41%; shimmer = 0.49 dB. The mean F_0 was considered substantially lower than expected. Patient MTD's jitter value was considerably higher than normative jitter values that are generally observed to be well below 1%. The increased jitter reflects increased perturbation in the periodicity of vocal fold vibration and was consistent with the perception of moderate hoarseness.

Phonational Range

Phonational range was measured at 10.63 semitones (171 to 316 Hz). Normal range for an adult female nonsinger may be expected in the 24 to 30 semitone range.

Respiratory and Durational Measures

The patient's vital capacity was measured at 2.95 L and was considered to be within normal expectations for her age and height (61 in.). Phonation quotient was measured at 368.75 ml/s; this result is consistent with increased airflow through the glottis and the perception of breathiness in this patient's voice quality. Both MPT (8 s; 0.4 ratio of measured to expected) and S/Z ratio (1.69) would be considered abnormal. These results are indicative of an inability to adequately valve the outgoing airstream at the vocal fold level.

Evaluation of Musculoskeletal Tension

Palpation of patient MTD's laryngeal and suprahyoid region (as described by Roy et al., 1997a) elicited verbalization of discomfort from the patient, particularly on the left side of her neck. In addition, the larynx was elevated such that detection of the thyrohyoid space was difficult. The presence of muscular rigidity made side-to-side manipulation of the larynx difficult.

By this point in the evaluation, the impression was that this patient had many characteristics consistent with MTD/ excessive laryngeal musculoskeletal tension. Although other factors in her history may also have contributed to her voice disorder (possible continuing effects of vocal nodules, vocal fold irritation secondary to reflux esophagitis), her descriptions of key characteristics such as tension in the laryngeal region, headaches, effortful voice, etc., led to the impression that MTD was playing a considerable role as a primary underlying physiological cause of her voice disorder.

Diagnostic Therapy Description

It has been previously stated that an essential diagnostic sign of the presence of MTD is the extent of voice improvement after tension reduction (Aronson, 1990a). Therefore, as part of the initial diagnostic session, patient MTD was treated with the laryngeal massage technique. The procedures used to relieve MTD were based on those previously described by Aronson (1990a). Patient MTD's sustained vowel productions after an initial 15-minute introduction to the laryngeal massage technique were perceived as being produced with reduced hoarse/breathy quality and with an increase in pitch. In addition, phonation was consistent with no intermittent periods of aphonia perceived. Recordings of the vowel samples played back to the patient by means of the computer sound card and speakers and results of voice analysis were visualized using the voice analysis software. The perceptual changes noted by the examiner were also evident to the patient. Circumlaryngeal massage was reintroduced several times so that (1) the patient could become accustomed to the feeling of producing improved voice with reduced tension and (2) so that the patient could become familiar with the laryngeal massage technique to such a degree that she would be able to apply it to herself outside of the voice therapy environment. After becoming comfortable with producing sustained vowels in a tension-free manner, patient MTD was instructed on extending the tension-free voice to syllable (CV and CVC syllables), word, and sentence productions.

At the end of the 45-minute diagnostic-therapy session, several acoustic measures from sustained vowels and continuous speech productions were repeated (see Table 6–1). Results after the introduction of the circumlaryngeal massage technique supported the perceptual impressions of improvement in voice characteristics and confirmed the impressions that MTD was a significant contributor to this patient's voice disorder.

A review of the before and after therapy results provided in Table 6–1 indicates the following.

1. An increase in this patient's speaking and sustained vowel F_0s was observed. It has been hypothesized that anterior-posterior squeezing of the larynx and/or tension focal to the vocal/thyroarytenoid muscles may cause F_0 to lower in cases of MTD. Therefore, it is hypothesized that the increases in vocal F_0 after therapy may have been due to the relief of excessive tension in the laryngeal region.

2. Reduced pitch sigma (reflective of long-term variability in this patient's voice) was observed in both continuous speech and sustained vowel production after circumlaryngeal massage. Increased control over vocal F_0 and reduced breathiness may contribute to this change.

3. Decreases in jitter and shimmer after circumlaryngeal massage indicate decreases in short-term variability (cycle-to-cycle variations in frequency and amplitude) and reflect the perception of improved voice quality (particularly in terms of decreased breathy quality).

After this initial diagnostic-therapy session, patient MTD received five more sessions of voice therapy over a 3-week period in which the primary goal was the reduction of excessive laryngeal musculoskeletal tension by circumlaryngeal massage techniques. Therapy sessions were similar in duration and content to the diagnostic-therapy session (approximately 45 minutes in duration). Therapy also incorporated computerized feedback (both visual and auditory) that appeared to be helpful in having patient MTD increase her awareness of changes in her voice.

Table 6–1 Voice Analysis Results Pre- and Postcircumlaryngeal Massage for a Patient Presenting with Characteristics of Muscle Tension Dysphonia (MTD)

	Pretherapy	Posttherapy	Change
Mean speaking frequency	194.9 Hz	201.77 Hz	+6.87 Hz
Pitch sigma (F_0 SD)	6.75 ST (37.5 Hz)	4.59 ST (26.6 Hz)	–2.16 ST (–10.9 Hz)
Mean frequency: vowel	174 Hz	208 Hz	+34 Hz
Pitch sigma (F_0 SD): vowel	1.42 ST (7.17 Hz)	0.61 ST (3.71 Hz)	–0.81 ST (–3.46 Hz)
Jitter	3.41%	1.2%	–2.21%
Shimmer	0.49 dB	0.18 dB	–0.31 dB

Application of Diagnostic Methods and Findings to Therapy

Although the discussion of methods such as laryngeal reposturing and circumlaryngeal massage has been provided primarily in terms of diagnostic use, therapy session data are provided for this case study to show (1) the direct carryover of diagnostic methods to the therapy situation and (2) to illustrate that the diagnostic procedures used in detecting MTD are *reactive* in nature (i.e., they have an effect on the patient's behavior; Schiavetti & Metz, 1997). Measurements of various voice parameters (mean F_0 [both sustained vowels and continuous speech], jitter, shimmer, phonational range) were conducted at the start (i.e., pretherapy) and at the end (i.e., posttherapy) of each therapy session (results are provided graphically in Figures 6–1 to 6–5). Because this is a single-case study, inferential statistics were not applied to the data. Instead, a more descriptive analysis of the observed changes in the various voice parameters will be provided. In addition to the raw data for the therapy and follow-up phases of this study, trend lines have been developed using a variation of the split-middle technique (White, 1974 in Kazdin, 1982). This technique permits examination of trends within each phase. Trend lines are developed by (1) identifying the median performance on the dependent variable (e.g., mean F_0) in each half of a particular phase and then (2) drawing a trend line that bisects the medians. These trend lines have also been referred to as celeration lines (Kazdin, 1982) and can be used to predict the direction of behavior change.

Vocal F_0: Continuous Speech and Sustained Vowels

Patient MTD showed consistent increases in her mean F_0 after the application of laryngeal massage in each of the therapy sessions for both continuous speech and sustained vowel productions (see Figures 6–6 and 6–7). In addition, F_0 was generally observed to progressively increase from session to session. This is reflected in the observation that

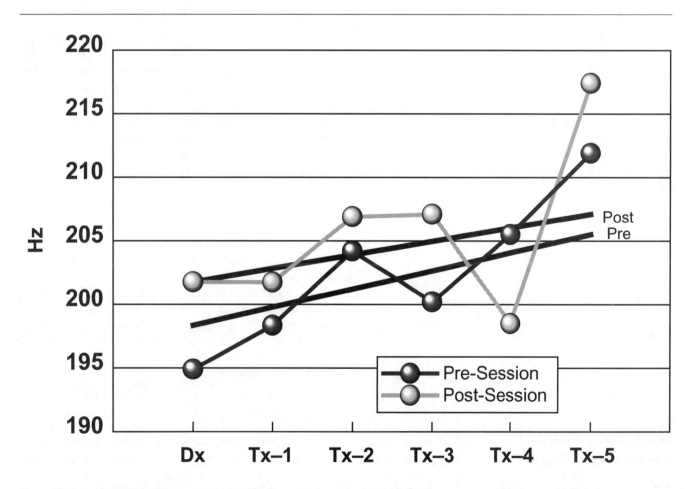

Figure 6–6 Patient MTD: Changes in Speaking Fundamental Frequency within and across Sessions (1 Diagnostic [Dx]; 5 Therapy [Tx]). Pre- and postsession trend lines are also provided.

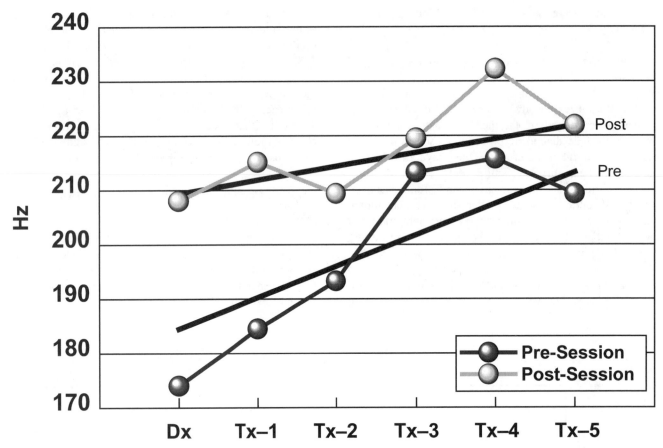

Figure 6–7 Patient MTD: Changes in Sustained Vowel Fundamental Frequency within and across Sessions (1 Diagnostic [Dx]; 5 Therapy [Tx]). Pre- and postsession trend lines are also provided.

the celeration lines for the presession and postsession data all have positive slopes. The celeration lines also indicate that, in general, postsession change in vocal F_0 was generally greater at the beginning of the therapy phase compared with the end of the therapy phase.

Vocal F_0: Phonational Range

Patient MTD showed consistent overall increases in her total phonation range (in semitones) across the six therapy sessions (see Figure 6–8). After application of laryngeal massage, increases in phonational range were noted in each of the first three therapy sessions. The final three sessions showed phonational range to be relatively stable from presession to postsession. The relatively small presession and postsession changes in phonational range are reflected in celeration lines that are quite similar in their predicted levels and slopes.

Jitter (%)

A drastic decrease in jitter (3.41% to 1.2%) was observed after the initial therapy session with the circumlaryngeal massage technique (see Figure 6–9). Reductions in jitter continued to be observed across the remaining therapy sessions, with jitter becoming relatively stable by the end of the therapy phase. This relative stability in jitter is reflected in the similarity and convergence of the presession and postsession celeration lines.

Shimmer (dB)

The interpretation of the shimmer data is somewhat more problematic than for the previously described variables (see Figure 6–10). The shimmer of patient MTD's sustained vowel productions was observed to decrease after laryngeal massage therapy during the first three sessions of the therapy

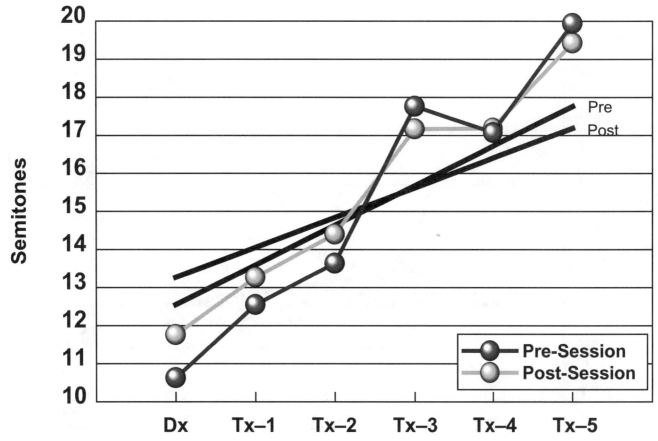

Figure 6–8 Patient MTD: Changes in Total Phonational Range (in Semitones) within and across Sessions (1 Diagnostic [Dx]; 5 Therapy [Tx]). Pre- and postsession trend lines are also provided.

phase. Celeration lines show a trend for pretherapy shimmer to decrease across the six sessions; however, the posttherapy celeration line shows a trend for increases in shimmer. Shimmer appears to have stabilized by the fifth and sixth sessions as reflected in the convergence of the celeration lines.

The aforementioned case study incorporated the circumlaryngeal massage technique based on the instructions of Aronson (1990a). However, Case (1996) believes that palpation of the extrinsic laryngeal musculature is a worthy addition to the voice diagnostic method "even if the stricter protocol of Aronson (1990) is not used" (p. 148). Case (1996) states that excessive tension in the extrinsic musculature probably mirrors that of the intrinsic musculature. Therefore, hyperfunctional voice use may be assumed in many cases from observation of tension in the extrinsic musculature solely.

RAPID COUNTING

In the previously presented case study, the patient was observed to have evident dysphonia and characteristics of MTD. However, there may be situations in which a patient comes in for a voice diagnostic, but tells the clinician, "My voice sounds pretty good today." Indeed, it may very well be that the patient's voice is perceived to be within normal limits in terms of pitch, loudness, and quality characteristics. This situation presents considerable difficulty for the voice clinician because he or she will be expected to provide appropriate recommendations to the patient on the basis of the patient's symptoms alone. Colton and Casper (1996) describe "symptoms" as the complaints/descriptions of the patient that may or may not be verified by the clinician. Once a symptom has been verified, it is referred to as a "sign" (Colton & Casper, 1996). It should be the clinician's goal to gather as many signs as possible concerning the patient's

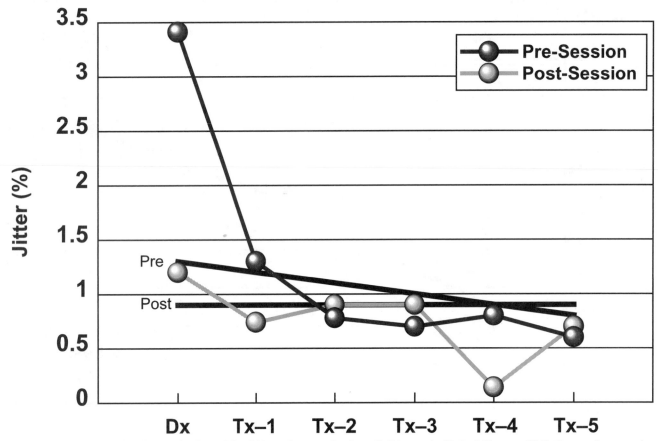

Figure 6–9 Patient MTD: Changes in Jitter (%) within and across Sessions (1 Diagnostic [Dx]; 5 Therapy [Tx]). Pre- and postsession trend lines are also provided.

voice characteristics. A diagnosis based on symptoms with little or no direct observation by way of signs would be considered much weaker than one supported by myriad signs and would most probably be more prone to error and misdirection.

The situation in which a patient presents with a voice that is considerably better than he or she reports under other circumstances makes verification difficult. Therefore, the clinician would be wise to *elicit* the disordered voice characteristics. An effective method of doing this is rapid counting (Prater & Swift, 1984; Weinberg, 1983). In this task, we simply ask patients to count as rapidly as they can from 1 to 100. The task is similar in nature to the maximum performance tasks discussed in the previous chapter in that this task "stresses" the speech mechanism. When the speech mechanism is stressed/taxed in this manner, we may observe the following:

1. Changes in voice characteristics (pitch, loudness, quality, duration) and their accompanying acoustic measures reflective of a breakdown in vocal capabilities
2. Patient compensation for impending vocal breakdown
3. No significant change in voice characteristics, indicating that either the patient's capabilities are within normal levels or may become disrupted only under very specific conditions or stresses beyond what may be used in the limited clinical setting

HOW TO DO IT: THE RAPID COUNTING TASK

Provide the following instructions to the patient. In addition, it is suggested that the clinician be prepared

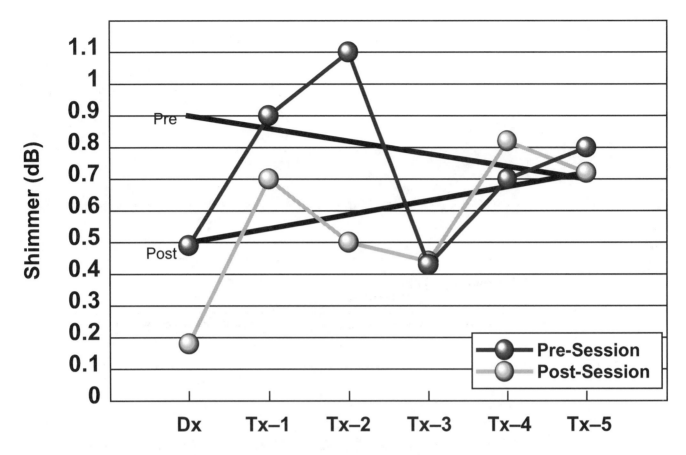

Figure 6–10 Patient MTD: Changes in Shimmer (dB) within and across Sessions (1 Diagnostic [Dx]; 5 Therapy [Tx]). Pre- and postsession trend lines are also provided.

to record and analyze voice samples (both sustained vowel and continuous speech productions) both before and immediately after the rapid counting task so that voice changes may be documented.

1. "I would like you to count as rapidly/quickly as you can from 1 to 100. You do not have to do this on one breath, but I want you to count as quickly as possible."

2. Listen closely to the patient during rapid counting for perceptual changes in voice characteristics (pitch, loudness, quality, duration). If you start to perceive changes near the end of the counting, ask the patient to continue on to 150 or 200. It is hoped that the added stress of continuing this task will elicit the voice change with more clarity.

3. Immediately after the counting task, ask the pa-

tient to sustain the vowel "ah" (use the chant method as previously described) and record for analysis of perturbation. In addition, have the patient read "The Rainbow Passage" at a comfortable pitch and loudness; also record and analyze.

WHAT TO EXPECT—CASE STUDY

I have found the rapid counting technique to be quite effective in eliciting voice change secondary to excessive musculoskeletal tension and other disorders in which hyperfunction is a core behavior (e.g., spasmodic dysphonia). Please refer to Case Study C (in Chapter 7), which provides an example of a patient referred with suspected spasmodic dysphonia in which rapid counting was an essential aspect of the voice diagnostic.

Conclusions and Case Studies

Having completed the various sections of the *VDP*, the clinician will have achieved the following:

- A comprehensive review of (1) patient case history, (2) possible causative factors and symptoms of the presenting voice problem, and (3) basic functioning of the speech and hearing mechanism
- An evaluation of the significant perceptual characteristics of the voice signal (various facets of pitch, loudness, quality, and duration)
- Extensive collection and review of key acoustic characteristics of the voice, including various measures of frequency, intensity, and perturbation and noise
- Various measures and estimates (perceptual, acoustic, and physiological) that have assessed the ability to control and coordinate both respiratory and laryngeal contributions to phonation.

The information gathered using the *VDP* is evaluated in light of the knowledge of *both* normal expectations and vocal physiology and abnormal expectations and pathophysiology. The multiple measures and observations incorporated into the *VDP* provide the clinician with valuable redundancy, in which consistency of findings related to specific types of underlying pathophysiology (e.g., multiple signs and symptoms indicative of hypoadduction, multiple signs and symptoms consistent with excessive muscle tension) helps to confirm a final differential diagnosis. Focus on the underlying pathophysiology that may be responsible for a patient's voice characteristics not only guides the clinician to an effective description of the possible causes of the voice problem but also relates specifically to the development of an effective treatment plan.

Figure 7–1 summarizes the key steps in the differential diagnosis of voice disorders.

Three case studies will be discussed in an effort to summarize much of the information presented in previous chapters of this book. In each case, key informational components will be highlighted and discussed in terms of possible underlying causes and physiology.

CASE STUDY A

Patient A was a **(1) woman in her mid 40s** who reported a **(2) "whisperlike" voice quality,** as well as **(3) decreased pitch** after a **(4) thyroidectomy** approximately 6 weeks before this evaluation. The patient reported **(5) no particular voice problems before thyroid surgery** and **(6) no history of previous neurological disease or insult**. After the thyroid surgery, she described her voice as "a little more than a whisper." She also described **(7) increased "tightness" in the laryngeal region, (8) necessity to take more frequent breaths and a feeling of "running out of breath" during speech, (9) "wheezing" during inhalation, (10) reduced pitch and loudness, (11) inability to produce a strong cough, (12) frequent headaches and "tightness" in the back of the neck and a feeling of a "lump in her throat."** Patient A also stated that her **(13) voice quality was better in the morning and worsened throughout the day**. The patient had received **(14) no previous voice therapy** for this problem.

After the case history session, formal evaluation of the patient's vocal capability was undertaken. The following observations were made.

Perceptual Assessment

Perceptual judgments regarding pitch, loudness, duration, and quality were made during conversational speech and sustained vowel production. The patient demonstrated **(15) consistent breathiness, (16) limited intonation, (17) decreased loudness, (18) inappropriately short breath groups,** and **(19) occasional inhalatory stridor**. Examples of patient A's continuous speech and sustained vowel pro-

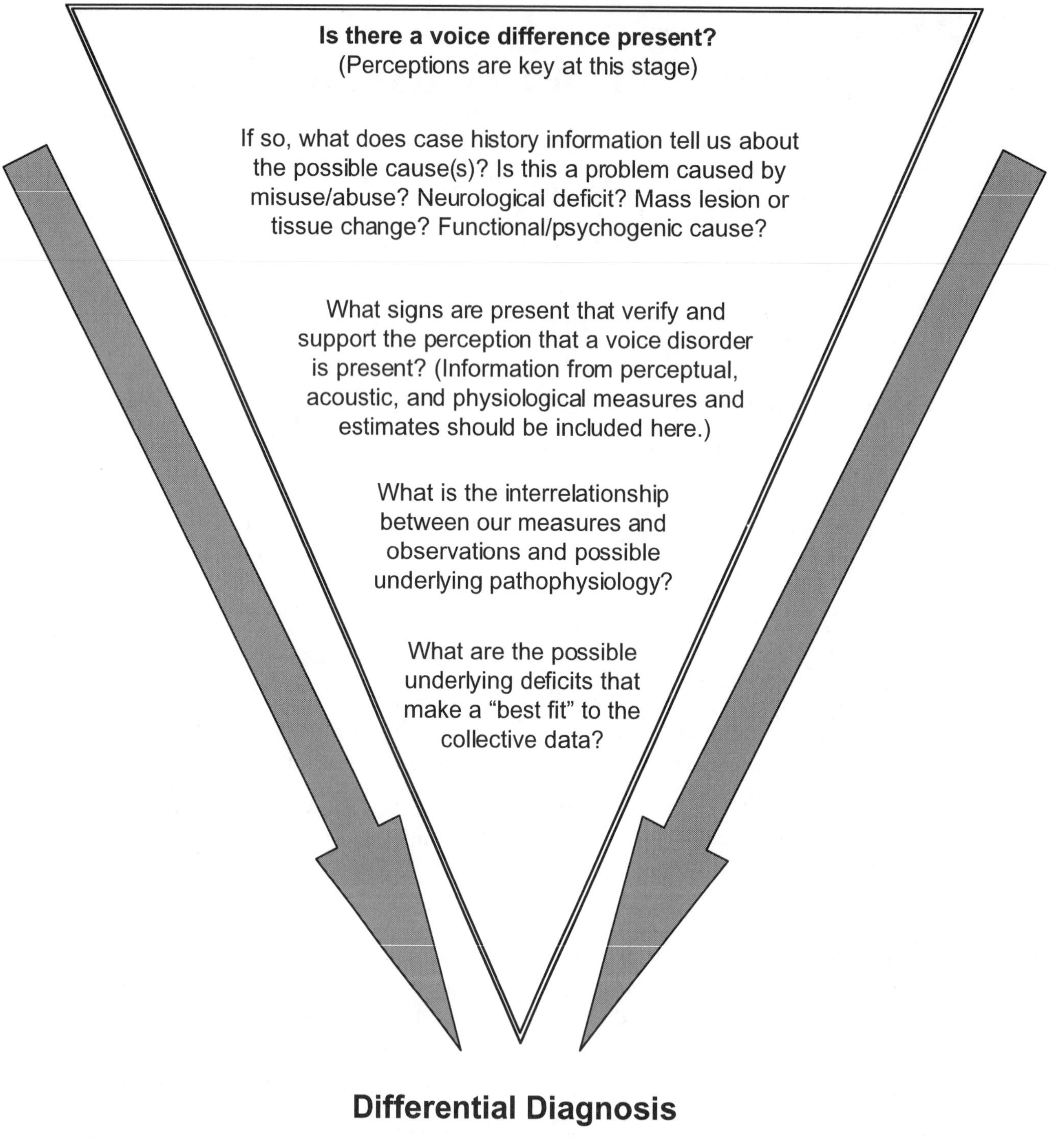

Is there a voice difference present?
(Perceptions are key at this stage)

If so, what does case history information tell us about
the possible cause(s)? Is this a problem caused by
misuse/abuse? Neurological deficit? Mass lesion or
tissue change? Functional/psychogenic cause?

What signs are present that verify and
support the perception that a voice disorder
is present? (Information from perceptual,
acoustic, and physiological measures and
estimates should be included here.)

What is the interrelationship
between our measures and
observations and possible
underlying pathophysiology?

What are the possible
underlying deficits that
make a "best fit" to the
collective data?

Differential Diagnosis

Figure 7–1 Possible Decision Outline for the Diagnosis of Voice Disorders

ductions may be heard by L. clicking on CS-A1.WAV (continuous speech sample) and CS-A2.WAV (sustained vowel) in the C:\VDP directory.

Speech Mechanism Examination

This examination was conducted to assess the structure and functioning of the speech production mechanism. Assessment of laryngeal posture revealed **(20) high laryngeal position and rigidity (inability to move the larynx laterally). (21) A weak voluntary cough was elicited, although, later in the evaluation, a strong reflexive cough was observed. (22) All other areas of the speech mechanism appeared adequate for speech production purposes.**

Acoustic Measures of Vocal Frequency and Noise

The **(23) patient's mean speaking F_0 was measured at 221.46 Hz ([24] SD = 7.65 Hz; pitch sigma = 1.19 semitones)**. In addition, the patient was asked to sustain the vowel /ɑ/ at a comfortable pitch and loudness for 2 to 3 seconds. Results from analysis of sustained vowel samples revealed the following: mean F_0 = 210.91 Hz **([25] SD = 6.75 Hz); (26) jitter = 3.88%; (27) Shimmer = 0.55 dB; (28) HNR = 8.59. (29) Total phonational range was measured at 8.70 semitones (204.61 to 338.15 Hz)**. Figures 7–2 and 7–3 provide examples of continuous speech and sustained vowel analysis results for patient A.

Vocal Intensity

(30) Intensity of conversational speech was measured at 60 dB (1-ft. mouth-to-microphone distance).

Respiratory and Durational Measures

The patient's **(31) vital capacity was measured at 3.1 L; (32) phonation quotient was measured at 258.33 ml/s. (33) MPT was measured to be 12 s (0.65 ratio of measured to expected)** and **(34) S/Z ratio was observed to be 1.50.**

Diagnostic Therapy

Laryngeal reposturing and massage techniques were performed on the client to investigate the possible effects of high laryngeal position and excessive musculoskeletal tension on this patient's voice function. During a 10- to 15-minute period of laryngeal massage, the larynx was felt to lower; lateral movement of the larynx was easily achieved. In addition, frequent sustained vowel phonations by the patient revealed improvements in perceived voice quality. **(35) After this period of laryngeal reposturing/massage, acoustic**

analysis of conversational and sustained vowel production revealed the following (see Tables 7–1 and 7–2).

Examples of patient A's continuous speech and sustained vowel productions after laryngeal reposturing and circumlaryngeal massage may be heard by L. clicking on CS-A3.WAV (continuous speech sample) and CS-A4.WAV (sustained vowel) in the C:\VDP directory.

CASE STUDY A: DISCUSSION OF KEY INFORMATIONAL COMPONENTS

(1) Female in her mid 40s: The possible effects of age on the voice must be taken into consideration by the clinician. This woman may be going through menopause, which may have ramifications for possible changes in voice characteristics (e.g., possible decreases in speaking F_0).

(2) "Whisperlike" voice quality: A "whispery" voice is often consistent with the perceptual sign of breathiness.

(3) Decreased pitch: The patient reports that she feels that the pitch of her voice has been lower than normal. If we accept the symptom as being accurate at this point, a number of possibilities for underlying problems may come to mind (e.g., natural voice changes caused by aging, endocrine imbalances, mass lesions that increase the vibratory mass of the vocal folds, neurological dysfunction such as flaccidity).

(4) Thyroidectomy: This is a very important piece of medical history information in the scope of this diagnostic case. The thyroid gland is found close to the nerve branches that innervate the intrinsic muscles of the larynx. It is possible that nerve damage or dysfunction (either temporarily or permanently) could underlie the patient's voice problems. Damage to the recurrent laryngeal nerve could result in flaccidity and inability to adequately valve the larynx (i.e., poor adductory capability). In addition to possible neurological dysfunction, functional dysphonias may be caused by the stress and anxiety associated with surgical procedures.

(5) No particular voice problems before thyroid surgery: This piece of information tells us that there was a relatively sudden onset to this voice disruption. Therefore, possibilities such as trauma to the larynx; sudden neurological disruption (e.g., cerebrovascular accident); or conversion dysphonia following psychological trauma should be considered.

(6) No history of neurological disease or insult: The patient was asked directly whether she had any significant neurological history that she was aware of, to which she replied "no."

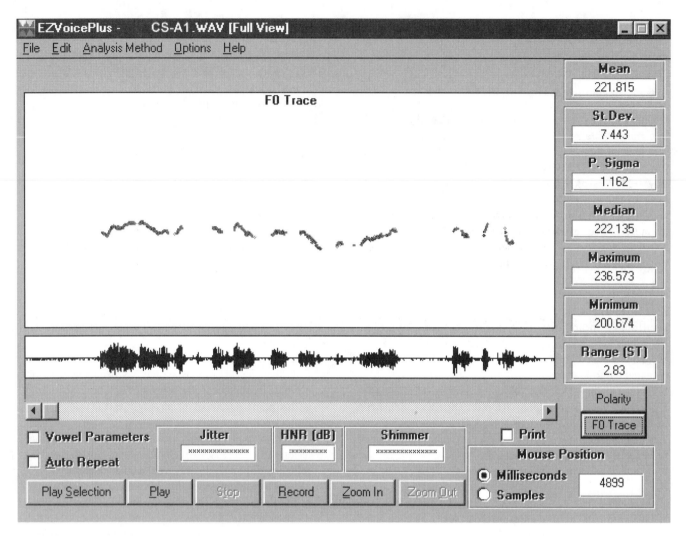

Figure 7–2 An Example of a Continuous Speech Sample for Patient A. Note the low F_0 standard deviation and pitch sigma consistent with the perception of limited intonation.

(7) Increased "tightness" in the laryngeal region: This symptom is often associated with muscle tension dysphonias (MTDs). The clinician must be aware that excessive musculoskeletal tension may be a primary cause of voice disorders or may be a secondary component in organic voice problems.

Table 7–1 Mean Changes in Several of Patient A's Continuous Speech Measurements After Laryngeal Reposturing and Circumlaryngeal Massage

Measures of Continuous Speech	Measurement	Postlaryngeal Reposturing/Massage Change
Mean speaking F_0	230.99 Hz	+9.53 Hz
Maximum speaking F_0	260.95 Hz	+24.41 Hz
Minimum speaking F_0	187.71 Hz	+13.81 Hz
Speaking range	5.70 STs	+2.95 STs
Pitch sigma	2.02 STs	+0.82 STs

Table 7–2 Mean Changes in Several of Patient A's Sustained Vowel Measurements After Laryngeal Reposturing and Circumlaryngeal Massage

Sustained Vowel Measures	Measurement	Postlaryngeal Reposturing/Massage Change
Jitter	0.24%	−3.64%
HNR	13.41%	+4.82 dB
Shimmer	0.32 dB	−0.23 dB
Pitch sigma	0.23 STs	−0.95 STs

(8) Necessity to take more frequent breaths and a feeling of "running out of breath" during speech: This patient had complained of a feeling of "losing her breath" easily during speech. A number of under-lying possibilities may be considered in relation to this symptom. The patient may have poor respiratory support for speech as a result of respiratory disease or neurological disruption. In addition, the patient may

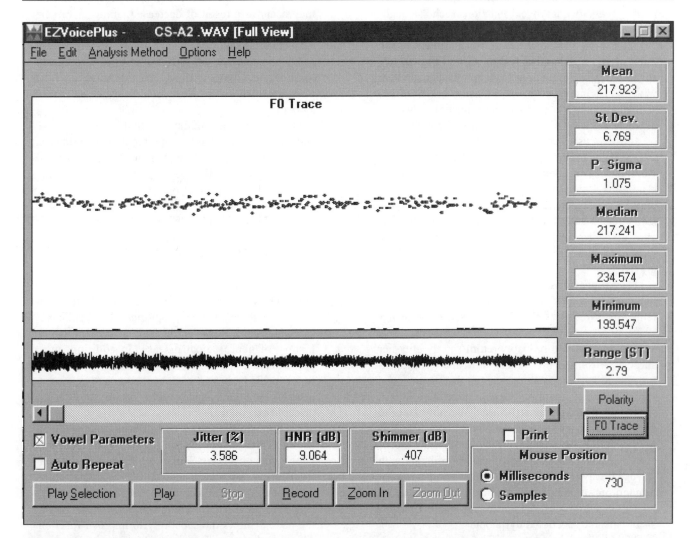

Figure 7–3 An Example of a Sustained Vowel Sample for Patient A. Increased perturbation and noise and randomly "splintered" F_0 contour are consistent with this patient's moderate breathy voice quality.

be experiencing difficulty controlling her expiratory airflow during speech because of poor laryngeal valving.

(9) "Wheezing" during inhalation: An important symptom that may indicate the presence of obstruction at the laryngeal level.

(10) Reduced pitch and loudness: Possible underlying causes of reduced pitch level have been discussed in No. 3. Decreased loudness level may be due to poor respiratory support and/or poor laryngeal valving. It is particularly the coordination between expiration and laryngeal valving that generates the increases in subglottal pressure necessary for increases in vocal loudness.

(11) Inability to produce a strong cough: A weak cough is often associated with laryngeal weakness, perhaps of neurological origin. In contrast, patients with functional dysphonias often are able to produce normal vegetative laryngeal functions such as coughing and throat clearing.

(12) Frequent headaches and "tightness" in the back of the neck and a feeling of a "lump in her throat": This combination of symptoms is consistent with MTD. Increased muscle tension has been described as both (1) a component of functional dysphonias and (2) a possible compensation for underlying organic deficits.

(13) Voice quality was better in the morning and worsened throughout the day: Worsening of voice symptoms with increased voice use through the day may be associated with (1) vocal fatigue (laryngeal myasthenia) associated with functional dysphonias and increased muscle tension and (2) progressive weakness of neurological origin (e.g., myasthenia gravis).

(14) No previous voice therapy: This patient had not sought any previous therapy for her voice problems since her physician had advised her that her voice problems were most likely temporary and normal voice would probably return shortly after her surgery. Although the patient did report some improvement in voice function, she felt that the time had come to consult regarding possible voice therapy.

(15) Consistent breathiness: We now start to gather signs to confirm patient symptoms. Breathiness is defined as audible airflow through the glottis and is associated with hypoadduction (difficulty with laryngeal valving). Some of the underlying causes of hypoadduction that may be considered are mass lesion(s), neurological dysfunction (vocal fold paralysis or paresis), functional dysphonias.

(16) Limited intonation: The patient was perceived as having a relatively "flat" intonation pattern. Limitations in speaking pitch variability and range may be associated with neurological dysfunction (weakness and limited range of motion), possible mass lesions that may restrict the ability to lengthen and tense the vocal folds, and functional dysphonias in which hypofunction is a key component (e.g., functional dysphonias associated with psychogenic dysfunction such as depression).

(17) Decreased loudness: A perceptual sign supporting the patient's symptom described in No. 10.

(18) Inappropriately short breath groups: The patient was perceived as producing inappropriately short utterances and observed to take breaths at inappropriate moments during an utterance. These are perceptual signs associated with factors such as poor respiratory support and/or poor control of expiratory airflow (i.e., the patient is losing air before completing the intended utterance). Poor control of airflow may occur as a result of decreased laryngeal valving ability (hypoadduction/hypofunction). Patients with hyperfunction may also have inappropriate breath groups but may be expected to have inappropriately long breath groups with speech extending past the point at which the speaker would be expected to take a breath.

(19) Occasional inhalatory stridor: A perceptual sign that confirms the patient symptom described in No. 9. Inhalatory stridor may be due to mass lesion(s) obstructing the glottis to some degree during inhalation, which create vibration or turbulence in the air stream; neurological dysfunction, such as a vocal fold paralyzed near the adducted position; or psychogenic disorders such as pseudoasthma.

(20) High laryngeal position and rigidity (inability to manipulate the larynx laterally): Rigidity in the extralaryngeal musculature is often associated with MTDs. Rigidity may also be found with neurological dysfunction such as spasticity or hypokinesia (parkinsonism). However, this patient has reported no history of neurological disease. In addition, most pyramidal/extrapyramidal disorders are not localized to a specific body part such as the phonatory mechanism (spasmodic dysphonia as a focal dystonia is the possible exception).

(21) A weak elicited cough was observed, although later in the evaluation, a strong reflexive cough was observed: This is an interesting observation during the speech mechanism examination. A weak cough is often associated with laryngeal weakness (see previous description in No. 11). However, the patient shows the capability to improve function. This may be an indication of hypofunction, perhaps as an avoidance of voice use since her surgery.

(22) All other areas of the speech mechanism appeared adequate for speech production purposes: The speech mechanism examination confirms that there are no evident neurological or structural deficits affecting other parts of the speech mechanism. Therefore, the underlying cause appears to be localized to the laryngeal mechanism.

(23) The patient's mean speaking F_0 was measured at 221.46 Hz: This measurement of the patient's speaking F_0 was considered well within normal limits for an adult woman, yet seems at odds with the patient's description of her "pitch" being lower than normal. Because the clinician cannot know what the patient sounded like before the onset of her voice problems, he or she should accept the patient's description of pitch change. However, this patient's pitch and speaking F_0 will probably not be among the highest priority goals in the event that voice therapy takes place. It should also be considered that the patient's perception of her own pitch level might be affected by the presence of noise in the voice signal.

(24) SD = 7.65 Hz; pitch sigma = 1.19: These acoustic measures confirm the perceptual sign of decreased pitch variability during the production of intonation patterns. As a general guideline, speaking F_0 standard deviation is often observed to be approximately 10% of the patient's mean speaking F_0; pitch sigma is approximately 3 to 6 semitones. Possible underlying causes for reduced pitch variability and "flat" intonation have been discussed in No. 16.

(25) SD = 6.75 Hz (sustained vowel production): The frequency of the voice should be held quite steady during a sustained vowel production. Average variability (i.e., the standard deviation) is generally observed to be ≤1% of the mean F_0 in sustained vowel production. Increased F_0 standard deviation in this task may indicate an inability to control F_0 perhaps because of underlying neurological problems and/or the addition of aperiodic components to the voice signal (consistent with breathy phonation in this case).

(26) Jitter = 3.88%: Jitter should be substantially less than 1% in normal voice production. This is a sign of increased cycle-to-cycle variability in F_0. Perturbation of this manner may be due to increased aperiodicity of vocal fold vibration and/or addition of turbulent noise from increased transglottal airflow.

(27) Shimmer = 0.55 dB: Shimmer should be substantially less than 1 dB (usually in the 0.2 to 0.3 dB region) in normal voice production. Increased shimmer indicates increases in the cycle-to-cycle amplitude of the voice signal. Although elevated, the patient's shimmer value is not as drastically affected as the jitter or HNR. This may be because the release of un-

modulated airflow may produce a relatively constant amplitude in the breathy voice signal.

(28) HNR = 8.59: This patient's HNR value is significantly lower than often observed in the normal voice (generally in the vicinity of 15 to 20 dB). This indicates that noise components are closely competing with harmonic components in terms of amplitude.

(29) Phonational range was measured at 8.70 semitones (204.61 to 338.15 Hz): The patient's total phonational range is significantly reduced compared with normal expectations (24 to 30 semitones in subjects without vocal training). Decreased phonational range may be due to an inability to substantially vary the length and tension of the vocal folds. Decreased phonational range is observed in a multitude of voice disorders such as hypofunction and hyperfunction, functional dysphonia (MTDs), neurological disturbances, and presence of mass lesions.

(30) Intensity of conversational speech was measured at 60 dB: Speaking vocal intensity is generally measured in the 65 to 70 dB range (1-ft. mouth-to-microphone distance). The patient's reduced vocal intensity confirms the perceptual signs and patient symptoms described in No. 10 and No. 17.

(31) Vital capacity was measured at 3.1 L: The vital capacity was considered to be within normal expectations considering this patient's age and height (64 in.; 1.63 m). The measure of vital capacity provides an indication of the patient's respiratory capability. Therefore, many of the aforementioned characteristics that had some association with respiratory deficit or laryngeal valving problems are most probably laryngeal in nature.

(32) Phonation quotient was measured at 258.33 ml/s: The patient's PQ level is elevated in comparison to normal expectations. The PQ is an estimate of transglottal airflow. Elevated PQs are associated with hypoadduction and the perception of breathiness. The underlying causes of breathiness have been discussed in No. 15.

(33) MPT was measured to be 12 s (0.65 ratio of measured to expected): The patient's MPT is substantially lower than normal expectations (generally in the vicinity of 20 s). Decreased MPT may be due to poor respiratory capacity and/or poor laryngeal valving. However, it would appear that this patient's respiratory capacity is adequate (see No. 31). Therefore, difficulty adducting the vocal folds during phonation is the likely underlying cause of this patient's low MPT. According to the formula of Beckett (1971), this patient would be expected to produce an MPT of approximately 18.29 s on the basis of her vital capacity. The ratio of her actual MPT to her expected

MPT is 0.65 (less than 0.70 indicates an abnormality in MPT).

(34) S/Z ratio was observed to be 1.50: Normal S/Z ratios are expected to be in the vicinity of 1.0 (or perhaps slightly lower than 1.0). An elevated S/Z ratio is consistent with problems with laryngeal valving (hypoadduction) and breathy phonation (see No. 15).

(35) Effects of laryngeal reposturing/massage: The patient had described several symptoms consistent with MTD. In addition, high, rigid laryngeal posture was noted during the speech mechanism examination. Therefore, a period of diagnostic therapy was incorporated into the session. Procedures for laryngeal reposturing and laryngeal massage were similar to those described previously.

After a 10- to 15-minute period of reposturing/massage, acoustic measures were conducted on continuous speech and sustained vowel samples. Representative results and degree of voice change after pretherapy are shown in Tables 7–1 and 7–2. Increases were observed in mean speaking F_0 and speaking range. Substantial improvements in pitch sigma were also observed. It was hypothesized that increased laryngeal tension was restricting this patient's ability to vary pitch for intonation purposes. Increases in speaking F_0 after laryngeal reposturing/massage are not uncommon because anterior-posterior squeezing of the larynx and/or increased tension focal to the thyroarytenoid/vocalis muscle may cause decreased speaking F_0. Therefore, relief of tension may cause an increase in observed speaking F_0 as well as range.

Posttreatment measures of perturbation and noise from the sustained vowel /ɑ/ reflect substantial improvements in voice quality that were perceived by both the patient and the clinician. Jitter and shimmer have both dropped to well within normal limits; HNR is still slightly reduced but much closer to normal expectations. In addition, pitch sigma (which should only be a small fraction [approximately 0.35 STs] of 1 semitone in sustained vowel productions) has also dropped considerably, reflecting a much steadier production in terms of F_0. Overall results (both perceptual and acoustic) appeared to indicate that excessive musculoskeletal tension was a contributing factor to this patient's voice problems.

The various perceptual and objective measures of pitch, loudness, quality, and duration conducted in this case must be combined with the pertinent aspects of the patient's case history, medical background, and speech mechanism examination results. On review and synthesis of all of the diagnostic observations, a number of particularly significant diagnostic points have consistently emerged as shown below.

- A consistent trend throughout the various observations is that this patient appears to have problems with laryngeal valving (i.e., inadequate adduction of the vocal folds to produce effective phonation and to control the outgoing airstream).

- This possible laryngeal valving problem has had a sudden onset and is associated with a particular episode of "trauma" (i.e., surgery in the laryngeal region). Because the surgery that was carried out (thyroidectomy) was on the external larynx, it is unlikely that trauma/damage to the vocal folds has directly occurred. Instead, it is possible that the cranial nerve (vagus nerve) branches serving the phonatory mechanism have been affected by the surgical procedure. Damage to a motor unit results in flaccidity, muscle weakness, and limited range. When affecting the larynx, this type of neurological damage characteristically results in the breathy voice quality perceived in the patient's voice. Of course, mass lesions could also result in many of the perceptual and acoustic characteristics mentioned in this case. However, this patient reported no history of vocal abuse or misuse, no history of smoking, and no history of chronic voice difficulties. It was previously discussed that the development of organized mass lesions (e.g., nodules) is generally a lengthy process resulting from consistent traumatic phonatory activity (an exception may be the vocal polyp, which has been associated with a sudden impact/trauma to the vocal fold mucosa). Although mass lesions could be present in this particular case study, it was believed that the history did not bear this out. The "weight of evidence" appears to indicate that this patient presents with laryngeal valving deficits (hypoadduction) as a result of neurological disruption focal to the larynx.

- A second factor in this patient's voice case also recurs, the presence of MTD. Various patient symptoms and clinician observations from the speech mechanism examination pointed toward the presence of excessive musculoskeletal tension. In addition, positive voice changes (both perceived and measured) after laryngeal reposturing and massage seem to confirm the hypothesis that MTD is a contributing factor in this patient's voice problems. Patients with organic deficits may develop increased laryngeal tension (1) subsequent to stress and anxiety related to the original voice disruption and/or (2) as a compensation for the decreased ability to produce effective phonation. In many cases, the addition of excessive musculoskeletal tension to the underlying organic deficit results in poorer phonatory functioning than if the voice would be affected solely by the original organic deficit alone. This appeared to be the case with this patient because voice produced after attempts to repose the larynx and relieve excessive laryngeal tension was markedly improved versus the voice characteristics before reposturing/laryngeal massage.

The identification of MTD in this patient had significant consequences in terms of recommended treatment goals and procedures. As an example, hypoadduction secondary to neurological dysfunction is often treated with methods that actually encourage hyperfunction (e.g., pushing, pulling, isometric exercises [Colton & Casper, 1996]). However, in this case, these types of treatment procedures would be contraindicated because excessive tension was already being used by the patient to detrimental effect. Instead, it was recommended that primary therapy tasks focus on the relief of excessive tension, with the underlying organic deficit to be addressed secondarily by means of (1) increased respiratory support and (2) its own natural resolution.

Impressions

The overall impression statement for this patient was the following: "Moderate dysphonia characterized by breathy voice quality; reduced vocal pitch and range; vocal fatigue. These deficits appear secondary to a possible laryngeal valving deficit (hypoadduction) of neurological/traumatic origin. In addition, the patient also shows signs and symptoms of muscle tension dysphonia."

In actual fact, a recent ENT visit had confirmed the presence of a L. vocal fold paresis. This informational point was reserved from the case study information so as not to bias the reader or detract from the formulation of possible clinical hypotheses on the basis of the voice diagnostic protocol information itself.

Recommendations

Voice therapy recommendations for the patient included (1) decreasing excessive musculoskeletal tension by means of laryngeal reposturing and massage and (2) improving breath support for speech and coordination of voicing with expiratory airstream. Therapy was to incorporate auditory and visual feedback regarding the patient's voice function into direct therapy tasks. A hydration program was also implemented in which the patient would strive to drink at least six to eight 8-oz. glasses of water or fruit juice per day. Finally, the patient was referred back to her otolaryngologist to monitor her status and any changes in her laryngeal functioning.

CASE STUDY B

Patient B was a **(1) 59-year-old female** who was referred by a local speech pathologist because of **(2) chronic** voice difficulty. This woman was a **(3) long-term smoker** (approximately 1 pack per day for the last 40 years), who reported that her voice had had a consistent hoarse voice quality for as long as memory served her. The patient reported no history of neurological disorder and no significant respiratory problems. The patient did report that she had felt some degree of recent stress and anxiety regarding her voice difficulties and possibility of cancer.

After the case history session, formal evaluation of the patient's vocal capability was undertaken. The following observations were made.

Perceptual Assessment

Perceptual judgments regarding pitch, loudness, duration, and quality were made during conversational speech and sustained vowel production. Voice was characterized as **(4) low in pitch**, with **(5) consistent hoarse quality**. The patient appeared to have **(6) inappropriately short breath groups**. Occasional episodes of **(7) inhalatory stridor** were also observed. Examples of patient B's continuous speech and sustained vowel productions may be heard by L. clicking on CS-B1.WAV (continuous speech sample) and CS-B2.WAV (sustained vowel) on the C:\VDP directory.

Speech Mechanism Examination

This examination was conducted to assess the structure and functioning of the speech production mechanisms. Results were unremarkable. No signs of extralaryngeal tension or poor laryngeal posture were observed.

Acoustic Measures of Vocal Frequency and Noise

The **(8) patient's mean speaking F_0 was measured at 116 Hz** (SD = 13 Hz; pitch sigma = 3.89 semitones). In addition, the patient was asked to sustain the vowel /ɑ/ at a comfortable pitch and loudness for 2 to 3 seconds. Results from analysis of sustained vowel samples revealed the following: **(9) jitter = 2.56%; shimmer = 0.7 dB; HNR = 11.5 dB. (10) Phonational range was measured at 11 semitones**. Figures 7–4 and 7–5 provide examples of continuous speech and sustained vowel analysis results for patient B.

Vocal Intensity

(11) Intensity of conversational speech was measured at 66 dB (1-ft. mouth-to-microphone distance).

Respiratory and Durational Measures

The patient's **(12) vital capacity was measured at 3.2 L; (13) phonation quotient was measured at 213.2 ml/s. (14)**

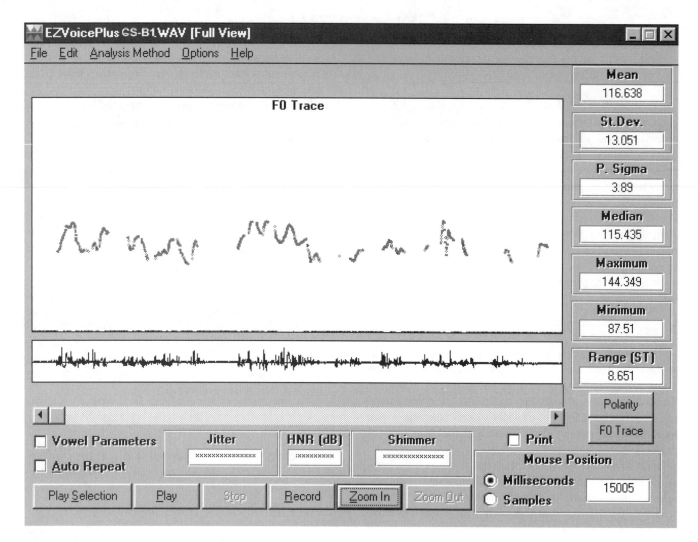

Figure 7–4 An Example of a Continuous Speech Sample for Patient B. Note the extremely low speaking F_0 for this adult female patient (59 years old).

MPT was measured to be 15 s (0.79 ratio of measured to expected) and (15) S/Z ratio was observed to be 1.32.

CASE STUDY B: DISCUSSION OF KEY INFORMATIONAL COMPONENTS

(1) **59-year-old woman:** Age may be a significant factor in this case. The woman is postmenopausal and, thus, may have undergone voice changes such as decrease in pitch and increased variability associated with possible endocrine imbalance and overall aging in women.

(2) **Chronic voice difficulty:** This patient reported that the voice difficulties had been present for "as long as she could remember." This component of her his-

tory would appear to rule out voice disorders related to sudden onsets such as laryngeal trauma, rapidly developing neurological insults (e.g., cerebrovascular accident), conversion dysphonias associated with psychological trauma). On the other hand, the possibility of disorders related to abuse/misuse (e.g., nodules, polypoid degeneration), progressive neurological disorders, long-term functional dysphonia and MTD, etc., must be considered by the clinician.

(3) **Long-term smoker:** This information is of major importance in consideration of possible underlying deficits in a voice disorder case. Smoking is not only an irritant of the vocal fold mucosa but is also associated with the development of laryngeal carcinoma. The clinician must consider the possibility

of benign changes in vocal fold structure (e.g., edema, polypoid degeneration), as well as lesions that may be malignant in nature.

(4) Low pitch: This patient was perceived by the clinician to have an abnormally low-pitch voice in comparison to similar age, gender, and body type peers. Low vocal pitch may be due to conditions that increase the mass of the vocal folds (lesions, edema) or that cause them to lose tension and, therefore, increase their effective mass (e.g., neurological deficits such as flaccidity). In addition, the clinician should remember that the perception of pitch might be influenced by vocal quality deviations (especially those presenting with roughness as a result of aperiodic vocal fold vibration).

(5) Consistent hoarse quality: This highly noticeable quality in this patient's voice was judged to be of moderate severity. Her voice was perceived as being hoarse (combined rough and breathy components), although intermittent periods of primarily rough voice were also perceived. The breathy component of a hoarse voice is associated with hypoadduction and increased transglottal airflow, whereas the rough/harsh quality is associated with aperiodic vocal fold vibration and possible hyperfunction.

(6) Inappropriately short breath groups: Patients who have poor respiratory support for speech and/or poor laryngeal valving may have inappropriately short breath groups.

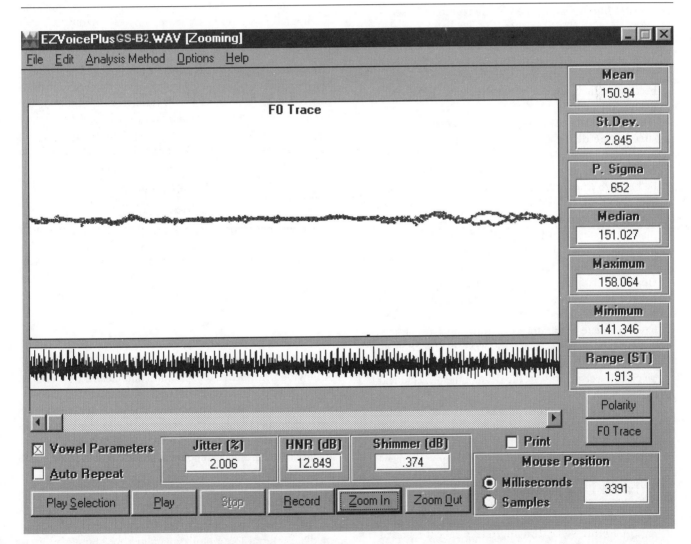

Figure 7–5 An Example of a Sustained Vowel Sample for Patient B. Evidence of diplophonia occurs near the end of this phonation, contributing to elevated jitter and F_0 standard deviation.

(7) Inhalatory stridor: This characteristic is associated with a possible glottal obstruction. "Noisy breathing" on inhalation may indicate the presence of a mass lesion or paralyzed fold creating turbulence in the airstream. The clinician should also consider the possibility of respiratory disorders as a possible source for stridor.

(8) Patient's mean speaking F_0 was measured at 116 Hz: This acoustic measure confirms the previous perceptual sign of low pitch. Although reductions in speaking F_0 may occur in postmenopausal women, this was believed to be substantially below expected levels. See No. 4 for possible underlying causes.

(9) Jitter = 2.56%; shimmer 0.7 dB; HNR = 11.5 dB: Jitter and shimmer are both abnormally high; HNR is abnormally low. These measures confirm the presence of a more than mild voice quality deviation.

(10) Phonational range was measured at 11 semitones: Total phonational range is generally expected in the 24 to 30 semitone range for patients with no vocal training. The patient may have a restricted ability to vary the length and tension of the vocal folds because of the presence of mass lesions, neurological dysfunction, etc.

(11) Intensity of conversational speech was measured at 66 dB: Vocal intensity and perceived loudness were judged to be adequate for this patient. Normal vocal intensity during speech is observed to be between 65 and 70 dB (1-ft. mouth-to-microphone distance).

(12) Vital capacity was measured at 3.2 L: During this diagnostic, it was originally hypothesized that this patient may have some reduction in respiratory capacity resulting from her long history of smoking. However, this measure of her vital capacity was considered well within normal expectations for her age and height (65 in.). Because the patient appeared to have adequate respiratory capability for speech and voice purposes, possible respiratory dysfunction as an underlying cause of her voice problems was now given a lower priority in the development of clinical hypotheses.

(13) Phonation quotient was measured at 213.2 ml/s: This estimate of transglottal airflow was considered to be on the high end of normal expectations. High PQ would be consistent with breathy voice quality and poor laryngeal valving (hypoadduction).

(14) MPT was measured to be 15 s (0.79 ratio of measured to expected): The patient's maximum phonation time was considered low normal. Because the patient showed adequate respiratory capacity (see No. 12), it was believed that this MPT may reflect some difficulty with laryngeal valving (hypoadduction).

(15) S/Z ratio was observed to be 1.32: The increased S/Z ratio is consistent with difficulty adducting the vocal folds and breathy voice quality.

As in the previous case study, we see that poor laryngeal valving (hypoadduction) is consistent with a number of observations (hoarse voice, elevated airflow estimate, increased S/Z ratio, decreased MPT, increased perturbation and noise in the voice). However, in this case, we have different underlying causes. This patient has a negative history for neurological disease, insult, or trauma and no significant signs of neurological disruption on speech mechanism examination. Therefore, the chance for an underlying neurological deficit to be the primary cause of her voice difficulties appears to be slim. On the other hand, the patient does have a history of vocal abuse (in terms of heavy smoking rather than behavioral use of the voice), chronic voice problems, and voice characteristics (decreased pitch and speaking F_0; limited F_0 range; increased perturbation and noise; stridor) consistent with the presence of mass lesion(s) at the vocal fold level. The presence of mass lesions could prevent adequate vocal fold adduction in the presence of normal neurological function and thus result in increased airflow, decreased MPT, increased S/Z ratio, etc. In addition, the presence of mass lesion(s) could result in aperiodicity of vocal fold vibration and a subsequent rough component to the voice (as well as the increased perturbation and noise measures).

Although the patient did relate some feelings of anxiety regarding the possibility of laryngeal cancer, possible signs and symptoms of MTD were not significant in this case. The patient did not report any specific symptoms associated with MTDs, and no significant extralaryngeal rigidity or high laryngeal position was observed during speech mechanism examination. Therefore, it was the opinion that increased muscle tension was not a significant factor in this patient's dysphonia.

Impression

The overall impression statement for this patient was the following: "Moderate dysphonia characterized by hoarse voice quality; decreased vocal pitch and range; inhalatory stridor. The observed voice characteristics in conjunction with the patient's history of long-term smoking lead to the impression that the observed voice difficulties may be secondary to the presence of possible mass lesion(s) at the vocal fold level."

Recommendations

The primary recommendation for this patient was an immediate referral to an otolaryngologist for complete laryngeal examination. Clearly the possibility of laryngeal carcinoma was a factor that needed medical assessment without delay. Any voice therapy for this patient was to be deferred until after the results of her ENT examination.

A laryngeal examination completed shortly after this voice diagnostic revealed the presence of Reinke's edema and chronic laryngitis affecting both vocal folds. The edema had caused the vocal folds to be grossly distended (increased mass and decreased vibratory frequency) and obstruct the glottis during inhalation (therefore, a source of inhalatory stridor). In addition, a significant longitudinal gap was observed during phonation (the source of increased airflow and breathiness). Stroboscopy revealed asymmetrical and aperiodic vocal fold vibration (the possible source of the rough component of this patient's voice quality).

CASE STUDY C

Patient C (a 40-year-old woman) was referred to our clinic for a suspected case of **(1) spasmodic dysphonia**. The patient related that she had been **(2) having problems with her voice for approximately 2 years**. The patient was not able to relate the initiation of her voice difficulties with any particular event; however, **(3) she did relate a history of emotional difficulties and anxiety**. When her voice problem occurs, **(4) she described it as sounding like a "helium" voice**. She also described **(5) difficulty in breathing when this voice change occurs**, as well as **(6) strain-struggle to produce voice**. She stated that she had been very worried that her voice difficulties were due to cancer but had been relieved because of a recent laryngeal examination by her otolaryngologist. The patient **(7) relates no history of neurological deficit** and is a nonsmoker.

After the case history session, formal evaluation of the patient's vocal capability was undertaken. The following observations were made.

Perceptual Assessment

Perceptual judgments of pitch, loudness, duration, and quality were made during conversational speech and sustained vowel production. Voice was characterized as **(8) slightly tense, with occasional roughness perceived at the ends of words**; pitch and loudness were judged as being within normal expectations. Although continuous speech was perceived as being relatively normal in characteristics, her sustained vowel production showed **(9) tremor and intermittent roughness**. Examples of patient C's continuous speech and sustained vowel productions may be heard by L. clicking on CS-C1.WAV (continuous speech sample) and CS-C2.WAV (sustained vowel) in the C:\VDP directory.

Speech Mechanism Examination

This examination was conducted to assess the structure and functioning of the speech production mechanisms. Re-

sults were unremarkable. No signs of extralaryngeal tension or poor laryngeal posture were observed.

Acoustic Measures of Vocal Frequency and Noise

The patient's mean speaking F_0 was measured at 192.10 Hz (SD = 16.6 Hz; pitch sigma = 3.00 semitones). In addition, the patient was asked to sustain the vowel /ɑ/ at a comfortable pitch and loudness for 2 to 3 seconds. Results from analysis of vowel samples revealed the following: **(10) jitter = 0.73%; shimmer 0.51 dB; HNR = 6.05 dB**. Figures 7–6 and 7–7 provide examples of continuous speech and sustained vowel analysis results for patient C.

Rapid Counting

The patient was next asked to count rapidly to 150. Approximately halfway through this task, the patient's voice changed to **(11) a strained, high-pitched voice quality with intermittent aphonia**. Recordings of continuous speech and sustained vowel samples were made immediately after this task. The patient's mean speaking F_0 was measured at 226.08 Hz (SD = 11.29 Hz; pitch sigma = 1.73 semitones). In addition, the patient was asked to sustain the vowel /ɑ/ at a comfortable pitch and loudness for 2 to 3 seconds. Results of analysis of vowel samples after rapid counting revealed the following: **(12) F_0 = 484.95 Hz (SD = 56.20 Hz; pitch sigma = 4.03 ST)**; jitter = 0.92%; shimmer 0.82 dB; HNR = 4.29 dB. Voice returned to normal after 2 to 3 minutes of rest. Examples of patient C's continuous speech and sustained vowel productions after the rapid counting task may be heard by L. clicking on CS-C3.WAV (continuous speech sample) and CS-C4.WAV (sustained vowel) in the C:\VDP directory. Figures 7–8 and 7–9 provide examples of continuous speech and sustained vowel analysis results after the rapid counting task.

CASE STUDY C: DISCUSSION OF KEY INFORMATIONAL COMPONENTS

(1) Spasmodic dysphonia: Often referred to as a focal dystonia, spasmodic dysphonia is a disorder in which the patient experiences intermittent periods of extreme hyperadduction (adductory spasmodic dysphonia) or periods in which the vocal folds involuntarily separate during voice production (abductory spasmodic dysphonia). There is controversy regarding the underlying cause of this disorder, with some seeing spasmodic dysphonia as a functional/psychogenic disorder versus those who regard it as an organic, neurologically based problem. This patient was referred for a suspected case of adductory spasmodic dysphonia.

(2) Having problems with her voice for approximately 2 years: Although the patient had experienced

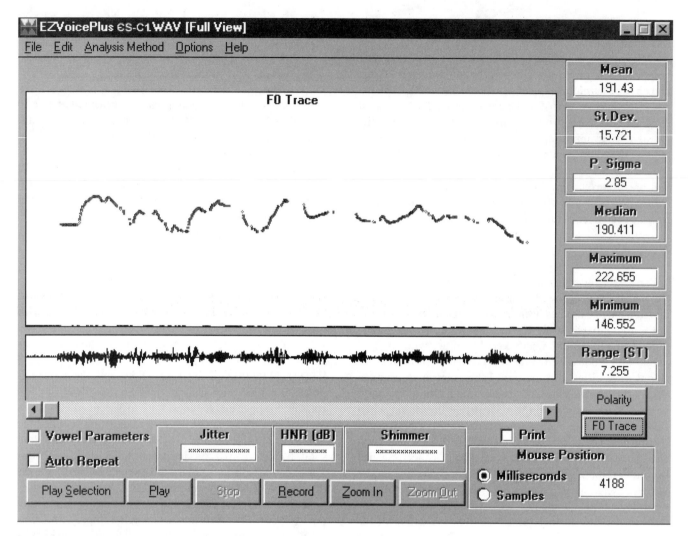

Figure 7–6 An Example of a Continuous Speech Sample for Patient C. The patient's F_0 standard deviation and pitch sigma are slightly low. Overall, F_0 characteristics are well within normal expectations.

her voice difficulties for some time, she only recently had seen an otolaryngologist for the problem. The patient was a cafeteria worker at a local hospital and related that her voice difficulties did not interfere with her work. The clinician should consider the possibility that the prognosis for success in therapy may be poorer for a patient who is relatively unaffected by his or her voice problem(s), regardless of severity.

(3) She did relate a history of emotional difficulties and anxiety: The patient related a recent history of marital difficulties and familial discontent that seemed to coincide with episodic voice problems. The clinician should consider that stress and anxiety may be reflected in physical consequences. This patient may have a significant psychogenic component to her voice problem.

(4) A "helium" voice: Occasionally, no matter what direction or cueing is provided by the clinician, personal history and characteristics of voice problem(s) as related by the patient may be quite vague. In this case, the description of a "helium" voice was unclear to the clinician as to precisely what symptoms the patient was describing. The vagueness of the description was further hindered by the fact that the patient's conversational voice characteristics on the date of the voice diagnostic were relatively normal (see No. 8).

(5) Difficulty in breathing when this voice change occurs: The patient reports breathing difficulty that coincides with the "helium" voice. Underlying respiratory and/or laryngeal valving difficulties (hyperadduction) should be considered by the clinician. Because the breathing difficulties appear to be related to phonation, extreme hyperadduction and laryngeal squeezing should be considered. If the vocal folds cannot adequately abduct during inspiration, the patient will not be able to sufficiently replenish the breath supply.

(6) A strain-struggle to produce voice: The patient reports extreme effort to produce voice during her "helium" voice episodes. This report is consistent with extreme hyperfunction in which increased effort is required to overcome the resistance of hyperadducted vocal folds.

(7) No history of neurological deficit: The patient's medical history (including that provided from her recent ENT examination) reported no history of neurological disease or insult. On the basis of this information, it would appear that overt neurological deficits (e.g., dysarthric effects resulting from cerebrovascular accident) may be ruled out and focus directed more toward disorders that may be functional in nature. However, because spasmodic dysphonia is a more covert disorder that may only reveal itself in particular situations, the presence of this disorder as an underlying cause of the patient's voice problems cannot be ruled out.

(8) Tense; occasional roughness perceived at the ends of words: A tense voice often has a "hard-edge" character to it and is associated with hyperfunction (Colton & Casper, 1996). Although tension was perceived, it was not perceived as a particularly conspicu-

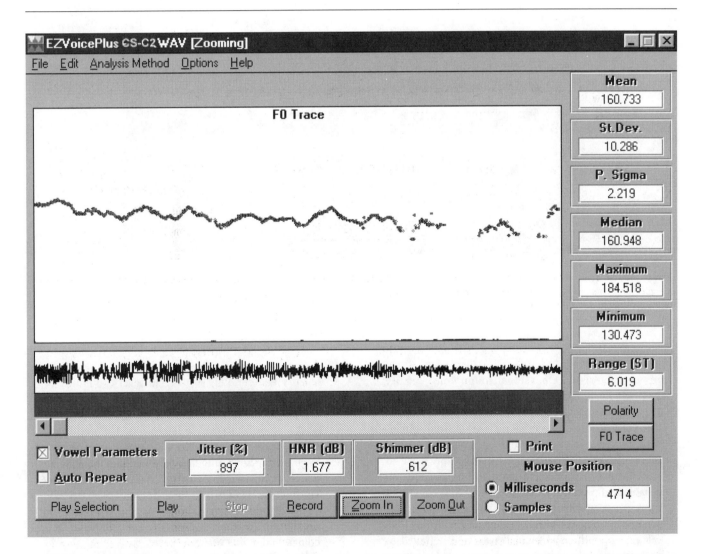

Figure 7–7 An Example of a Sustained Vowel Sample for Patient C. Evidence of tremor occurs throughout this production. In addition, vocal instability occurs near the end of this phonation. The combination of these factors contributes to highly aberrant measures of perturbation, noise, and variability.

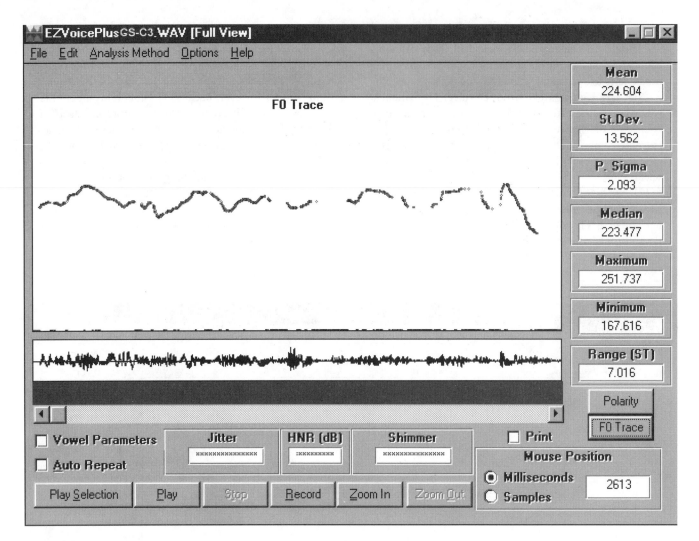

Figure 7–8 An Example of a Continuous Speech Sample for Patient C after the Rapid Counting Task. The patient's speaking F_0 has increased approximately 30 Hz compared with earlier in the diagnostic session. In addition, F_0 standard deviation and pitch sigma are reduced, consistent with the perception of limited intonation.

ous characteristic. Occasional rough voice quality was perceived near the ends of words and on unstressed syllables. Roughness is associated with aperiodic vocal fold vibration that may result from sources such as hyperfunctional voice use (both functional and neurological [organic] in origin) or presence of mass lesions. However, rough quality on unstressed syllables may also be an element of vocal/glottal fry register, which may be considered normal under these conditions. Overall, although roughness was perceived by the clinician, it was also believed to be a relatively minor characteristic of the patient's speaking voice. The patient's speaking voice characteristics were judged to be relatively mild in terms of

severity and certainly not of the severity implied by the patient's descriptions of her voice problem.

(9) Tremor and intermittent roughness: The patient's voice characteristics were considered much more severe in her sustained vowel productions. Tremor (rhythmic fluctuations in pitch and/or loudness) was perceived, indicative of possible underlying neurological dysfunction (e.g., hyperkinesia) and also a possible characteristic observed in spasmodic dysphonia. In addition to the tremor, a rough quality was again noted in this patient's voice.

(10) Jitter = 0.73%; shimmer 0.51 dB; HNR = 6.05 dB: Acoustic analysis of the patient's sustained vowel sample shows slightly elevated jitter and shimmer but substantially reduced HNR compared with normal expectations (15 to 20 dB). The HNR reflects the tremor and pitch variability in the patient's voice, as well as rough quality (aperiodic vibration) near the end of her phonation. Jitter is slightly elevated compared with norms (often in the 0.4% to 0.6% range) but is not affected as much by rhythmic variation in vocal pitch because the actual cycle-to-cycle variations in frequency are relatively small. The patient's conversational speech analysis (mean F_0 and standard deviation) was within normal expectations for her age and gender.

(11) Strained, high-pitched voice quality with intermittent aphonia: Although the patient's symptoms were consistent with episodes of extreme hyperfunc-

tion and possible spasmodic dysphonia, to this point in the diagnostic, very few signs of significant voice disorder had been observed. Without directly observing the characteristics of the patient's voice disorder, the development of a comprehensive clinical hypothesis would be tentative at best and, perhaps, not the best fit for the patient's actual characteristics. Therefore, in an attempt to elicit the patient's voice disorder, the patient was asked to count rapidly from 1 to 100. This task attempts to "stress" the speech and phonatory mechanisms. The hope is that speech/voice characteristics that may be elusive under normal speech conditions will reveal themselves under extraordinary circumstances. In this particular case, as the patient progressed with the rapid counting task, dramatic changes

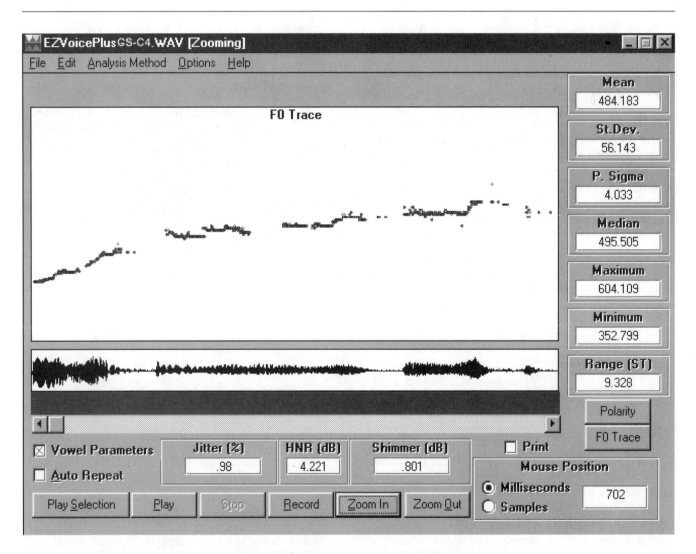

Figure 7–9 An Example of a Sustained Vowel Sample for Patient C after the Rapid Counting Task. Note the exceptionally high mean F_0 and evidence of phonation breaks during extreme hyperadduction of the vocal folds.

were perceived in her voice; significantly increased pitch (particularly in sustained vowel productions), extreme effort, and occasional periods of aphonia were noted. It appeared that this was the "helium" voice as previously described by the patient (the patient confirmed this). The patient had perceived her voice change as similar to the "Donald Duck" qualities of someone who speaks after inhaling a small amount of helium gas. The patient was asked to continue counting up to 150 to provide more time for the clinician to observe perceptual signs. At the end of counting, samples of the patient's continuous speech and sustained vowel productions were recorded.

(12) F_0 = 484.95 Hz (SD = 56.20 Hz; pitch sigma = 4.03 ST): These acoustic measures affirm and document the perception of voice change during and after the rapid counting task. The patient was perceived as producing falsetto phonation during the sustained vowel production and also showed tremendous pitch variability (as documented by the standard deviation and pitch sigma measures). Although not as drastic, significant increases in speaking F_0 were also observed after the rapid counting task.

In this particular case example, it was evident that stress played a significant role in triggering her voice change. Because the patient had no significant history of overt neurological disturbance and no signs of mass lesions (no breathiness or hoarseness, no history of abuse/misuse, a nonsmoker), it was believed that the best clinical hypothesis to explain this patient's symptoms was that the underlying cause was extreme hyperfunction derived from stress and anxiety reaction. The observation of tremor during her sustained vowel production and description of breathing difficulties would be consistent with the diagnosis of adductor spasmodic dysphonia; however, it may be more effective for the clinician to focus on the underlying physiological effects of stress and anxiety rather than the particular label by which we should categorize her disorder. The focus on underlying physiology directs the clinician toward therapy goals with much greater clarity than a diagnostic label.

Impression

Mild-to-moderate dysphonia is characterized by episodes of highly effortful speech and voice; strain; tense, rough voice quality; and substantially increased pitch level. These characteristics may be a result of intermittent spasmodic dysphonia of the adductory type, although the effects of anxiety and stress on this patient's voice appear to be highly significant.

Recommendations

The primary reason that this patient had been referred for this voice evaluation was that her ENT specialist was requesting advice in regard to whether this patient would benefit from botulin toxin injections for her possible spasmodic dysphonia. It was the clinician's impression that the patient would be a better candidate for voice therapy because there appeared to be a substantial psychogenic component to this patient's voice problem.

References

Anders, L.C., Hollien, H., Hurme, P., Sonninen, A., & Wendler, J. (1988). Perception of hoarseness by several classes of listeners. *Folia Phoniatrica*, 40(2), 91–100.

Andrews, M. (1995). *Manual of voice treatment: Pediatrics through geriatrics.* San Diego, CA: Singular Publishing Group, Inc.

Andrews, M.L., & Schmidt, C.P. (1997). Gender presentation: Perceptual and acoustical analyses of voice. *Journal of Voice*, 11(3), 307–313.

Aronson, A. (1973). *Psychogenic voice disorders: An interdisciplinary approach to detection, diagnosis, and therapy: audio seminars in speech pathology.* Philadelphia: W.B. Saunders Co.

Aronson, A. (1985). *Clinical voice disorders* (2nd ed.). New York: Thieme Medical Publishers.

Aronson, A.E. (1990a). *Clinical voice disorders: An interdisciplinary approach* (3rd ed.). New York: Thieme Medical Publishers.

Aronson, A.E. (1990b). Importance of the psychosocial interview in the diagnosis and treatment of "functional" voice disorders. *Journal of Voice*, 4(4), 287–289.

Askenfelt, A., & Hammarberg, B. (1986). Speech waveform perturbation analysis: A perceptual-acoustical comparison of seven measures. *Journal of Speech and Hearing Research*, 29, 50–64.

Awan, S.N. (1989). *Phonetographic assessment of voice characteristics in young adults with and without vocal training* (Dissertation). Kent, OH: Kent State University.

Awan, S.N. (1991). Phonetographic profiles and F_0-SPL characteristics of untrained versus trained vocal groups. *Journal of Voice*, 5(1), 41–50.

Awan, S.N. (1993). Superimposition of speaking voice characteristics and phonetograms in untrained and trained vocal groups. *Journal of Voice*, 7(1), 30–37.

Awan, S.N. (1999). The relief of excessive laryngeal tension: Clinical case studies. Paper presented at the American Speech Language Hearing Association Convention, San Francisco, CA.

Awan, S.N., & Coy, K. (1992). Quantitative assessment of the voice in female smokers and nonsmokers. Paper presented at the American Speech Language Hearing Association Convention, San Antonio, TX.

Awan, S.N., Coy, K., & Riley, S. (1990). Comparison of five estimation methods of optimum frequency: Clinical implications. Paper presented at the American Speech Language Hearing Association Convention, Seattle, WA.

Awan, S.N., & Frenkel, M.L. (1994). Improvements in estimating the harmonics-to-noise ratio of the voice. *Journal of Voice*, 8(3), 255–262.

Awan, S.N., & Knych, C. (2000). The effects of smoking on the acoustic characteristics of the voice in young adults. Paper presented at the 29th Annual Symposium: Care of the Professional Voice, Philadelphia, PA.

Awan, S.N., & Mueller, P.B. (1990). Comment on "Methodological variables affecting phonational frequency range in adults." *Journal of Speech and Hearing Disorders*, 55, 799–806.

Awan, S.N., & Mueller, P.B. (1992). Speaking fundamental frequency characteristics of centenarian females. *Clinical Linguistics and Phonetics*, 6(3), 249–254.

Awan, S.N., & Mueller, P.B. (1996). Speaking fundamental frequency characteristics of white, African American and Hispanic kindergartners. *Journal of Speech and Hearing Research*, 39, 573–577.

Awan, S.N., Mueller, P.B., Larson, G., & Summers, P. (1991). Frequency and intensity measures of black, white, and Hispanic kindergartners. Paper presented at the Texas Speech-Language-Hearing Association Convention, Houston, TX.

Awan, S.N., & Scarpino, S. (1999). A comparison of computerized speech/voice analysis programs. In B. Maassen & P. Groenen (Eds.), *Pathologies of speech & language: Advances in clinical phonetics and linguistics* (pp. 322–332). London: Whurr Publishers.

Awan, S.N., & Ziminsky-Ammon, R. (1996). The aging female voice: Acoustic and respiratory data. Paper presented at the American Speech Language Hearing Association Convention, Seattle, WA.

Baken, R.J. (1987). *Clinical measurement of speech and voice.* Boston: Little, Brown and Company.

Baldwin, E.DeF., Courand, A., & Richards, D.W., Jr. (1948). Pulmonary insufficiency. *Medicine*, 27, 243–276.

Bassich, C.J., & Ludlow, C.L. (1986). The use of perceptual methods by new clinicians for assessing voice quality. *Journal of Speech and Hearing Disorders*, 51, 125–133.

Bastian, R.W., Keidar, A., & Verdolini-Marston, K. (1990). Simple vocal tasks for detecting vocal fold swelling. *Journal of Voice*, 4(2), 172–183.

Beckett, R. (1971). The respirometer as a diagnostic and clinical tool in the speech clinic. *Journal of Speech and Hearing Disorders*, 36, 235–241.

Behrman, A., & Orlikoff, R.F. (1997). Instrumentation in voice assessment and treatment: What's the use? *American Journal of Speech-Language Pathology*, 6, 9–16.

Bell Telephone Laboratories. (1940). *High speed pictures of the human vocal cords.* (Motion Picture). New York: Bell Telephone Laboratories Bureau of Publications.

Bennett, S. (1983). A 3-year longitudinal study of school-aged children's fundamental frequencies. *Journal of Speech and Hearing Research*, 26, 137–142.

Bielamowicz, S., Kreiman, J., Gerratt, B.R., Dauer, M.S., & Berke, G. S. (1996). Comparison of voice analysis systems for perturbation measurement. *Journal of Speech and Hearing Research*, 39, 126–134.

Blaugrund, S., Taira, T., & Isshiki, N. (1991). Laryngeal manual compression in the evaluation of patients for laryngeal framework surgery. In J. Gauffin & B. Hammarberg (Eds.), *Vocal fold physiology acoustic, perceptual and physiological aspects of voice mechanisms* (pp. 207–212). San Diego, CA: Singular Publishing Group, Inc.

Bless, D.M., & Hicks, D.M. (1996). Diagnosis and measurement: Assessing the "whs" of voice function. In W. Brown, B. Vinson, & M. Crary (Eds.), *Organic voice disorders assessment and treatment* (pp. 119–170). San Diego, CA: Singular Publishing Group, Inc.

Blood, G.W. (1994). Efficacy of a computer-assisted voice treatment protocol. *American Journal of Speech-Language Pathology*, 3(1), 57–66.

Bohme, G., & Stuchlik, G. (1995). Voice profiles and standard voice profile of untrained children. *Journal of Voice*, 9(3), 304–307.

Boltezar, I.H., Burger, Z.R., & Zargi, M. (1997). Instability of voice in adolescence: Pathologic condition or normal developmental variation? *The Journal of Pediatrics*, 130(2), 185–190.

Boone, D. (1977). *The voice and voice therapy*. Englewood Cliffs, NJ: Prentice-Hall.

Boone, D. (1980). Voice disorders. In T. Hixon, L. Shriberg, & J. Saxman (Eds.), *Introduction to communication disorders* (pp. 312–351). Englewood Cliffs, NJ: Prentice-Hall.

Boone, D., & McFarlane, S. (1977; 1988). *The voice and voice therapy* (3rd & 4th eds.). Englewood Cliffs, NJ: Prentice Hall.

Borden, G.J., Harris, K.S., & Raphael, L.J. (1994). *Speech science primer: Physiology, acoustics, and perception of speech* (3rd ed.). Baltimore: Williams & Wilkins.

Boshoff, P. (1945). The anatomy of the South African Negro larynges. *South African Journal of Medical Sciences*, 10, 35–50.

Bouhuys, A., Proctor, D., & Mead, J. (1966). Kinetic aspects of singing. *Journal of Applied Physiology*, 21, 483–496.

Brown, W., & McGlone, R. (1974). Aerodynamic and acoustic stress in sentence production. *Journal of Acoustical Society of America*, 56, 971–974.

Campbell, D.T., & Stanley, J.C. (1966). *Experimental and quasi-experimental designs for research*. Chicago: Rand McNally.

Cannito, M.P. (1991). Emotional considerations in spasmodic dysphonia: Psychometric quantification. *Journal of Communication Disorders*, 24, 313–329.

Canter, G. (1963). Speech characteristics of patients with Parkinson's disease. I. Intensity, pitch and duration. *Journal of Speech and Hearing Disorders*, 28, 221–229.

Canter, G. (1965). Speech characteristics of patients with Parkinson's disease: Physiological support for speech. *Journal of Speech and Hearing Disorders*, 30, 44–49.

Caruso, A.J., Mueller, P.B., & Xue, A. (1994). Relative contributions of voice and articulation to listener judgements of age and gender: Preliminary data and implications. *Voice*, 3, 1–9.

Case, J. (1996). *Clinical management of voice disorders*. Austin, TX: PRO-ED.

Coleman, R. (1969). Effect of median frequency levels upon the roughness of jittered stimuli. *Journal of Speech and Hearing Research*, 12, 330–336.

Coleman, R.F. (1993). Sources of variation in phonetograms. *Journal of Voice*, 7(1), 1–14.

Coleman, R.F., & Markham, I.W. (1991). Normal variations in habitual pitch. *Journal of Voice*, 5(2), 173–177.

Coleman, R., & Mott, J. (1978). Fundamental frequency and sound pressure level profiles of young female singers. *Folia Phoniatrica*, 30, 94–102.

Colton, R. (1973). Vocal intensity in the modal and falsetto registers. *Folia Phoniatrica*, 25, 62–70.

Colton, R., & Casper, J. (1996). *Understanding voice problems: A physiological perspective for diagnosis and treatment* (pp. 186–240). Baltimore: Williams & Wilkins.

Countryman, S., Hicks, J., Ramig, L.O., & Smith, M.E. (1997). Supraglottal hyperadduction in an individual with Parkinson disease: A clinical treatment note. *American Journal of Speech-Language Pathology*, 6(6), 74–84.

Damste, H. (1970). The phonetogram. *Practica-Oto-Rhino-Laryngologica*, 32, 185–187.

Darley, F.L., Aronson, A.E., & Brown, J.R. (1975). *Motor speech disorders*. Philadelphia: W.B. Saunders Company.

Davis, S.B. (1981). Acoustic characteristics of laryngeal pathology. In J.K. Darby (Ed.), *Speech Evaluation in Medicine*. New York: Grune & Stratton, Inc.

de Callatay, A. (1986) *Natural and artificial intelligence: Processor systems compared to the human brain*. Amsterdam: Elsevier Science.

de Krom, G. (1994). Consistency and reliability of voice quality ratings for different types of speech fragments. *Journal of Speech and Hearing Research*, 37, 985–1000.

Deem, J.F., Manning, W.H., Knack, J.V., & Matesich, J.S. (1989). The automatic extraction of pitch perturbation using microcomputers: Some methodological considerations. *Journal of Speech and Hearing Research*, 32, 689–697.

Denes, P., & Pinson, E. (1973). *The speech chain*. New York: Doubleday.

Dockery, D.W., Ware, J.H., Ferris, B.G., Jr., Glicksberg, M.E.F., Spiro, A. III, & Speizer, F.E. (1985). Distribution of forced expiratory volume in one second and forced vital capacity in healthy, white, adult never-smokers in six U.S. cities. *American Review of Respiratory Disease*, 131, 511–520.

Dromey, C., Ramig, L.O., & Johnson, A.B. (1995). Phonatory and articulatory changes associated with increased vocal intensity in Parkinson disease: A case study. *Journal of Speech and Hearing Research*, 38, 751–764.

Dwire, A., & McCauley, R. (1995). Repeated measures of vocal fundamental frequency perturbation obtained using the Visi-Pitch. *Journal of Voice*, 9(2), 156–162.

Dworkin, J., & Culatta, R. (1980) *Dworkin-Culatta oral mechanism examination*. Nicholasville, KY: Edgewood Press.

Dworkin, J., & Meleca, R. (1997). *Vocal pathologies: Diagnosis, treatment, and case studies*. San Diego, CA: Singular Publishing Group, Inc.

Dworkin, J.P. (1991). *Motor speech disorders: A treatment guide*. St. Louis, MO: Mosby.

Eckel, F.C., & Boone, D.R. (1981). The s/z ratio as an indicator of laryngeal pathology. *Journal of Speech and Hearing Disorders*, 46, 138–146.

Eguchi, S., & Hirsh, I.J. (1969). Development of speech sounds in children. *Acta Otolaryngologica Suppl.*, 257, 5–43.

Enright, P.L., Vaz Fragoso, C.A., & Sly, R.M. (1996). A concise guide to office spirometry. *Patient Care*, 46–67.

Eskanazi, L., Childers, D.G., & Hicks, D.M. (1990). Acoustic correlates of vocal quality. *Journal of Speech and Hearing Research*, 33, 298–306.

Eustace, C.S., Stemple, J.C., & Lee, L. (1996). Objective measures of voice production in patients complaining of laryngeal fatigue. *Journal of Voice*, 10(2), 146–154.

Faaborg-Andersen, K. (1957). Electromyographic investigation of intrinsic laryngeal muscles in humans. *Acta Physiologica Scandinavica*, 41, 140.

Fairbanks, G. (1960). *Voice and articulation drill book* (2nd ed.). New York: HarperCollins Publishers.

Fant, G. (1970). *Acoustic theory of speech production.* Mouton: The Hague.

Fendler, M., & Shearer, W.M. (1988). Reliability of the s/z ratio in normal children's voices. *Language, Speech, and Hearing Services in Schools*, 19, 2–4.

Fex, S. (1992). Perceptual evaluation. *Journal of Voice*, 6(2), 155–158.

Finnegan, D.E. (1984). Maximum phonation time for children with normal voices. *Journal of Communication Disorders*, 17, 309–317.

Fisher, K., & Swank, P.R. (1997). Estimating phonation threshold pressure. *Journal of Speech, Language, and Hearing Research*, 40, 1122–1129.

Fitch, J.L., & Holbrook, A. (1970). Modal vocal fundamental frequency of young adults. *Archives in Otolaryngology*, 92, 379–382.

Flanagan, J. (1958). Some properties of the glottal sound source. *Journal of Speech and Hearing Research*, 1, 99–116.

Fletcher, W. (1950). *A study of internal laryngeal activity in relation to vocal intensity.* PhD Thesis. Chicago: Northwestern University.

Folkins, J., & Kuehn, D. (1982). Speech production. In Lass, N., McReynolds, L., Northern, J., & Yoder, D. (Eds.), *Speech, language, and hearing, Vol. 1: Normal processes.* Philadelphia: W.B. Saunders Company.

Gauffin, J., & Sundberg, J. (1980). Data on the glottal voice source behavior in vowel productions. Speech Transmission Lab., *Quarterly Progress Status Report*. Stockholm: Royal Institute of Technology, 2–3, 60–70.

Gelfer, M. (1986). The stability of total phonational frequency range. *Journal of Acoustical Society of America*, 79, Suppl. 1, S83.

Gelfer, M.P. (1993). A multidimensional scaling study of voice quality in females. *Phonetica*, 50, 15–27.

Gelfer, M.P. (1995). Fundamental frequency, intensity, and vowel selection: Effects on measures of phonatory stability. *Journal of Speech and Hearing Research*, 38, 1189–1198.

Gelfer, M.P., Andrews, M.L., & Schmidt, C.P. (1991). Effects of prolonged loud reading on selected measures of vocal function in trained and untrained singers. *Journal of Voice*, 5(2), 158–167.

Gelfer, M.P., & Fendel, D.M. (1995). Comparisons of jitter, shimmer, and signal-to-noise ratio from directly digitized versus taped voice samples. *Journal of Voice*, 9(4), 378–382.

Gilbert, H.R., & Weismer, G.G. (1974). The effects of smoking on the fundamental frequency of women. *Journal of Linguistic Research*, 3(3), 225–231.

Glaze, L., Bless, D., & Susser, R. (1990). Acoustic analysis of vowel and loudness differences in children's voice. *Journal of Voice*, 4, 37–44.

Goldman, S.L., Hargrave, J., Hillman, R.E., Holmberg, E., & Gress, C. (1996). Stress, anxiety, somatic complaints, and voice use in women with vocal nodules: Preliminary findings. *American Journal of Speech-Language Pathology*, 5, 44–52.

Goodglass, H., & Kaplan, E. (1983). *The assessment of aphasia and related disorders* (2nd ed.). Baltimore: Lea & Febiger.

Gould, W. (1977). The effect of voice training on lung volumes in singers and the possible relationship to the damping factor of Pressman. *Journal of Research in Singing*, 1, 3–15.

Gould, W., & Okamura, H. (1974). Respiratory training of the singer. *Folia Phoniatrica*, 26, 275–286.

Gramming, P. (1988). *The Phonetogram: An experimental and clinical study.* (Dissertation). Department of Otolaryngology, University of Lund, Malmo General Hospital, Malmo, Sweden.

Gramming, P., & Sundberg, J. (1988). Spectrum factors relevant to phone-

togram measurement. *Journal of Acoustical Society of America*, 83, 2352–2360.

Gramming, P., Sundberg, J., Ternstrom, S., Leanderson, R., & Perkins, W. (1988). Relationship between changes in voice pitch and loudness. In P. Gramming, *The Phonetogram: An experimental and clinical study.* (Dissertation). Department of Otolaryngology, University of Lund, Malmo General Hospital, Malmo, Sweden.

Hall, K.D., & Yairi, E. (1992). Fundamental frequency, jitter, and shimmer in preschoolers who stutter. *Journal of Speech and Hearing Research*, 35, 1002–1008.

Hammarberg, B., Fritzell, B., Gauffin, J., Sundberg, J., & Wedin, L. (1980). Perceptual and acoustic correlates of abnormal voice qualities. *Acta Otolaryngologica*, 90, 441–451.

Harden, J.R., & Looney, N.A. (1984). Duration of sustained phonation in kindergarten children. *International Journal of Pediatric Otorhinolaryngology*, 7, 11–19.

Hartelius, L., Buder, E.H., & Strand, E.A. (1997). Long-term phonatory instability in individuals with multiple sclerosis. *Journal of Speech, Language, and Hearing Research*, 40, 1056–1072.

Haynes, W., Pindzola, R., & Emerick, L. (1992). *Diagnosis and evaluation in speech pathology.* New York: Simon & Schuster.

Heiberger, V.L., & Horii, Y. (1982). Jitter and shimmer in sustained phonation. In N.J. Lass (Ed.), *Speech and language: Advances in basic research and practice* (pp. 299–332). New York: Academic Press.

Hewlett, N., Topham, N., & McMullen, C. (1996). The effects of smoking on the female voice. In M.J. Ball & M. Duckworth (Eds.), *Advances in clinical phonetics* (pp. 227–235). Philadelphia: John Benjamins Publishing Company.

Heylen, L., Wuyts, F.L., Mertens, F., De Bodt, M., Pattyn, J., Croux, C., & Van de Heyning, P. (1998). Evaluation of the vocal performance of children using a voice range profile index. *Journal of Speech-Language-Hearing Research*, 41, 232–238.

Higgins, M.B., Chait, D.H., & Schulte, L. (1999). Phonatory air flow characteristics of adductor spasmodic dysphonia and muscle tension dysphonia. *Journal of Speech, Language, and Hearing Research*, 42, 101–111.

Hill, D.P., Meyers, A.D., & Scherer, R.C. (1990). A comparison of four clinical techniques in the analysis of phonation. *Journal of Voice*, 4(3), 198–204.

Hillenbrand, J. (1987). A methodological study of perturbation and additive noise in synthetically generated voice signals. *Journal of Speech and Hearing Research*, 30, 448–461.

Hirano, M. (1981). The function of the intrinsic laryngeal muscles in singing. In K. Stevens & M. Hirano (Eds.), *Vocal fold physiology.* Tokyo: University of Tokyo Press.

Hirano, M. (1989). Objective evaluation of the human voice: Clinical aspects. *Folia Phoniatrica*, 41, 89–144.

Hirano, M. (1991). Clinical applications of voice tests. In *Assessment of Speech and Voice Production: Research and Clinical Application.* National Institute on Deafness and Other Communication Disorders (NIDCD) Monograph, 1, 5–16.

Hirano, M., Koike, Y., & von Leden, H. (1968). Maximum phonation time and air usage during phonation. *Folia Phoniatrica*, 20, 185–201.

Hirano, M., Mori, K., Tanaka, S., & Fujita, M. (1995). Vocal function in patients with unilateral vocal fold paralysis before and after silicone injection. *Acta Otolaryngologica*, 115, 553–559.

Hirano, M., Ohala, J., & Vennard, W. (1969). The function of the laryngeal muscles in regulating fundamental frequency and intensity of phonation. *Journal of Speech and Hearing Research*, 12, 616–628.

Hirano, M., Tanaka, S., Fujita, M., & Terasawa, R. (1991). Fundamental frequency and sound pressure level of phonation in pathological states. *Journal of Voice*, 5(2),120–127.

Hixon, T.J., Goldman, M.D., & Mead, J. (1973). Kinematics of the chest wall during speech production: Volume displacements of the rib cage, abdomen, and lung. *Journal of Speech and Hearing Research*, 16, 78–115.

Hixon, T., Hawley, J.L., & Wilson, K. (1982). An around-the-house device for the clinical determination of respiratory driving pressure: A note on making simple even simpler. *Journal of Speech and Hearing Disorders*, 47, 413–415.

Hixon, T., & Hoffman, C. (1978). Chest wall shape in singing. *Professional Voice*, 9–10.

Hixon, T., Klatt, D., & Mead, J. (1971). Influence of forced transglottal pressure changes on vocal fundamental frequency. *Journal of Acoustical Society of America*, 49A, 105(A).

Hixon, T.J., & Hoit, J.D. (1998). Physical examination of the diaphragm by the speech language pathologist. *American Journal of Speech-Language Pathology*, 7, 37–45.

Hollien, H. (1983). In search of vocal frequency control mechanisms. In D. Bless & J. Abbs (Eds.), *Vocal fold physiology: Contemporary research and clinical issues*. San Diego, CA: College Hill Press.

Hollien, H., Dew, D., & Philips, P. (1971). Phonational frequency ranges of adults. *Journal of Speech and Hearing Research*, 14, 755–760.

Hollien, H., & Jackson, B. (1973). Normative data on the speaking fundamental frequency characteristics of young adult males. *Journal of Phonetics*, 1, 117–120.

Hollien, H., & Malcik, E. (1967). Evaluation of cross-sectional studies of adolescent voice change in males. *Speech Monographs*, 34, 80–84.

Hollien, H., Michel, J., & Doherty, E.T. (1973). A method of analyzing vocal jitter in sustained phonation. *Journal of Phonetics*, 1, 85–91.

Hollien, H., & Moore, P. (1960). Measurements of the vocal folds during changes in pitch. *Journal of Speech and Hearing Research*, 3, 157–165.

Hollien, H., & Shipp, T. (1972). Speaking fundamental frequency and chronologic age in males. *Journal of Speech and Hearing Research*, 15, 148–154.

Holmes, T.H., & Rahe, H.B. (1967). The social readjustment rating scale. *Journal of Psychosomatic Research*, 11, 213–218.

Honda, K. (1983). Relationship between pitch control and vowel articulation. In D.M. Bless & J.H. Abbs (Eds.), *Vocal fold physiology: Contemporary research and clinical issues* (pp. 286–297). San Diego, CA: College-Hill.

Honjo, I., & Isshiki, N. (1980). Laryngoscopic and voice characteristics of aged persons. *Archives in Otolaryngology*, 106, 149–150.

Horii, Y. (1975). Some statistical characteristics of voice fundamental frequency. *Journal of Speech and Hearing Research*, 18, 192–201.

Horii, Y. (1979). Fundamental frequency perturbation observed in sustained phonation. *Journal of Speech and Hearing Research*, 22, 5–19.

Horii, Y. (1980). Vocal shimmer in sustained phonation. *Journal of Speech and Hearing Research*, 23, 202–209.

Horii, Y. (1982a). Jitter and shimmer differences among sustained vowel phonations. *Journal of Speech and Hearing Research*, 25, 12–14.

Horii, Y. (1982b). Some voice fundamental frequency characteristics of oral reading and spontaneous speech by hard of hearing young women. *Journal of Speech and Hearing Research*, 25, 608–610.

Horii, Y. (1983). Some acoustic characteristics of oral reading by ten- to twelve-year-old children. *Journal of Communication Disorders*, 16, 257–267.

Horii, Y. (1985). Jitter and shimmer in sustained vocal fry phonation. *Folia Phoniatrica*, 37, 81–86.

Huang, D., Lin, S., & O'Brien, R. (1995). *Dr. Speech for Windows, Version 3, User's Guide.* Seattle, WA: Tiger Electronics, Inc.

Hudson, A., & Holbrook, A. (1982). Fundamental frequency characteristics of young black adults: Spontaneous speaking and oral reading. *Journal of Speech and Hearing Research*, 25, 25–28.

Hudson, A.I., & Holbrook, A. (1981). A study of the reading fundamental vocal frequency of young black adults. *Journal of Speech and Hearing Research*, 24, 197–201.

Hufnagle, J., & Hufnagle, K. (1984). An investigation of the relationship between speaking fundamental frequency and vocal quality improvement. *Journal of Communication Disorders*, 17, 95–100.

Hufnagle, J., & Hufnagle, K.K. (1988). S/z ratio in dysphonic children with and without vocal nodules. *Language, Speech, and Hearing Services in Schools*, 19, 418–422.

Hutchinson, B.B., Hanson, M.L., & Mecham, M.J. (1979). *Diagnostic handbook of speech pathology.* Baltimore: Williams & Wilkins.

Isshiki, N. (1964). Regulatory mechanism of voice intensity variation. *Journal of Speech and Hearing Research*, 7, 7–16.

Isshiki, N. (1965). Vocal intensity and airflow rate. *Folia Phoniatrica*, 17, 92–104.

Isshiki, N., Yanagihara, N., & Morimoto, M. (1966). Approach to the objective diagnosis of hoarseness. *Folia Phoniatrica*, 18, 393–400.

Iwata, S., & von Leden, H. (1970). Phonation quotient in patients with laryngeal diseases. *Folia Phoniatrica*, 22, 117–128.

Jiang, J., Lin, E., & Hanson, D.G. (1998). Effect of tape recording on perturbation measures. *Journal of Speech, Language, and Hearing in Schools*, 41, 1031–1041.

Johansson, C., Sundberg, J., & Willbrand, H. (1983). X-ray study of articulation and formant frequencies in two male singers (pp. 203–218). Proceedings of the Stockholm Music Acoustics Conference. Stockholm: Royal Swedish Academy of Music.

Kahane, J.C., (1990). Age-related changes in the peripheral speech mechanism: Structural and physiological changes. *Proceedings of the Research Symposium on Communication Sciences and Disorders and Aging*, No. 19, 75–87.

Kaplan, H. (1960). *Anatomy and physiology of speech.* New York: McGraw-Hill.

Kane, M., & Wellen, C.J. (1985). Acoustical measurements and clinical judgements of vocal quality in children with vocal nodules. *Folia Phoniatrica*, 37, 53–57.

Karnell, M.P. (1991). Laryngeal perturbation analysis: Minimum length of analysis window. *Journal of Speech and Hearing Research*, 34, 544–548.

Karnell, M.P., Hall, K.D., & Landahl, K.L. (1995). Comparison of fundamental frequency and perturbation measurements among three analysis systems. *Journal of Voice*, 9(4), 383–393.

Kazdin, A.E. (1982). *Single-case research designs: Methods for clinical and applied settings.* New York: Oxford University Press.

Keidar, A., Hurtig, R., & Titze, I. (1987). The perceptual nature of vocal register change. *Journal of Voice*, 1(3), 223–233.

Kelley, A. (1977). Fundamental frequency measurements of female voices from 20–90 years of age. Unpublished manuscript. Chapel Hill, NC: University of North Carolina.

Kent, J.F., Kent, R.D., Rosenbek, J.C., Weismer, G., Martin, R., Sufit, R., & Brooks, B.R. (1992). Quantitative description of the dysarthria in women with amyotrophic lateral sclerosis. *Journal of Speech and Hearing Research*, 35, 723–733.

Kent, R., Kent, J.F., & Rosenbek, J.C. (1987) Maximum performance tests of speech production. *Journal of Speech & Hearing Research*, 52, 367–387.

Kent, R., & Rosenbek, J. (1982). Prosodic disturbance and neurologic lesion. *Brain and Language*, 15, 259–291.

Kent, R.D. (1976). Anatomical and neuromuscular maturation of the speech mechanism: Evidence from acoustic studies. *Journal of Speech and Hearing Research*, 19, 421–447.

Kent, R.D. (1994). *Reference manual for communicative sciences and disorders: Speech and language.* Austin, TX: PRO-ED.

Kinzl, J., Biebl, W., & Rauchegger, H. (1988). Function aphonia: Psychosomatic aspects of diagnosis and therapy. *Folia Phoniatrica*, 40(3), 131–137.

Kitajima, K. (1981). Quantitative evaluation of the noise level in the pathologic voice. *Folia Phoniatrica*, 33, 115–124.

Klatt, D.H., & Klatt, L.C. (1990). Analysis, synthesis, and perception of voice quality variations among female and male talkers. *Journal of Acoustical Society of America*, 87(2), 820–857.

Klingholtz, F. (1990). Acoustic recognition of voice disorders: A comparative study of running speech versus sustained vowels. *Journal of Acoustical Society of America*, 87(5), 2218–2224.

Koike, Y., & Hirano, H. (1968). Significance of vocal velocity index. *Folia Phoniatrica*, 20, 285–296.

Kojima, H., Gould, W.J., Lambiase, A., & Isshiki, N. (1980). Computer analysis of hoarseness. *Acta Otolarygologica*, 89, 547–554.

Komiyama, S., Watanabe, H., & Ryu, S. (1984). Phonographic relationship between pitch and intensity of the human voice. *Folia Phoniatrica*, 36, 1–7.

Koufman, J.A., & Blalock, P.D. (1982). Classification and approach to patients with functional voice disorders. *Annals of Otolaryngology Rhinology and Laryngology*, 91, 372–377.

Kreiman, J., Gerratt, B., Kempster, G.B., Erman, A., & Berke, G.S. (1993). Perceptual evaluation of voice quality: Review, tutorial, and a framework for future research. *Journal of Speech and Hearing Research*, 36, 21–40.

Kreul, E.J. (1972). Neuromuscular control examination (NMC) for Parkinsonism: Vocal prolongation and diadochokinetic and reading rates. *Journal of Speech and Hearing Research*, 15, 72–83.

Krogman, W. (1972). *Child growth.* Ann Arbor: The University of Michigan Press.

Large, J. (1971). Observations on the vocal capacity of singers. *NATS Bulletin*, 28, 34–35.

Large, J., Baird, E., & Jenkins, T. (1980). Studies of male high voice mechanisms. *Journal Research Singing*, 3, 26–33.

Larson, G.W., Mueller, P.B., & Summers, P.A. (1991). The effect of procedural variations on the s/z ratio of adults. *Journal of Communication Disorders*, 24, 135–140.

Laures, J.S., & Weismer, G. (1999). The effects of a flattened fundamental frequency on intelligibility at the sentence level. *Journal of Speech, Language, and Hearing Research*, 42, 1148–1156.

Leff, J., & Abberton, E. (1981). Voice pitch measurements in schizophrenia and depression. *Psychological Medicine*, 11, 849–852.

Lewis, K., Casteel, J., & McMahon, J. (1982). Duration of sustained /ɑ/ related to the number of trials. *Folia Phoniatrica*, 34, 41–48.

Lindblom, B.A., & Sundberg, J. (1971). Acoustical consequences of lip, tongue, jaw, and larynx movement. *Journal of Acoustical Society of America*, 50, 1166–1179.

Linville, S. (1987). Maximum phonational frequency range capabilities of women's voices with advancing age. *Folia Phoniatrica*, 39, 297–301.

Linville, S. (1988). Intraspeaker variability in fundamental frequency stability: An age-related phenomenon? *Journal of Acoustical Society of America*, 83(2), 741–745.

Linville, S., & Fisher, H. (1985). Acoustic characteristics of women's voices with advancing age. *Journal of Gerontology*, 40, 324–330.

Linville, S., Skarin, B.D., & Fornatto, E. (1989). The interrelationship of measures related to vocal function, speech rate, and laryngeal appearance in elderly women. *Journal of Speech and Hearing Research*, 32, 323–330.

Liss, J., Weismer, G., & Rosenbek, J.C. (1990). Selected acoustic characteristics of speech production in very old males. *Journal of Gerontology: Psychological Sciences*, 45, 35–45.

Logemann, J.A. (1998). *Evaluation and treatment of swallowing disorders.* Austin, TX: PRO-ED.

Luchsinger, R., & Arnold, G. (1965). Physiology and pathology of respiration and phonation. In R. Luchsinger & G. Arnold (Eds.), *Voice-speech-language. clinical communicology: Its physiology and pathology.* Belmont, CA: Wadsworth Publishing Co.

Ludlow, C.L., Bassich, C.J., Conner, N.P., Coulter, D.C., & Lee, Y.J. (1987). The validity of using phonatory jitter and shimmer to detect laryngeal pathology. In T. Baer, C. Sasaki, & K. Harris, *Laryngeal function in phonation and respiration* (pp. 492–507). Boston: College-Hill Press.

Martin, D., Fitch, J., & Wolfe, V. (1995). Pathologic voice type and the acoustic prediction of severity. *Journal of Speech and Hearing Research*, 38, 765–771.

Mayo, R., & Manning, W.H. (1994). Vocal tract characteristics of African-American and European-American adult males. *Texas Journal of Audiology and Speech Pathology*, XX, 33–36.

McGlone, R., & McGlone, J. (1972). Speaking fundamental frequency of eight-year-old girls. *Folia Phoniatrica*, 24, 313–317.

Mendoza, E., Valencia, N., Munoz, J., & Trujillo, H. (1996). Differences in voice quality between men and women: Use of the long-term average spectrum. *Journal of Voice*, 10(1), 59–66.

Michel, J., & Wendahl, R. (1971). Correlates of voice production. In L. Travis (Ed.), *Handbook of speech pathology and audiology.* Englewood Cliffs, NJ: Prentice Hall.

Milenkovic, P. (1987). Least mean square measures of voice perturbation. *Journal of Speech and Hearing Research*, 30, 529–538.

Milenkovic, P.H., Bless, D.M., & Rammage, L.A. (1991). Acoustic and perceptual characterization of vocal nodules. In J. Gauffin & B. Hammarberg (Eds.), *Vocal fold physiology: Acoustic, perceptual, and physiological aspects of voice mechanisms* (pp. 265–272). San Diego, CA: Singular Publishing Group, Inc.

Monsen, R.B. (1979). Acoustic qualities of phonation in young hearing-impaired children. *Journal of Speech and Hearing Research*, 22, 270–288.

Moore, G.P. (1971). Voice disorders organically based. In L.E. Travis (Ed.), *Handbook of speech pathology and audiology* (pp. 535–569). Englewood Cliffs, NJ: Prentice-Hall.

Moran, M., & Gilbert, H. (1984). Relationship between voice profile ratings and aerodynamic and acoustic parameters. *Journal of Communication Disorders*, 17, 245–260.

Morris, R. (1997). Speaking fundamental frequency characteristics of 8- through 10-year-old white and African-American boys. *Journal of Communication Disorders*, 30, 101–116.

Morris, R.J., & Brown, W.S. (1994a). Age-related differences in speech intensity among adult females. *Folia Phoniatrica*, 46, 64–69.

Morris, R.J., & Brown, W.S. (1994b). Age-related differences in speech variability among women. *Journal of Communication Disorders*, 27, 49–64.

Morris, R.J., & Brown, W.S. (1996). Comparison of various automatic means for measuring mean fundamental frequency. *Journal of Voice*, 10(2), 159–165.

Morris, R.J., Brown, W.S., Hicks, D.M., & Howell, E. (1995). Phonational profiles of male trained singers and nonsingers. *Journal of Voice*, 9(2), 142–148.

Morrison, M.D. (1997). Pattern recognition in muscle misuse voice disorders: How I do it. *Journal of Voice*, 11, 108–114.

Morrison, M.D., & Rammage, L.A. (1993). Muscle misuse voice disorders: Description and classification. *Acta Otolaryngologica*, 113, 428–434.

Mueller, P.B. (1978). *Communicative disorders in a geriatric population.* Paper presented at the Annual Convention of the American Speech Language Hearing Association, San Francisco, CA.

Mueller, P.B. (1982). Voice characteristics of octogenarians and nonagenarian persons. *Ear, Nose, and Throat Journal*, 61, 33–37.

Mueller, P.B. (1993). Maximum durations of /s/ and /z/ and the s/z ratio of elderly subjects. *Voice*, 2, 49–54.

Mueller, P.B. (1997). The aging voice. *Seminars in Speech and Language*, 18(2), 159–169.

Mueller, P.B. (1998). Voice ageism. *Contemporary Issues in Communication Science and Disorders*, 25, 62–64.

Mueller, P.B., Larson, G.W., & Summers, P.A. (1991). S/z ratio variability in normal children and adults. *Texas Journal of Audiology and Speech Pathology*, 17, 43–45.

Mueller, P.B., & Xue, A. (1996). Variability of fundamental frequency measures. *Logopedics Phoniatrics Vocology*, 21, 64–67.

Murphy, C.H., & Doyle, P.C. (1987). The effects of cigarette smoking on voice fundamental frequency. *Otolaryngology–Head and Neck Surgery*, 97(4), 376–380.

Murry, T. (1978). Speaking fundamental frequency characteristics associated with voice pathologies. *Journal of Speech and Hearing Disorders*, 43, 374–379.

Murry, T. (1982). Phonation: Assessment. In N. Lass, L. McReynolds, J. Northern, & D. Yoder (Eds.), *Speech, language, and hearing* (Vol. II; pp. 477–488). Philadelphia: W.B. Saunders Company.

Murry, T. (1990). Pitch-matching accuracy in singers and nonsingers. *Journal of Voice*, 4(4), 317–321.

Murry, T., Brown, W., & Morris, R. (1995). Patterns of fundamental frequency for three types of voice samples. *Journal of Voice*, 9(3), 282–289.

Murry, T., & Doherty, E.T. (1980). Selected acoustic characteristics of pathologic and normal speakers. *Journal of Speech and Hearing Research*, 23, 361–369.

Neiman, G.S., & Edeson, B. (1981). Procedural aspects of eliciting maximum phonation time. *Folia Phoniatrica*, 33, 285–293.

Newby, H. (1979). *Audiology* (4th ed.). Englewood Cliffs, NJ: Prentice Hall.

Nicolosi, L., Harryman, E., & Kresheck, J. (1989). *Terminology of communication disorders speech-language-hearing* (3rd ed.). Baltimore: Williams & Wilkins.

Nittrouer, S., McGowan, R.S., Milenkovic, P.H., & Beehler, D. (1990). Acoustic measurements of men's and women's voices: A study of context effects and covariation. *Journal of Speech and Hearing Research*, 33, 761–775.

Nordstrom, P. (1977). Female and infant vocal tracts simulated from male area functions. *Journal of Phonetics*, 5, 81–92.

Olsen, B., Perez, D., Burk, K.W., & Platt, L.J. (1969). Respirometric-phonatory study of children with and without vocal nodules. Paper presented at the American Speech and Hearing Association Convention, Chicago, IL.

Omori, K., Kojima, H., Kakani, R., Slavit, D.H., & Blaugrund, S.M. (1997). Acoustic characteristics of rough voice: Subharmonics. *Journal of Voice*, 11(1), 40–47.

Orlikoff, R.F. (1990). The relationship of age and cardiovascular health to certain acoustic characteristics of male voices. *Journal of Speech and Hearing Research*, 33, 450–457.

Orlikoff, R.F., Dejonckere, P.H., Dembowski, J., Fitch, J., Gelfer, M.P., Gerratt, B.R., Haskell, J.A., Kreiman, J., Metz, D.E., Schiavetti, N., Watson, B.C., & Wolfe, V. (1999). The perceived role of voice perception in clinical practice. *Phonoscope*, 2(2), 89–104.

Orlikoff, R.F., & Kahane, J.C. (1991). Influence of mean sound pressure level on jitter and shimmer measures. *Journal of Voice*, 5(2), 113–119.

Pabon, J.P., & Plomp, R. (1988). Automatic phonetogram recording supplemented with acoustical voice-quality parameters. *Journal of Speech and Hearing Research*, 31, 710–722.

Papamichalis, P.E. (1987). *Practical approaches to speech coding.* Englewood Cliffs, NJ: Prentice-Hall.

Pedersen, M.F., Moller, S., & Bennett, P. (1990). Voice characteristics compared with phonetograms, androgens, oestrogens and puberty stages in 8–19 year old choir girls. *Journal of Research in Singing and Applied Vocal Pedagogy*, 13, 1–10.

Pedersen, M.F., Moller, S., Krabbe, S., & Bennett, P. (1986). Fundamental voice frequency measured by electroglottography during continuous speech. A new exact secondary sex characteristic in boys in puberty. *International Journal of Pediatric Otorhinolaryngology*, 11, 21–27.

Peifang, C. (1991). Massage for the treatment of voice ailments. *Journal of Traditional Chinese Medicine*, 11, 209–215.

Peppard, R.C. (1996). Management of functional voice disorders in adolescents. *Language, Speech, and Hearing Services in Schools*, 27, 257–270.

Perkins, W. (1985). Assessment and treatment of voice disorders: State of the art. In J. Costello (Ed.), *Speech disorders in adults*. San Diego, CA: College Hill Press.

Perkins, W., & Yanagihara, N. (1968). Parameters of voice production: Some mechanisms for the regulation of pitch. *Journal of Speech and Hearing Research*, 11, 246–267.

Peterson, H., & Marquardt, T. (1990). *Appraisal and diagnosis of speech language disorders*. Englewood Cliffs, NJ: Prentice Hall.

Pressman, J. (1942). Physiology of the vocal cords in phonation and respiration. *Archives of Otology*, 35, 378.

Prater, R., & Swift, R. (1984). *Manual of voice therapy.* Boston: Little, Brown and Company.

Proctor, D. (1974). Breathing mechanisms during phonation and singing. In *Ventilatory and phonatory control systems*. London: Oxford University Press.

Pruszewicz, A., Obrebowski, A., Swidzinski, P., Demenko, G., Wika, T., & Wojciechowska A. (1991). Usefulness of acoustic studies on the differential diagnostics of organic and functional dysphonia. *Acta Otolaryngologica*, 111, 414–419.

Ptacek, P.H., & Sander, E.K. (1963). Maximum duration of phonation. *Journal of Speech and Hearing Disorders*, 28(2), 171–182.

Ptacek, P.H., & Sander, E.K. (1966). Age recognition from voice. *Journal of Speech and Hearing Research*, 9, 273–277.

Ptacek, P.H., Sander, E.K., Maloney, W.H., & Jackson, C. (1966). Phonatory and related changes with advanced age. *Journal of Speech and Hearing Research*, 9, 353–360.

Rabinov, C.R., Kreiman, J., Gerratt, B., & Bielamowicz, S. (1995). Comparing reliability of perceptual ratings of roughness and acoustic measures of jitter. *Journal of Speech and Hearing Research*, 38, 26–32.

Ramig, L.O., & Ringel, R.L. (1983). Effects of physiological aging on selected acoustic characteristics of voice. *Journal of Speech and Hearing Research*, 26, 22–30.

Ramig, L.O., Scherer, R.C., Klasner, E.R., Titze, I.R., & Horii, Y. (1990). Acoustic analysis of voice in amyotrophic lateral sclerosis: A longitudinal case study. *Journal of Speech and Hearing Disorders*, 55, 2–14.

Rastatter, M.P., & Hyman, M. (1982). Maximum phoneme duration of /s/ and /z/ by children with vocal nodules. *Language, Speech, and Hearing Services in Schools*, 13, 197–199.

Rau, D., & Beckett, R. (1984). Aerodynamic assessment of vocal function using hand held spirometers. *Journal of Speech and Hearing Research*, 49, 183–188.

Reich, A.R., Mason, J.A., & Polen, S.B. (1986). Task administration variables affecting phonation-time measures in third-grade girls with normal voice quality. *Language, Speech, and Hearing Services in School*, 17, 262–269.

Reich, A.R., & McHenry, M.A. (1987). Respiratory volumes in cheerleaders with a history of dysphonic episodes. *Folia Phoniatrica*, 39, 71–77.

Renout, K.A., Leeper, H.A., Bandur, D.L., & Hudson, A.J. (1995). Vocal fold diadochokinetic function of individuals with amyotrophic lateral sclerosis. *American Journal of Speech-Language Pathology*, 4, 73–79.

Ringel, R.L., & Chodzko-Zajko, W.J. (1987). Vocal indices of biological age. *Journal of Voice*, 1, 31–37.

Roy, N., & Bless, D.M. (1998). Manual circumlaryngeal techniques in the assessment and treatment of voice disorders. *Current Opinion in Otolaryngology & Head and Neck Surgery*, 6, 151–155.

Roy, N., Bless, D.M., Heisey, D., & Ford, C.N. (1997a). Manual circumlaryngeal therapy for functional dysphonia: An evaluation of short- and long-term treatment outcomes. *Journal of Voice*, 11(3), 321–331.

Roy, N., Ford, C.N., & Bless, D.M. (1996). Muscle tension dysphonia and spasmodic dysphonia: The role of manual laryngeal tension reduction in diagnosis and management. *Annals of Otology Rhinology and Laryngology*, 105, 851–856.

Roy, N., & Leeper, H.A. (1993). Effects of the manual laryngeal musculoskeletal tension reduction technique as a treatment for functional voice disorders: Perceptual and acoustic measures. *Journal of Voice*, 7(3), 242–249.

Roy, N., McGrory, J.J., Tasko, S.M., Bless, D.M., Heisey, D., & Ford, C.N. (1997b). Psychological correlates of functional dysphonia: An investigation using the Minnesota Multiphasic Personality Inventory. *Journal of Voice*, 11(4), 443–451.

Ryan, W. (1972). Acoustic aspects of the aging voice. *Journal of Gerontology*, 27(4), 265–268.

Ryan, W., & Burke, K. (1974). Perceptual and acoustic correlates of aging in the speech of males. *Journal of Communication Disorders*, 7, 181–192.

Sapienza, C., & Dutka, J. (1996). Glottal airflow characteristics of women's voice production along an aging continuum. *Journal of Speech and Hearing Research*, 39, 322–328.

Sapienza, C.M. (1997). Aerodynamic and acoustic characteristics of the adult African American voice. *Journal of Voice*, 11(4), 410–416.

Sapienza, C.M., & Stathopoulos, E.T. (1994). Respiratory and laryngeal measures of children and women with bilateral vocal fold nodules. *Journal of Speech and Hearing Research*, 37, 1229–1243.

Sawashima, M. (1974). Laryngeal research in experimental phonetics. In Sebok, T. (Ed.), *Current Trends in Linguistics*, Volume 12. The Hague: Mouton.

Sawashima, M., Gay, T., & Harris, K. (1969). Laryngeal muscle activity during vocal pitch and intensity changes. Haskins Laboratories Status Report on Speech Research, SR-19/20, 211–220.

Sawashima, M., & Hirose, H. (1983). Laryngeal gestures in speech production. In P. MacNeilage (Ed.), *The production of speech*. New York: Springer-Verlag.

Scherer, R.C., Vail, V.J., & Guo, C.G. (1995). Required number of tokens to determine representative voice perturbation values. *Journal of Speech and Hearing Research*, 38, 1260–1269.

Schiavetti, N., & Metz, D.E. (1997). *Evaluating research in communicative disorders*. Needham Heights, MA: Allyn & Bacon.

Schutte, H., & Seidner, W. (1983). Recommendations by the Union of European Phoniatricians (UEP): Standardizing voice area measurement/phonetography. *Folia Phoniatrica*, 35, 286–288.

Shanks, S., & Mast, D. (1977). Maximum duration of phonation objective tool for assessment of voice. *Perceptual and Motor Skills*, 45, 1315–1322.

Shanks, S.J. (1966). *An investigation of the nature of vocal fold diadochokinesis of adult subjects and of the effect of pitch, intensity, and aging upon the performance of this phonatory task.* Doctoral dissertation. Baton Rouge, LA: Louisiana State University.

Shipp, T., Qi, Y., Huntley, R., & Hollien, H. (1992). Acoustic and temporal correlates of perceived age. *Journal of Voice*, 6(3), 211–216.

Sodersten, M., & Lindestad, P. (1990). Glottal closure and perceived breathiness during phonation in normally speaking subjects. *Journal of Speech and Hearing Research*, 33, 601–611.

Sorensen, D., & Horii, Y. (1982). Cigarette smoking and voice fundamental frequency. *Journal of Communication Disorders*, 15, 135–144.

Sorenson, D.N., & Parker, P.A. (1992). The voiced/voiceless phonation time in children with and without laryngeal pathology. *Language, Speech. and Hearing in Schools*, 23, 163–168.

Sperry, E.E., & Klich, R.J. (1992). Speech breathing in senescent and younger women during oral reading. *Journal of Speech and Hearing Research*, 35, 1246–1255.

Spielberger, C.D., Gorsuch, R.L., Lushene, R., Vagg, P.R., & Jacobs, G.A. (1983). *Manual for the State-Trait Anxiety Inventory (Form Y) ("Self-evaluation questionnaire")*. Palo Alto, CA: Consulting Psychologists Press.

Stemple, J. (1993). *Voice therapy: Clinical studies*. St. Louis, MO: Mosby.

Stemple, J.C., Stanley, J., & Lee, L. (1995). Objective measures of voice production in normal subjects following prolonged voice use. *Journal of Voice*, 9(2), 127–133.

Stevens, K., & House, A. (1955). Development of a quantitative description of vowel articulation. *Journal of Acoustical Society of America*, 27, 484–493.

Stevens, K., & House, A. (1961). An acoustic theory of vowel production and some of its implications. *Journal of Speech and Hearing Research*, 4, 303–320.

Stoicheff, M. (1981). Speaking fundamental frequency characteristics of nonsmoking female adults. *Journal of Speech and Hearing Research*, 24, 437–441.

Stone, R.E. (1983). Issues in clinical assessment of laryngeal function: Contraindications for subscribing to maximum phonation time and optimum fundamental frequency. In G.M. Bless & J.H. Abbs (Eds.), *Contemporary Research and Clinical Issues* (pp. 410–424). San Diego: College Hill Press.

Stone, R., Bell, C., & Clack, T. (1978). Minimum intensity of voice at selected levels within pitch range. *Folia Phoniatrica*, 30, 113–118.

Stone, R.E., & Ferch, P.A.K. (1982). Intra-subject variability in F_0-SPL_{min} voice profiles. *Journal of Speech and Hearing Disorders*, 47, 134–137.

Stone, R.E., & Rainey, C.L. (1991). Intra- and intersubject variability in acoustic measures of normal voice. *Journal of Voice*, 5(3), 189–196.

Sulter, A.M., Wit, H.P., Schutte, H.K., & Miller, D.G. (1994). A structured approach to voice range profile (phonetogram) analysis. *Journal of Speech and Hearing Research*, 37, 1076–1085.

Sundberg, J. (1987). *The science of the singing voice*. Dekalb, IL: N. Illinois University Press.

Sundberg, J., & Leanderson, R. (1987). Phonatory breathing—physiology behind vocal pedagogy. *Journal of Research in Singing*, 10, 3–21.

Sussman, J.E., & Sapienza, C. (1994). Articulatory developmental, and gender effects on measures of fundamental frequency and jitter. *Journal of Voice*, 8(2), 145–156.

Tait, N.A., Michel, J.F., & Carpenter, M.A. (1980). Maximum duration of sustained /s/ and /z/ in children. *Journal of Speech and Hearing Disorders*, 45, 239–246.

Takahashi, H., & Koike, Y. (1975). Some perceptual dimensions and acoustical correlates of pathologic voices. *Acta Otolaryngologica (Stockholm)*, 338, 1–24.

Tanaka, S., Hirano, M., & Terasawa, R. (1991). Examination of air usage during phonation: Correlations among test parameters. *Journal of Voice*, 5(2), 106–112.

Thomas-Kersting, C., & Casteel, R.L. (1989). Harsh voice: Vocal effort perceptual ratings and spectral noise levels of hearing-impaired children. *Journal of Communication Disorders*, 22, 125–135.

Titze, I. (1989). Physiological and acoustic differences between male and female voices. *Journal of Acoustical Society of America*, 85(4), 1699–1707.

Titze, I. (1991). Acoustics inverse filter. Paper presented at the American Speech Language Hearing Association Scientific Advances in the Treatment of Voice Workshop, Madison, WI.

Titze, I. (1994). *Principles of voice production*. Englewood Cliffs, NJ: Prentice-Hall.

Titze, I., Horii, Y., & Scherer, R. (1987). Some technical considerations in voice perturbation measurements. *Journal of Speech and Language Research*, 21, 240–249.

Titze, I., & Liang, H. (1993). Comparison of F_0 extraction methods for high-precision voice perturbation measurements. *Journal of Speech and Hearing Research*, 36, 1120–1133.

Tonkova-Yampol'skaya, R.V. (1968). Ravitie re chevoi intonatsii u detei pervykh dvukh let zhini (The development of speech intonation in children during the first two years of life). *Vop. Psikhiat.*, 14, 94–101. Also in Fergusson, C.A., & Slobin, D.A. (1973) (Eds.), *Studies of child language development* (pp. 128–138). Orlando, FL: Holt, Rinehart and Winston.

Troup, G. (1981). The physics of the singing voice. *Journal of Research in Singing*, 1–26.

Trudeau, M.D., & Forrest, L.A. (1997). The contributions of phonatory volume and transglottal airflow to the s/z ratio. *American Journal of Speech Language Pathology*, 6, 65–69.

Trullinger, R., & Emanuel, F. (1989). Airflow, volume, and duration characteristics of sustained vowel productions of normal-speaking children. *Folia Phoniatrica*, 41, 297–307.

Van Oordt, H., & Drost, H. (1963). Development of the frequency range of the voice in children. *Folia Phoniatrica*, 15, 289–298.

Verdolini, K. (1994). Voice disorders. In J.B. Toblin, H.L. Morris, & D.C. Spriesterbach (Eds.), *Diagnosis in speech-language pathology* (pp. 247–305). San Diego, CA: Singular Publishing Group, Inc.

Walton, J., & Orlikoff, R.F. (1994). Speaker race identification from acoustic cues in the vocal signal. *Journal of Speech and Hearing Research*, 37, 738–745.

Watson, P., & Hixon, T. (1985). Respiratory kinematics in classical (opera) singing. *Journal of Speech and Hearing Research*, 28, 104–122.

Weinberg, B. (1983). Diagnosis of phonatory based voice disorders. In I. Meitus & B. Weinberg (Eds.), *Diagnosis in speech language pathology* (pp. 151–182). Baltimore: University Park Press.

Weiner, J.B., Lee, L., Cataland, J., & Stemple, J.C. (1996). An assessment of pitch-matching abilities among speech-language pathology graduate students. *American Journal of Speech-Language Pathology*, 5, 91–95.

Wendahl, R.W. (1963). Laryngeal analog synthesis of harsh voice quality. *Folia Phoniatrica*, 15, 241–250.

Wheat, M.C., & Hudson, A.I. (1988). Spontaneous speaking fundamental frequency of 6-year-old black children. *Journal of Speech and Hearing Research*, 31, 723–725.

White, O.R. (1974). The "split middle" a "quickie" method of trend estimation. Seattle, WA: University of Washington, Experimental Education Unit, Child Development and Mental Retardation Center.

Wilcox, K., & Horii, Y. (1980). Age and changes in vocal jitter. *Journal of Gerontology*, 35, 194–198.

Winholtz, W., & Titze, I. (1997). Conversion of a head-mounted microphone signal into calibrated SPL units. *Journal of Voice*, 11(4), 417–421.

Winholtz, W., & Titze, I. (1998). Suitability of minidisc recordings for perturbation analysis. *Journal of Voice*, 12(2), 138–142.

Wit, J., Maassen, B., Gabreels, F.J.M., & Thoonen, G. (1993). Maximum performance tests in children with developmental spastic dysarthria. *Journal of Speech and Hearing Research*, 36, 452–459.

Wolfe, V., Fitch, J., & Cornell, R. (1995). Acoustic prediction of severity in commonly occurring voice problems. *Journal of Speech and Hearing Research*, 38, 273–279.

Wolfe, V., Fitch, J., & Martin, D. (1997). Acoustic measures of dysphonic severity across and within voice types. *Folia Phoniatrica et Logopaedica*, 49, 292–299.

Wolfe, V., & Martin, D. (1997). Acoustic correlates of dysphonia: Type and severity. *Journal of Communication Disorders*, 30, 403–416.

Wolfe, V., & Ratusnik, D.L. (1988). Acoustics and perceptual measurements of roughness influencing judgments of pitch. *Journal of Speech and Hearing Disorders*, 53, 15–22.

Wolfe, V., & Steinfatt, T.M. (1987). Prediction of vocal severity within and across voice types. *Journal of Speech and Hearing Research*, 30, 230–240.

Yanagihara, N., Koike, Y., & von Leden, H. (1966). Phonation and respiration. *Folia Phoniatrica*, 18, 323–340.

Yumoto, E. (1983). The quantitative evaluation of hoarseness: A new harmonics to noise ratio method. *Archives in Otolaryngology*, 109, 48–52.

Yumoto, E. (1987). Quantitative assessment of the degree of hoarseness. *Journal of Voice*, 1, 310–313.

Yumoto, E., Gould, W.J., & Baer, T. (1982). Harmonics-to-noise ratio as an index of the degree of hoarseness. *Journal of Acoustical Society of America*, 71, 1544–1550.

Yumoto, E., Sasaki, Y., & Okamura, H. (1984). Harmonics-to-noise ratio and psychophysical measurement of the degree of hoarseness. *Journal of Speech and Hearing Research*, 27, 2–6.

Zemlin, W.R. (1988). *Speech and hearing science: Anatomy and physiology*. Englewood Cliffs, NJ: Prentice-Hall.

Zwirner, P., Murry, T., & Woodson, G. (1991). Phonatory function of neurologically impaired patients. *Journal of Communication Disorders*, 24, 287–300.

Zyski, B.J., Bull, G.L., McDonald, W.E., & Johns, M.E. (1984). Perturbation analysis of normal and pathologic larynges. *Folia Phoniatrica*, 36, 190–198.

Contact Information for Various Software and Equipment Manufacturers

VOICE ANALYSIS SOFTWARE

CSpeech/CSpeechSP
Dr. P. Milenkovic
3623 Engineering Hall
1415 Engineering Drive
Madison, WI 53706
Telephone: (608) 262-3892
E-mail: milenkovic@engr.wisc.edu

Dr. Speech 4
Tiger DRS, Inc.
PO Box 75063
Seattle, WA 98125
Telephone: (206) 499-5757
Fax: (206) 367-2672
Website: www.drspeech.com
E-mail: tiger-electronics@worldnet.att.net

EZVoice/EZVoicePlus
VoiceTek Enterprises
909 Fair Street
Nescopeck, PA 18635
E-mail: sawan@bwkip.com

IVANS (The Interactive Voice Analysis System)
AVAAZ Innovations Inc.
PO Box 8040
1225 Wonderland Road North
London, Ontario, Canada N6G 2B0
Telephone: (519) 472-7944
Fax: (519) 472-7814
Website: www.avaaz.com

Multi-Speech Model 3700 & Computerized Speech Lab (CSL)
Kay Elemetrics Corp.
2 Bridgewater Lane
Lincoln Park, NJ 07035
Telephone: (973) 628-6200
Fax: (973) 628-6363
Website: www.kayelemetrics.com

SoundScope
GW Instruments Inc.
35 Medford Street
Somerville, MA 02143
Telephone: (617) 625-4096
Fax: (617) 625-1322
Website: www.gwinst.com
E-mail: info@gwinst.com

SPIROMETERS

MicroPlus Spirometer
Micro Medical Ltd.
PO Box 6
Rochester, Kent, United Kingdom ME1 2AZ
Telephone: +44 (0) 1634 360044
Fax: +44 (0) 1634 360055
E-mail: sales@micromedical.co.uk

SOUND LEVEL METERS, MICROPHONES, AMPLIFIERS, ETC.

Radio Shack Online Catalog
Website: www.radioshack.com

RECORDING EQUIPMENT

MiniDisc
Website: www.minidisc.org

Perceptual Evaluation of the Voice: Record Form

Patient Name: _____ Date: _____ Clinician: _____

Overall Severity Level

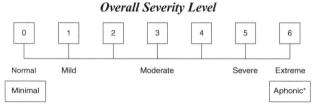

Habitual Pitch

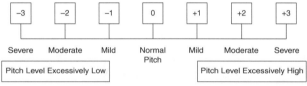

Pitch Variability

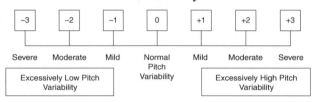

Habitual Loudness

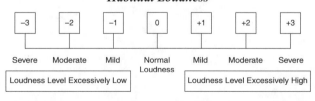

Loudness Variability

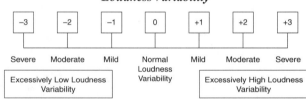

Vocal Quality

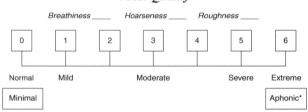

Durational Aspects

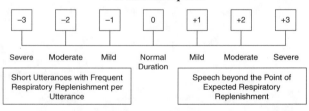

Mild: Although the listener experienced in the perceptual characteristics of the disordered voice would consider the voice abnormal, the untrained listener may consider the voice to be only unusual in nature and within normal expectations. The voice characteristic is not distracting, and the ability to effectively communicate is not affected. The dysphonia does not interfere with phonation.

Moderate: Both trained and untrained listeners would consider the voice abnormal. There may be intermittent periods in which the voice characteristic is highly distracting. The ability to effectively communicate is noticeably affected under certain conditions (e.g., noisy environments). The dysphonia may occasionally cause phonation to cease or become highly effortful.

Severe: Both trained and untrained listeners would consider the voice extremely abnormal. The voice characteristic is highly distracting. The ability to effectively communicate is consistently affected. The dysphonia causes phonation to be mainly absent or extremely effortful.

Quantitative Evaluation of the Voice: Record Form

Patient Name: _____ Date: _____ Clinician: _____

Frequency Evaluation

Continuous Speech ("*The Rainbow Passage*")

Mean Speaking F_0:	_____ Hz
F_0 Standard Deviation:	_____ Hz
Pitch Sigma:	_____ ST
Maximum F_0:	_____ Hz
Minimum F_0:	_____ Hz
Speaking Range:	_____ Hz or ST

Instructions: "I would like you to read this passage in your normal speaking voice." Record and analyze the 2nd sentence. Average results from 3 trials are recommended.

Expectations: Adult Males (100–150 Hz); Adult Females (180–230 Hz); Prepubertal Children (250 Hz or higher)—Consult Norms.

Total Phonational Range

Highest F_0:	_____ Hz
Lowest F_0:	_____ Hz
F_0 Range:	_____ ST

Comments:

Instructions: "I am going to ask you to hold out the sound "ah" (/ɑ/) at several different notes or pitches. Starting at a comfortable pitch level, I would like you to go down in steps to the lowest note you can hold out without your voice breaking or cracking. It will be similar to singing down a scale, such as…" (provide example for your patient here).

"Starting at a comfortable pitch level, I would like you to go up in steps to the highest note you can hold out without your voice breaking or cracking, including falsetto voice—falsetto is a high, thin, reedy voice such as… (provide example). It will be similar to singing up a scale, such as…" (provide example for your patient here).

An average result from 3 trials is recommended.

Expectations: At least 20–24 semitones (musical range).

Intensity Evaluation

Continuous Speech ("*The Rainbow Passage*")

Mean Speaking Intensity:	_____ dB
Max. Speaking Intensity:	_____ dB
Min. Speaking Intensity:	_____ dB
Speaking Range:	_____ dB

Instructions: "I would like you to read this passage in your normal speaking voice." The patient should read the entire 1st paragraph of "The Rainbow Passage." Use the intensity-by-count method. A 12-inch (30-cm) mouth-to-microphone distance is recommended.

Expectations: Adult males and females (mean speaking intensity of 65–70 dB).

Results of High Pitch/Quiet Phonation or Phonetogram

Comments:

Quality-related Measures

Sustained Vowel (/ɑ/)

Mean F_0	_____ Hz
F_0 Standard Deviation:	_____ Hz
Pitch Sigma:	_____ ST
Jitter:	_____
Shimmer:	_____
HNR:	_____ dB

Comments:

Instructions: "I want you to repeat the numbers "one, two, three, four." I would like you to chant them like this:"

$$\rightarrow \quad \rightarrow \quad \rightarrow \quad \rightarrow$$
One, two, three, four

(These words have a horizontal arrow over them to imply a flat intonation pattern.)

"I want you to sustain the "or" of the number "four" and then match it with a vowel /ɑ/. You will sustain the vowel /ɑ/ for at least 2–3 seconds at a comfortable loudness level."

The average result from 3 trials is recommended.

Expectations: Jitter (considerably less than 1%); Shimmer (less than 0.5 dB); HNR (15–20 dB)—Consult Norms.

Durational Measures

Vital Capacity:	_____ ml

Instructions: "I want you to take a deep breath and blow out as long and as hard as possible into the spirometer tube." Maximum performance from 3 trials is recommended.

Expectations: Adult Males (4000–5000 ml); Adult Females (3000–4000 ml)—Consult Norms.

Max. Phonation Time:	_____ seconds

Instructions: "I want you to take a deep breath and sustain/hold out the vowel "ah" (/ɑ/) as long as possible." The clinician should model the MPT task for the patient. Maximum performance from 3 trials is recommended.

Expectations: Adult males and females should be in the vicinity of 20 s or greater (Expected MPT/Observed MPT > 0.70)—Consult Norms.

Max. /s/ Duration:	_____ seconds
Max. /z/ Duration:	_____ seconds
S/Z Ratio:	_____ seconds

Instructions: "I want you to take a deep breath and hold out the sound /s/ ("Sssss…") as long as possible." "Now I want you to take a deep breath and sustain the sound /z/ ("Zzzzz…") as long as possible."

The clinician should provide a model for the patient. Time and record the duration using a stopwatch. As with previous tasks (VC and MPT), it is useful to verbally encourage the patient into sustaining the productions for as long as possible.

Elicit 3 trials of maximally sustained /s/ and /z/ in the following order: /s, z/ /s,z/ /s,z/

Calculate the S/Z ratio using the single longest /s/ and single longest /z/ durations from the 3 trials.

Expectations: S/Z Ratio ≈ 1.0; Durations of /s/ and /z/ phonemes should be in the vicinity of 20 s in adults—Consult Norms.

Phonation Quotient:	_____ ml/sec.

Instructions: Calculate PQ from the maximum VC and maximum MPT.

Comments:

Expectations: Adult Males (mean PQ of 145 ml/s, with measures less than 69 ml/s or greater than 307 ml/s considered abnormal); Adult Females (mean PQ of 137 ml/s, with measures less than 78 ml/s or greater than 241 ml/s considered abnormal) (*Source:* Hirano, Koike, & von Leden, 1968)—Consult Norms.

Evaluation of Effects of Muscle Tension

Effects of Rapid Counting (1 to 100):

Instructions: The clinician should closely observe for changes in voice characteristics after (a) inducing stress or (b) attempts to relieve muscle tension. Voice recordings following these tasks are useful in documenting effects of stress and/or relief of excessive muscle tension on the voice.

Effects of Laryngeal Reposturing/Circumlaryngeal Massage:

Comments:

The Rainbow Passage

(First paragraph)

When the sunlight strikes raindrops in the air, they act like a prism and form a rainbow. The rainbow is a division of white light into many beautiful colors. These take the shape of a long round arch, with its path high above, and its two ends apparently beyond the horizon. There is, according to legend, a boiling pot of gold at one end. People look, but no one ever finds it. When a man looks for something beyond his reach, his friends say he is looking for the pot of gold at the end of the rainbow (Fairbanks, 1960).

Using the Hertz-to-Semitone Converter Program

A program entitled VDP-UTIL.EXE is provided on CD-ROM for the use of the reader. Figure E–1 provides a screen shot of the program.

The VDP-UTIL program allows the user to quickly calculate three clinically useful measures:

- *Semitone Range:* Most voice analysis programs will provide a measure of F_0 range in Hz. However, as described in Chapter 2, it is often advisable to convert F_0 range in Hz to semitones because (1) range reported on a musical note scale has more relation to the perceptual judgment of pitch, and (2) by converting to semitones, F_0 range is "normalized" for different voice types (adult male, adult female, child voices).

To calculate the range (e.g., total phonational range) of your patient's voice, follow these steps.

1. Using your mouse, select the Semitone Range calculation (left click on the selection box to the left of "Semitone Range"). You should now see a check mark (✔) in the selection box.

Figure E–1 Screen Shot of the VDP-UTIL Program

2. Next, left click on the text box located under the word "Maximum," then type in the patient's maximum vocal F_0 in Hz (for example, 494).

3. Next, left click on the text box located under the word "Minimum," then type in the patent's minimum vocal F_0 in Hz (for example, 123).

4. Click on the button labeled "OK." You will now see the range (in semitones) between the patient's maximum and minimum vocal F_0s in the textbox located under the word "Semitones" (for example, 24.07 semitones).

- **Pitch Sigma:** A measure of the average variability of the vocal F_0 has been used as a measure of the long-term instability of the voice. Voice analysis programs will commonly report average variability in terms of the F_0 standard deviation (in Hz). However, for the same reasons as discussed regarding Semitone Range, it is often advisable to convert F_0 standard deviation in semitones. This conversion is referred to as the Pitch Sigma.

Pitch sigma may be calculated from either continuous speech or sustained vowel samples. To calculate the pitch sigma of the patient's voice, follow these steps.

1. Using your mouse, select the Pitch Sigma calculation (left click on the selection box to the left of "Pitch Sigma"). You should now see a check mark (✔) in the selection box.

2. Next, left click on the text box located under the word "Mean," then type in the patent's mean vocal F_0 in Hz as reported for the sustained vowel or continuous speech sample (for example, 210).

3. Next, left click on the text box located under the word "Std. Deviation," then type in the patient's F_0 standard deviation in Hz (for example, 21).

4. Click on the button labeled "OK." You will now see the pitch sigma (in semitones) for the patient's continuous speech or sustained vowel sample reported in the textbox located under the word "Pitch Sigma" (for example, 3.47 semitones).

Calculations for both Semitone Range and Pitch Sigma are derived via a formula described by Baken (1987). See Chapter 2 for this equation.

- **Z-Score:** When assessing a patient's score/result on a particular voice task (e.g., mean speaking F_0, speaking intensity, MPT, etc.), it is useful to have an objective means to establish exactly how different the patient's score is from a comparable normative sample. Most behaviors, including respiratory and voice function, have

some degree of normal variation both above and below mean performance. Therefore, a score that is higher or lower than a published average does not necessarily mean that the score is abnormal.

The Z-score is a simple statistical measure that allows the clinician to measure how many standard deviations a patient's score is above or below a comparative mean (the Z-score can, therefore, be a positive [+] or negative [–] number). The Z-score formula is as follows:

$$z = \frac{Patient's\ Score - Normative\ Mean}{Normative\ Standard\ Deviation}$$

To use the VDP-UTIL program to quickly calculate a Z-score, follow these steps:

1. Using your mouse, select the Z-Score calculation (left click on the selection box to the left of "Z-Score"). You should now see a check mark (✔) in the selection box.

2. Next, left click on the text box located under the word "Pts. Score," then type in the patient's score/result for a particular task (for example, if an adult male patient produces a mean speaking F_0 of 125 Hz, type in "125" for the Pts. Score).

3. Next, left click on the text box located under the word "Sample Mean," then type in the sample mean for a comparable normative sample (compare to a mean derived from a sample similar to your patient in terms of variables such as age, gender, race, etc.). As an example, we could compare this patient's mean F_0 to the data of Horii (1975) as presented in Table 2–2 in Chapter 2. In this case, type in "112.5" for the Sample Mean.

4. Next, left click on the text box located under the word "Sample S.D.," then type in the sample standard deviation for the normative sample. To continue with our example, type in "17.3" for the Sample S.D. (from Horii [1975], as presented in Table 2–2 in Chapter 2).

5. Click on the button labeled "OK." You will now see the Z-score reported in the text box located under the word "Z-Score." In this case, the Z-score would be approximately + .72, meaning that your patient's mean F_0 was .72 standard deviations above the mean as published by Horii (1975).

Conservatively, 2 standard deviations above or below a mean is considered abnormal. However, for clinical purposes, many use ±1.5 standard deviations or even as low as ±1 standard deviation (Verdolini, 1994) as indicative of abnormal performance. In the example that was provided, a Z-score of +.72 would be considered well within normal expectations. Finally, the clinician should be aware that (1) the normative data sample to which you are comparing should be normally distributed (ideally, the authors will establish this); (2) the units for the mean and standard deviation from the normative sample should be the same (e.g., F_0 data in which the mean is reported in Hz and the standard deviation is reported in semitones (ST) cannot be used in the Z-score calculation); and (3) the larger the comparative sample, the better the estimate of normality as derived by means of the Z-score.

Index